Medicine

PRESERVING THE PASSION IN THE 21ST CENTURY

Also by Lois DeBakey, Ph.D.
The Scientific Journal: Editorial Policies and Practices

Springer
New York
Berlin
Heidelberg
Hong Kong
London
Milan
Paris
Tokyo

Medicine

PRESERVING THE PASSION IN THE 21ST CENTURY

SECOND EDITION

Phil R. Manning, M.D.

Professor of Medicine Emeritus

Paul Ingalls Hoagland-Hastings Foundation Professor of Continuing Medical Education

Former Associate Vice President for Health Affairs

Former Associate Dean for Postgraduate Affairs

Keck School of Medicine of the University of Southern California

Los Angeles, California

Lois DeBakey, Ph.D.

Professor of Scientific Communication

Baylor College of Medicine

Houston, Texas

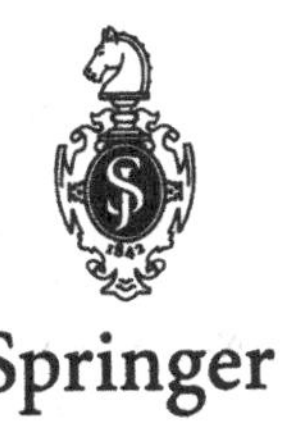

Springer

PHIL R. MANNING, M.D.
Keck School of Medicine
University of Southern California
1975 Zonal Avenue
Los Angeles, CA 90033
USA

LOIS DEBAKEY, PH.D.
Professor of Scientific Communication
Baylor College of Medicine
One Baylor Plaza
Houston, Texas 77030
USA

• • •

LIBRARY OF CONGRESS CATALOGING-IN-PUBLICATION DATA
Manning, Phil R., 1921–
Medicine: preserving the passion in the 21st century / Phil R. Manning, Lois DeBakey.—
2nd ed.
p. ; cm.
Rev. ed. of: Medicine: preserving the passion. c1987.
Includes bibliographical references and index.
ISBN 0-387-0046-2 (h/c : alk. paper) ISBN 0-387-00427-0 (s/c : alk. paper)
1. Medicine—Study and teaching (Continuing education) I. DeBakey, Lois.
II. Manning, Phil R., 1921—Medicine: preserving the passion. III. Title.
[DNLM: 1. Education, Medical, Continuing—trends. W 20 M284m 2003]
R845.M36 2003
610'.71'5—dc21 2003042484

PRINTED ON ACID-FREE PAPER.

ISBN 0-387-00426-2 (hardcover)
ISBN 0-387-00427-0 (softcover)

Text design by Steven Pisano.

PRINTED IN THE UNITED STATES OF AMERICA.

9 8 7 6 5 4 3 2 1 SPIN 10908273 (hardcover) SPIN 10908280 (softcover)

www.springer-ny.com

Springer-Verlag New York Berlin Heidelberg
A member of BertelsmannSpringer Science+Business Media GmbH

Dedicated to

practicing physicians,

who have invested many years

in medical school and graduate training,

often at great personal and financial sacrifice,

and who place the highest priority

on the health and welfare

of their patients.

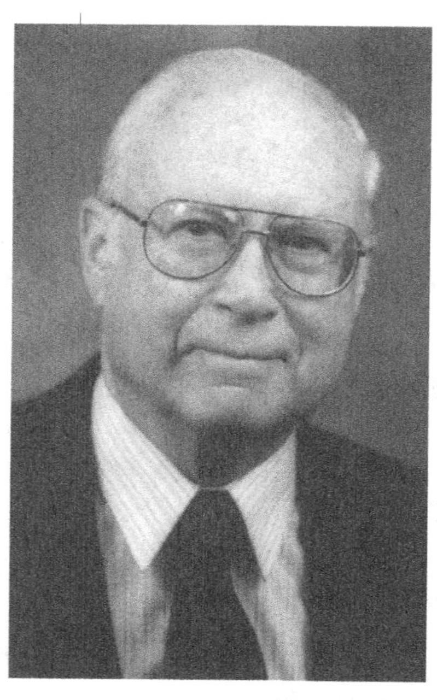

The outstanding advances in information technology are simplifying and encouraging independent, practice-related study, making it easier for physicians to enhance learning in the practice environment.

Phil R. Manning, M.D.

An inquiring, analytical mind; an unquenchable thirst for new knowledge; and a heartfelt compassion for the ailing—these are prominent traits among the committed clinicians who have preserved the passion for medicine, even with the advent of "managed" care.

Lois DeBakey, Ph.D.

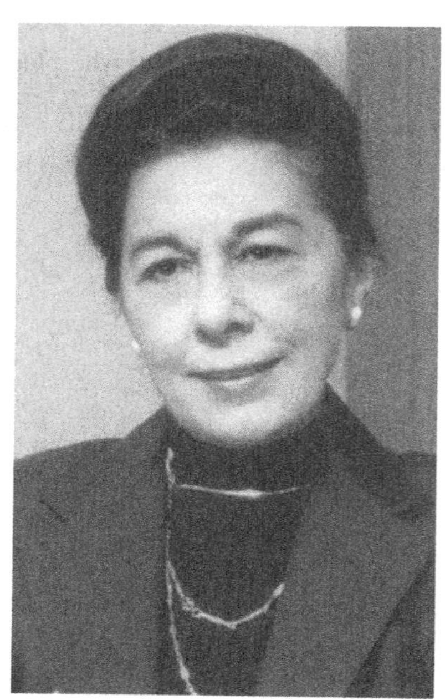

The education of the doctor which goes on after
he has his degree is, after all,
the most important part of his education.

JOHN SHAW BILLINGS
Boston Med Surg J. 1894; 131:140.

• • •

The art of medicine cannot be inherited,
nor can it be copied from books . . . .

PARACELSUS
Foreword, *Das zweite Buch der Grossen Wundarznei,* 1536 (verso of leaf b, ed. 1562)

• • •

[T]he student begins with the patient,
continues with the patient,
and ends his studies with the patient,
using books and lectures as tools,
as means to an end.

WILLIAM OSLER
Aequanimitas, with Other Addresses,
"The Hospital as a College," 1903

Foreword

• • •

The Association of American Medical Colleges recently recommended that the traditional model for lifelong learning, which focused on attendance at courses, should be replaced by individualized study closely related to personal medical practice. Phil R. Manning has dedicated almost all of his professional life to demonstrating that continual medical education should occur precisely in this fashion. Lois DeBakey has devoted much of her professional life to instructing physicians and biomedical researchers in critical reasoning and its companion, clarity of thought, writing, and speech. Together, they have created a highly readable book that shows physicians how to gain the most from their clinical experience and, in doing so, preserve their passion for clinical practice and lifelong education.

The authors describe techniques used by highly successful clinicians and academicians to achieve these goals, synthesizing lessons from their clinical experience with reading of medical publications and discussions of clinical problems with colleagues. Personal essays and reflections by distinguished physicians are woven into the text. The book's emphasis is on immersion in practice, with tips on how to live with this commitment.

Chapters discuss the remarkable advances in information technology and medical library services that facilitate the active approach to learning. In fact, Manning insists that "With the current information services, there is no excuse for a physician not to remain current."

On the other hand, the traditional mental model of "information retrieval" as equivalent to "staying current" runs aground fairly quickly when the current medical advances outpace the doctor's education and understanding. Few practitioners today attended medical school lectures on introns, exons, transposons, or epigenetics (to name just a few of the bewildering concepts in the most recent medical journals). Consequently, the highly fragmented research papers that reach us so quickly via computer searches must fail to educate us if we have not—somehow, somewhere—gotten a satisfactory understanding of the scientific theories and assumptions that underlie the "current" progress. This is difficult. Manning and DeBakey include an emphasis on a physician's continuing need to be part of the profession, part of a network of colleagues. The computer can, indeed, retrieve facts with great facility. Yet for us to advance our understanding of difficult areas needs the interplay of minds. Here, too, this update of the popular first edition of *Medicine: Preserving the Passion in the 21st Century* gives the reader a good start in getting both understanding and facts.

DONALD A. B. LINDBERG, M.D.
Director
National Library of Medicine

Preface

• • •

Since the first edition of *Medicine: Preserving the Passion* was published in 1987, the practice of medicine has changed notably and so, therefore, has the physician's approach to lifelong learning. The spread of managed care has discouraged many physicians for several reasons: (1) they must often obtain approval from healthcare organizations for certain procedures, (2) because employers often shop for more economical health plans, patients may be required to change physicians, (3) paperwork has increased, and (4) physicians must see more patients to maintain their income. On a more positive note, healthcare organizations routinely collect data on individual practices for financial reasons, and these data can be used to identify educational needs of practitioners.

Unprecedented educational opportunities on the Internet are revolutionizing physicians' access to information, both reliable and unreliable. Although the rapid growth of electronic services precludes precise predictions of such resources during the next five years, it is safe to say that the Internet services will continue to expand and improve, making it ever easier for physicians to remain current. Information sources include easy access to MEDLINE, and range from brief news reports and summaries of recent developments to abstracts or entire journal articles online. The potential is promising for quick and accurate information at the time and place a physician sees patients. Prompt access, coupled with improved methods for the study of clinical practice and collegial discussions of patient problems, should facilitate education and thus enhance patient care.

We describe the experiences of physicians who use new approaches as an adjunct to traditional methods, such as reading medical textbooks and journals, attending conferences, and holding informal discussions with colleagues. For methods that rely on recording experiences on paper, ledgers, and note cards, computer software is usually available to simplify the input and analysis of legible data. We address the recent emphasis on avoiding medical errors, and we review the meaning and state of professionalism.

Rather than rely solely on our experience and study of medical publications, we have organized this edition, like the first, using interviews and written materials sent to us by academic and practicing physicians who have described their successful learning techniques. Thus, we are emphasizing the practical rather than the theoretical.

We maintain our belief that the implementation of the highest ideals of the science and art of medicine and the opportunity to serve patients combine to make the practice of medicine the most fulfilling and gratifying of all professions. Medicine will be most rewarding to physicians who immerse themselves in the profession and who practice the principles found on the following pages. And it is those principles that will preserve the passion.

PHIL R. MANNING, M.D.
LOIS DEBAKEY, PH.D.

Acknowledgments

PHIL R. MANNING, M.D.

• • •

I have always been motivated to discover how outstanding scholars, and especially medical practitioners, maintain their interest in lifelong learning and how they go about it. Although I have diligently studied educational principles, my true interest has always been what actually goes on in the field. This interest, I believe, sprang from my Father, a perpetual student who studied two to three hours each night almost until his death at 104 years. He was, in addition, a very practical man who cut through jargon and got to the basis of performance as quickly as anyone I have met. My Mother's persistence in my receiving a good education impressed on me from childhood the importance of continuing education for life.

The numerous outstanding clinicians and academicians who provided real-life examples of the methods they use to continue their education throughout life form the basis of this book. We all can be grateful to them for their descriptions of the techniques that facilitated their careers.

I owe a great deal to my colleagues and students at the University of Southern California School of Medicine, now the Keck School of Medicine of the University of Southern California. The opportunity to discuss educational and medical problems with outstanding professionals has surely been one of my greatest assets. The continued support I have received from the medical school administration has enabled me to pursue my investigations to improve methods of lifelong learning.

The experience I gained working with colleagues and staff in the American College of Physicians as a Regent and as chairman of several educational committees of the American College of Cardiology greatly enriched my understanding of medical practice and the importance of specialty societies. My friends in the Society of Academic Continuing Medical Education have enhanced my professional life and have added to my enjoyment of learning, as have my colleagues at the American College of Medical Informatics.

Of course, the support I received from my wife Mary, our daughter Carol and her husband Mark Boettger, our son Robert, and now our grandchildren David and Linda Boettger has added to my satisfaction and enhanced my passion for life and enthusiasm for lifelong learning.

I shall always be indebted to my coauthor, Lois DeBakey, for her diligence in achieving excellence. Lois sees through fuzzy thinking and provides precision in the written and spoken word. The clarity that I believe the reader will find throughout the book is her doing. If there are passages that are not clearly expressed, I am probably the culprit.

I appreciate the work of the Postgraduate Division staff of the Keck School of Medicine for its excellent organizing of educational programs for the practicing physician.

My special appreciation goes to Mr. David Arriola, who typed successive drafts of the manuscript and kept everything in order. He did much more than this by providing constructive criticism, detecting errors, verifying references, offering suggestions, and keeping calm during the various emendations the authors found it necessary to make.

I am also indebted to the Hastings Foundation, which supported much of my career by creating an endowed chair in continuing education and naming me the Paul Ingalls Hoagland-Hastings Foundation Professor of Continuing Medical Education.

Acknowledgments

LOIS DEBAKEY, PH.D.

• • •

Medicine: Preserving the Passion in the 21st Century is a clear example of the benefits of collegiality. This book grew out of a professional relationship with Phil Manning that dates some years back when we both served on a committee of the National Library of Medicine. Shared standards of excellence in medical education and medical communication and a shared interest in ethical and human values led to what has been a rewarding and productive collegial association of many years.

Phil, a leading international expert in lifelong medical education, conceived the basis for the book, and because I had observed and admired his ardent dedication to the highest principles of medicine and ethics, I eagerly agreed to collaborate. As with the first edition, I have benefited from my co-author's intellectual acuity and expertise, and from the knowledge and wisdom contained in the contributions of various distinguished physicians and surgeons.

I am indebted to those who led me into a scholarly career, primarily my beloved family. Even before I began my formal schooling, my parents stimulated my intellectual curiosity about the wonders of the world and introduced me to the delight of learning, the pleasure of reading, and the excitement of opening the mind to new knowledge and new ideas. They fully supported my undergraduate and postgraduate studies and endorsed my choice of an academic career. My debt to them is incalculable, not only because they were peerless models of love, intelligence, altruism, and probity, but also because they instilled in their children the reach for excellence and provided the opportunities to achieve that goal. My brothers, Michael and Ernest, both distinguished surgeons, and my sisters all served as strong role models to whom I am deeply and affectionately grateful for their encouragement and support of all my scholarly endeavors. My brothers' lofty standards as surgeons, their noble character, and their many silent humanitarian deeds, like those of my parents, have been a lifelong inspiration. My brother Michael directed my sister Selma and me into a truly exciting and fulfilling career. A man of vision, dedication, and ingenuity, he recognized the need for instruction in medical writing, editing, and speech, and he encouraged us to establish this new discipline. To Selma—my preceptor and *alter ego*—goes my unbounded gratitude, not only for her sage counsel during the preparation of this and all my other publications, but for her superb tutelage, unstinting support, and sororal devotion throughout my life.

We thank our publisher, Springer-Verlag, for assistance in processing our manuscript. To David Arriola, we are indebted for his outstanding professional efforts throughout the successive drafts and final manuscript of the second edition; his dedication to accuracy, precision, and excellence made the authors' work much easier. To Janice Brookes, I am deeply grateful for meticulous proofreading of the various drafts, her diligent reference verification, and her superb assistance in scrutinizing the proof.

We are especially indebted to all the physicians who granted us the benefit of their academic and clinical experience. Their raw material provided a basis for our analysis, interpretation, and commentary. Finally, to you, our readers, we are grateful for your own service to humanity and your intellectual curiosity. We hope that you will feel rewarded for your investment in reading this book.

Contents

• • •

Photographs

• • •

Introduction

• • •

No one denies that physicians must be lifelong students. Self-directed and practice-linked learning are also well accepted in principle, but techniques that enhance their execution have not been emphasized in medical schools. By the time physicians enter residency training and practice, many have become too busy to develop their own methods. As a result, they lose the opportunity to profit maximally from their experience. Classroom instruction has therefore been called upon to perform functions that it is ill-equipped to do.

Since the turn of the century, the classroom has dominated continuing medical education in the United States. In 1906, the American Medical Association (AMA) sent J. N. McCormack to several states to stimulate interest in postgraduate education. Under this stimulus, several states began to organize courses. At the request of the AMA, John Blackburn, Director of the Bowling Green County

Society in Kentucky, submitted a national plan and designed weekly programs on basic sciences and therapy for use by county medical societies.[1]

By 1909, about 350 county societies were sponsoring programs,[2] but because of a decline in attendance, these were ultimately discontinued. In 1916, W. S. Rankin, a North Carolina state health officer, developed circuit courses that took education to rural physicians. The instructors traveled to various communities delivering lectures and discussing the diagnosis and treatment of patients brought in by class attendees.[3]

In 1927, the University of Michigan established the first department of postgraduate medicine within a medical school.[1] Eight years later, John B. Youmans, under the aegis of the Commonwealth Fund, made surprise visits to 30 physicians in small towns and rural communities of Tennessee who had completed formal postgraduate courses at Vanderbilt University School of Medicine and graded them against a standard developed to assess improved quality of practice.[4] Although there was no precourse visit for comparison, Youmans decided that practical programs dealing with patients and technical procedures were more beneficial than didactic lectures.

In 1932, the Commission on Medical Education of the Association of American Medical Colleges concluded that "Continued education of physicians is synonymous with good medical practice . . ." and called for cooperation of medical associations, medical schools, and hospitals in conducting comprehensive programs of postgraduate education.[5] In 1936, the University of Minnesota constructed the first permanent center to house continuing medical education. Four years later, in accordance with a resolution adopted by the Advisory Board for Medical Specialties, the Commission on Graduate Medical Education was organized. The Commission, led by Willard C. Rappleye, concluded that undergraduate medical education did not strongly motivate busy practitioners to pursue continuing education.[6]

After World War II, the W. K. Kellogg Foundation awarded grants to 18 medical schools to broaden and innovate continuing medical education.[7] Since then, the growth of formal continuing medical education has been explosive, with hospitals, medical societies, and medical schools acting as the main sponsors. Mandatory continuing medical education and accreditation of organizations offering courses further stimulated the growth of postgraduate classroom instruction. Thus, the emphasis on formal classroom courses has overshadowed individual methods linking education more directly to the physician's own practice. The concept of lifelong learning, in fact, has seemed almost locked in the classroom.

Despite the continued emphasis on classroom education, various authorities, including Osler Peterson,[8] George Miller,[9] John Williamson,[10] and Clement Brown,[11] have demonstrated the limitations of formal continuing education. Miller and his followers have advocated that physicians analyze their practices to identify specific educational needs and thus direct their own education efficiently. In Miller's words, "... the practitioner-learner must progress steadily from listener to questioner to participant to contributor."[9]

Medicine: Preserving the Passion in the 21st Century calls attention to the systematic methods that physicians have used to continue their learning, hone their skills, and benefit maximally from their experience. Although traditional classroom approaches will continue to be useful, we expect a major shift in emphasis, if not a revolution, away from the conventional classroom enterprise to individual techniques devised by physicians to address their own educational requirements. The major advances in information technology have converted self-directed, practice-linked continuing medical education from a desirable dream to a reality within our grasp. With the advent of "managed" care, lifelong learning is more important than ever, not only for optimal healthcare delivery but also to preserve the passion for medicine.

PHIL R. MANNING, M.D.
LOIS DEBAKEY, PH.D.

REFERENCES

1. Bruce JD. Postgraduate education in medicine. *J Mich State Med Soc.* 1937; 36:369–377.

2. The American Medical Association, Council on Medical Education and Hospitals. *Graduate Medical Education in the United States: I—Continuation Study for Practicing Physicians 1937 to 1940.* Chicago: American Medical Association; 1940:216.

3. Adams FD. The North Carolina extension plan: an experiment in postgraduate medical teaching. *JAMA.* 1923; 80:1714–1717.

4. Youmans JB. Experience with a postgraduate course for practitioners: evaluation of results. *J Assoc Am Med Coll.* 1935;10:154–173.

5. Commission on Medical Education. Postgraduate medical education. In: *Final Report of the Commission on Medical Education.* New York: Office of the Director of Study; 1932:136.

6. Commission on Graduate Medical Education (W. C. Rappleye, Chm.). *Graduate Medical Education.* Chicago: Univ of Chicago Press; 1940:168.

7. Shepherd GR. History of continuation medical education in the United States since 1930. *J Med Educ.* 1960; 35:740–758.

8. Peterson OL, Andrews LP, Spain RS, Greenberg BG. An analytical study of North Carolina general practice 1953–54. Part 2. *J Med Educ.* 1956;31:1–8.

9. Miller GE. Continuing education for what? *J Med Educ.* 1967;42:324.

10. Williamson JW, Alexander M, Miller GE. Continuing education and patient care research: physician response to screening test results. *JAMA.* 1967;201:118–122.

11. Brown CR, Uhl HSM. Mandatory continuing education: sense or nonsense? *JAMA.* 1970;213:1660–1668.

1

Enjoying the Struggle

• • •

> In a highly regimented, regulated, or restrictive environment, medical practice can frustrate, oppress, and enslave—unless the physician holds his noble purpose uppermost in mind. In a humanitarian and intellectually stimulating environment, on the other hand, medicine can be intriguing, exhilarating, and engrossing. It is the continual search for ways to maintain or restore health and well-being to patients and the achievement of that goal that preserve the passion for medicine.
>
> LOIS DEBAKEY, PH.D.

At once one of the most demanding and most rewarding of all professions, medicine can be tyrannizing or exhilarating. If the pressing responsibilities, sensitive interpersonal relationships, and strenuous time pressures in caring for patients are allowed to escalate to tedium or drudgery, the passion for medical practice will vanish. If patient care becomes overly demanding, onerous, or boring, enthusiasm and pleasure will fade, and both patient and physician will suffer. But that does not have to happen. The practice of medicine is admittedly a strict taskmaster, requiring daily decisions about puzzling, often life-threatening illnesses, as well as constant awareness of the newest, most authentic information. But medicine also offers endless opportunities for enjoyment, satisfaction, and exhilaration through intellectual advancement and service to patients.

Can physicians organize their daily work to make the practice of medicine more gratifying? Our extensive communications indicate that those who immerse themselves most deeply in clinical work derive the greatest fulfillment. Such engagement includes daily reading and interacting with colleagues about medical problems, continually examining the nature and results of practice, and modifying performance accordingly. Physicians who practice such immersion base their continuing education largely on the puzzling problems that arise in their practice (individual patients as well as aggregate practice) and the defects they uncover in their performance. And they take prompt remedial steps. The result is improved patient care, gratification, and gusto.

We are not advocating that physicians limit their potential for fulfillment and satisfaction to medical practice, since family, friends, the arts, sports, and hobbies all offer additional rewards. Physicians cannot, however, escape spending inordinate time in practice, so it behooves them to find ways to make the long hours more pleasurable and gratifying. Patients of physicians who enjoy their work, moreover, receive the best care. This book shows how some outstanding physicians have kept the flame of professional fervor alive despite excessive demands on their time and energy.

THE NEED FOR LIFELONG LEARNING

All good physicians realize that they must perpetually revise their knowledge base; they must discard and add continually. Underlying lifelong study are the need to remain aware of the state of medicine, the need to find solutions to specific problems in practice, and the desire for intellectual stimulation, with its attendant personal and social pleasure. The patient is the ultimate beneficiary of all.[1,2] In Garrett Lynch's words, "Lifelong learning is indispensable to maintaining zest for medical practice. One of the greatest joys of medicine is its dynamism, continuously building on, and adding to, previous knowledge—an exciting phenomenon to experience daily. And to see a patient with a metastatic testicular malignancy, for example, finish college, establish a career, and have children makes all the diligent, time-consuming work worthwhile."

REWARDS FROM LEARNING FROM EXPERIENCE

Some of the benefits of lifelong learning are subtle, whereas others are more obvious.

Confidence, Self-respect, and Pride

A primary reward of an expanded intellect is greater self-confidence. As Osler wrote, "If you do not believe in yourself how can you expect other people to do so? If you have not an abiding faith in the profession you cannot be happy in it."[3] Paul Sanazaro agreed: "You need the motivation that stems from pride and security in your knowledge. You must know what you are doing and how it compares with the best you can do; any discrepancy should prompt you to do better." A driving force among the outstanding physicians whom we interviewed is their pride in performance—a desire never to be or seem professionally inadequate.

Enjoyment

Since people tend to invest more of themselves in what is enjoyable, patients benefit when physicians like their work. Emphasizing the salutary relationship of work and pleasure, George Bernard Shaw, in *John Bull's Other Island*, looked forward to a commonwealth where "work is play and play is life."[4] Osler was fond of quoting John Locke's definition of education as a relish for knowledge. "Get early this relish," Osler advised, "this clear, keen joyance in work, with which languor disappears and all shadows of annoyance flee away."[5]

Irvine Page described the engrossing quality of medicine thus: "Medicine makes life worthwhile. If you lose that attitude at any point in your life, you have essentially lost your life. You can combat that danger by remembering that medicine is a grand and rapidly possessive discipline that requires a lifelong interest in things human. If you give that up at any time in your practice, you are lost."

"The method a physician selects for lifelong learning must give pleasure or other rewards," said Eugene Stead, "because human beings will not continue a program that does not have tangible dividends." To make lifelong learning enjoyable, physicians need to organize their time and practice to allow for regular, but not necessarily rigidly scheduled, study in a pleasant, relaxed atmosphere—one that is comfortable, uninterrupted, and unhurried.

The merging of personal and professional pleasure is not uncommon among eminent physicians. To some physicians, the greatest pleasure in medicine comes from seeing a patient improve, and that pleasure is dependent on steady learning. As Michael DeBakey put it, "In medicine, helping others while solving complex intellectual puzzles is our special reward."

ATTRIBUTES TO BE NURTURED

Curiosity

> Curiosity is, in great and generous minds, the first passion and the last. . . .
>
> SAMUEL JOHNSON[6]

"In research," said Baruch Blumberg, "and probably also in practice, maintaining and fostering curiosity—the ability to ask questions each time a new phenomenon occurs—is indispensable." Most physicians we interviewed considered an insatiable curiosity to be innate or to be established in early childhood, but they also recognized the need to nourish it. The drama and complexity of medicine, by providing opportunities for the thrill of discovery, can arouse curiosity despite the inhibitory effect of time pressures. Not being satisfied with an immediate answer, but wanting to go beyond is the mark of the intellectually curious. As Lazar Greenfield said, "In the quest for lifelong learning, we are usually interested in the answer to a question, but that answer will often raise more questions. The result is the opportunity to discover new knowledge, upon which all advances are based. Curiosity will always be the mother of discovery."

Jean Hamburger of Paris related an incident in medical history that illustrates how curiosity can guide genius, allowing a researcher to explain an experimental result that others may dismiss. "In 1879–1880, Pasteur and his coworkers studied the fowl cholera germ. It was a most virulent agent, killing all exposed hens within 24 to 48 hours. After some time, however, some cultures of the germ were unable to kill the animals. 'I am possibly responsible for this failure,' said someone in the laboratory, 'since I left the cultures exposed to air for several days before using them. I shall not repeat this mistake, and the next experiment will be made with fresh cultures.' So the same hens were inoculated some weeks later with germs that were supposed to be very virulent. But Pasteur's coworkers were astonished to find that again the hens did not succumb. 'We are sorry,' they said to Pasteur. 'Something must be wrong with our technique or with the hens we use.' But Pasteur turned the negative results to advantage, and out of this 'failed' experiment came the discovery of vaccination with attenuated germs."

Alfredo Sadun recalled an incident involving David Glendenning Cogan, Chief at the Massachusetts Eye and Ear Infirmary of Harvard Medical School. "Dr. Cogan lived in a large townhouse on Beacon Hill, one of the most exclusive areas but not far from where the drunks reside. One evening the doorbell rang, and when Mrs. Cogan opened the door, she found a drunk who was asking for money. He behaved obstreperously, and when she found it difficult to get rid of him, she enlisted Dr. Cogan's help. Mrs. Cogan then returned to the kitchen. An hour later, she realized that she had not heard from her husband. Unable to find him in the apartment, she feared he may have come to harm in turning away the drunk. Frantically, she left her apartment and raced down the stairs, only to find Dr. Cogan sitting on the street curb next to the drunk under a street light. Scattered around them were a variety of prisms, which Dr. Cogan was using to measure the extent of the drunk's alcohol-induced strabismus. Dr. Cogan was having the drunk fixate (on dollar bills) at varying distances and was then measuring the induced esotropia. He was carefully logging all the data. This incident illustrates the master clinician's child-like curiosity and the constant enthusiasm, which transcend the oddest situation. Even in the most unclinical setting, David Cogan saw an opportunity for gaining further understanding of a subject of interest."

Stimulating Curiosity. You can promote curiosity by engaging in academic interests; relating knowledge to experience; associating with stimulating colleagues, mentors, and students; carefully delineating questions rather than seeking immediate answers to ill-defined problems; and developing pet interests in medicine. The burden of too much to do in too short a time, however, is sure to stifle curiosity.

Associating with intellectually inquisitive people stimulates curiosity. Curiosity thrives in an open atmosphere that permits absolute intellectual honesty. Exposure to medical students, residents, fellows, and young colleagues who challenge traditional concepts can also excite curiosity.

Artful teachers nurture curiosity, especially at the bedside, and teachers who continually ask "Why?" arouse curiosity in their students. Students and house officers who ask provocative questions can have a similar effect on their teachers.

The pursuit of knowledge in a field of special interest and the thrill of resolving previously unanswered or unasked questions are remarkably energizing. To formulate a theoretical answer and then to validate it scientifically provide genuine excitement. Concern about peer judgment and an intense desire to compete with peers for higher levels of knowledge also kindle intellectual curiosity.

Discipline, Diligence, and Determination

Lifelong learning, like the study and training leading to an M.D. degree, requires discipline, diligence, and determination. Charles Brunicardi believes that "Staying current is essential to optimal medical practice, and principles of time management can help establish a disciplined program for learning. Learning should be a daily priority; by incorporating learning techniques into your daily work routine, you will ensure currency in the rapidly changing medical advances."

"No matter how much you read or know," said Norton Greenberger, "you have to keep refurbishing your information. In 1958, when I was a senior medical student at the Massachusetts General Hospital, I went on rounds with the Chief Resident, John Knowles. He seemed to know everything about everything. I asked him how he became so smart, and he replied that he had gotten into the habit of reading every day. If you read ten pages a day, that is about 3,000 pages a year, the equivalent of a textbook."

The challenge of teaching stimulates physicians to study and to organize their thoughts. Having a target date encourages reserving time to review and master a topic. In fact, the most effective way to ensure self-discipline, according to Saul Farber, is to make teaching a part of your daily life.

Compassion and a Sense of Service

In dedicated physicians, an encounter with sick or troubled patients triggers empathy and stimulates the desire to serve. Truly compassionate physicians hone their skills continually to serve their patients better. Willis Hurst considers competence to be an important sign of the physician's compassion, for the compassionate physician cares enough about the patient to seek answers to the clinical questions posed by the patient's illness. The methods described in this book permit the physician to channel his compassion into action benefiting his patients.

The importance of compassion becomes evident when one considers the vulnerability of patients and the trust they place in their physicians. As Sir Berkeley Moynihan wrote: "A patient can offer you no higher tribute than to entrust you with his life and his health, and, by implication, with the happiness of all his family. To be worthy of this trust we must submit for a lifetime to the constant discipline of unwearied effort in the search of knowledge, and of most reverent devotion to every detail in every operation that we perform."[7]

When asked if he took his work home with him, Michael DeBakey responded: "Of course I take my work home with me. Any physician who doesn't should not be practicing medicine. There may be five or six open-heart operations scheduled the next day. All represent individual lives to me. I care about every patient; I worry about them. I think about all of them—their families and their hopes. I may be having dinner with you and talking about baseball, but my mind is with those patients. I wouldn't be a real physician if I didn't do that." We observed the same concern, compassion, and caring in all the outstanding physicians we interviewed, and we are convinced that, because of these noble human qualities, they are able to perform above the average in ministering to their patients.

LEARNING FROM EXPERIENCE

> To study the phenomena of disease without books is to sail an uncharted sea, while to study books without patients is not to go to sea at all.
>
> WILLIAM OSLER, M.D.[8]

All physicians have experiences from their own practices that reinforce Osler's views. Observations made under the pressure and excitement of patient care are usually remembered. Physicians can recall for decades lessons learned from specific patients and their problems. To be most reliable, the memory must, of course, be substantiated by a review of records and notes and must be integrated into current observations.

Robert Manning related an anecdote illustrating the value of such experience. "One of Dr. Richard Vilter's former residents mustered his courage, approached Dr. Vilter, and asked, 'Dr. Vilter, you are such a marvelous clinician. To what do you attribute your success?' Vilter replied, 'Good judgment.' The questioner thought for a moment and, not completely satisfied with the response, asked, 'But Dr. Vilter, to what do you attribute your good judgment?' Vilter replied: 'Experience.' Still not satisfied, the questioner pursued it one step further. 'But Dr. Vilter, how does one gain experience?' Vilter's response: 'Bad judgment.' "

In subsequent chapters, we describe conventional as well as idiosyncratic methods used by practicing physicians and academic clinicians to submerge themselves in their professional work and to gain maximal benefit from their experience. But, first, let us review the underlying philosophic principles. The methods used by our interviewees to gain the most from experience and from reading, conferences, and colleagues represent a blending of study and first-hand experience, as advocated by Osler.

First-hand Knowledge

> First-hand knowledge is the ultimate basis of intellectual life. To a large extent book-learning conveys second-hand information, and as such can never rise to the importance of immediate practice.
>
> ALFRED NORTH WHITEHEAD[9]

Mortimer Adler underscored the importance of experience when he wrote: "[T]he difference between a man and a child is a difference wrought by experience, pain and suffering, by hard knocks. It cannot be produced by schooling."[10] William Osler echoed that idea when he admonished physicians: "Let not your conception of the manifestations of disease come from words heard in the lecture room or read from the book. See, and then reason and compare and control. But see first."[11] Oliver Wendell Holmes concurred: "The most essential part of a student's instruction is obtained . . . not in the lecture-room, but at the bedside. Nothing seen there is lost; the rhythms of disease are learned by frequent repetition; its unforeseen occurrences stamp themselves indelibly in the memory."[12]

Wu Jieping, Honorary President of the Chinese Academy of Medical Sciences, stresses the importance of physicians summarizing and documenting their clinical experiences, as well as keeping up with medical progress through reading and attending conferences. These are complementary. Masterful physicians emphasize skills in the physician–patient relation and a high standard of ethics, both of which are integral to lifelong learning.

Somerset Maugham, who studied medicine, noted his vivid memories of clinical experiences. "Even now that forty years have passed I can remember certain people so exactly that I could draw a picture of them. Phrases that I heard then still linger on my ears. I saw how men died. I saw how they bore pain. I saw what hope looked like, fear and relief; I saw the dark lines that despair drew on a face; I saw courage and steadfastness. I saw faith shine in the eyes of those who trusted in what I could only think was an illusion and I saw the gallantry that made a man greet the prognosis of death with an ironic joke because he was too proud to let those about him see the terror of his soul."[13]

"Clearly at the heart of continuing medical education," said James Young, "is the passion for learning about disease, patients, and healthcare. This is difficult in today's harried patient-care environment, but it is the surest way to nurture the passion. One cannot help being awestruck in the clinic with the resilience of patients, as well as their occasional imprudence and intransigence. The human spirit is remarkable—undaunted and unparalleled. Even the most seemingly mundane patient can spark a question in the physician's mind: Will I see benefit from a particular procedure or medication? What if I change the treatment protocol? Can the treatment plan be simplified? These questions can stimulate the physician to search for answers, and that search is what I enjoy most about my profession: the total unpredictability of what the day will bring, along with the certainty of learning something new from each patient. Often, it is searching out nuances of a patient's personality, or that of a relative or friend, that can make a perverse interaction pleasant and rewarding. By turning difficult encounters into golden moments with smiles and questions, the stage is set to explore both scientific and personally introspective continuing medical education."

Monitoring One's Own Practice. The most fruitful education for a profession, Cyril Houle wrote, "occurs when its practitioners constantly monitor their own work, making judgments about success or failure and subsequently altering behavior as a consequence."[2] Such monitoring requires techniques that permit analysis of what the physician actually does in the aggregate and the lessons learned from puzzling individual patients. When physicians know the types of problems seen, the drugs prescribed, and the procedures performed, they can direct their study for maximal benefit to their patients. Medical school faculties, despite lip service to the contrary, still emphasize the didactic transfer of information, and most physicians have therefore not been taught to organize their practices in a way to produce objective data that can direct their education. Fortunately, there are simple ways of organizing and analyzing everyday work, and we describe these throughout the book.

Self-directed Learning. Malcolm Knowles cited accumulating evidence that "Whatever people learn through their own initiative, they understand better, internalize more effectively, apply more generally, and retain longer than anything they are taught didactically." Since the most valuable continuing education is linked to practical experience and since each physician has individual experiences, physicians can direct their own learning best from an analysis of their practice.

George Miller wrote: "There is ample evidence to support the view that adult learning is not most efficiently achieved through systematic subject instruction; it is accomplished by involving learners in identifying problems and seeking ways to solve them. It does not come in categorical bundles but in a growing need to know."[14]

Harold Jeghers summarized the basic premises of lifelong learning in medicine thus: "The secret is to learn to educate oneself. One remembers best what one learns by personal effort. Strong initiative and motivation are important. Reading should be directed primarily toward solving a problem with a specific goal in mind. Since patient care is basic to the practice of medicine, reading and learning are most effective when they involve discussion and solution of clinical problems. Beyond formal education, a well-developed personal medical information center supports continued personal education."

On July 1, 2000, Jordan Cohen, President of the Association of American Medical Colleges (AAMC), distributed a document entitled "Association of American Medical Colleges Statement on Life-long Professional Development and Maintenance of Competence," which was developed by the Council of Academic Societies Administrative Board in association with AAMC Division of Medical Education.[15] A relevant passage reads: "Recent evidence suggests that to be effective, CME [continuing medical education] should be highly self-directed with content, learning methods, and learning resources selected specifically for the purpose of maintaining or improving the knowledge, skills, and attitudes which physicians need on a regular basis in their practices. Individual CME activities should incorporate interactive learning formats, and include practice enabling and reinforcing strategies. To the degree possible, the learning experiences should be accessible within physicians' practice or work settings. In order for CME to be effective, physicians must recognize the knowledge, skills, and attitudes they need to maintain competence in their specialty or practice, and participate in CME activities designed specifically for that purpose.

"The AAMC believes that specialty societies and specialty boards are best able to assist physicians in their efforts to maintain their clinical competence. To this end, the societies and boards should set forth on a regular basis the attributes that are needed to practice medicine on a specialty-specific basis, and should identify for physicians the valid kinds of CME activities that will allow them to maintain or acquire those attributes. The societies and boards also must develop new assessment methods that will allow them to determine whether or not individual physicians have developed and maintained the attributes needed for practice. While some specialty boards are in the process of actually implementing new assessment methodologies to achieve this purpose, the majority of boards are not."

Make the Most of Your Situation

Some physicians fail to become immersed in their practice because they allow it to become too routine. This is primarily an attitudinal problem, for almost any practice environment can be made stimulating. Mansell Pattison uses his regular resident clinical case conference to stimulate forays into "forgotten and new paths of clinical investigation." "My teacher, Dr. Maury Levine of Cincinnati," he recalled, "used to admonish us that each clinical case is a research project. I similarly ask my residents to look for the unanswered research question in every routine case. The rewards have been ample. In just the past year, 'routine' cases uncovered interesting information. A depressed patient with porphyria led to a literature review and the discovery that porphyric psychosis is omitted from current textbooks of medicine; a case of pseudo-seizure led to the demonstration of a basic linkage in the thought-speech process; a case of self-mutilation led to the description of a new clinical syndrome; a case of dissociation led to the analysis of visceral brain components of consciousness. Four simple cases led to four major research projects. That is surely enough excitement in one year to keep a jaded administrator alive and enthusiastically on his toes to see what the next 'routine case' will turn up."

COMPANIONSHIP IN MEDICINE

Self-directed learning does not, of course, require isolation. In medicine, the collegial network provides strong support for physicians by allowing them to share experiences, knowledge, and inspiration in an atmosphere of fellowship while remaining responsible for their own learning. Discussions with colleagues about patients and medical problems afford excellent opportunities to gain information enjoyably.

"Encouragement of medical companionship is important," said Sherman Mellinkoff, "whether in group practice, participation in rounds, attendance at courses to update important subjects, or attendance at medical meetings. When a complicated problem needs clarification, I sometimes go to the library, but I usually turn to one of my colleagues for a consultation. It is so useful for doctors to have little groups or affinities that provide someone near at hand with whom to exchange ideas and discuss patients or published articles. Such interaction makes learning more vibrant and useful."

"One reason we academicians like our work," noted Norton Greenberger, "is that we learn a lot by osmosis. We go to conferences, and we seek out people who have the answers to our questions. So my advice to young physicians is to surround yourself with people who can educate you."

REDUCING RELIANCE ON MEMORY

Acquiring knowledge when it is needed is more effective than memorizing facts that may not be used for weeks or months. "I have never tried to convert medical students into textbooks," said Eugene Stead. "If we did, we would clearly be forced to lower tuition, since the best composite of medical knowledge can be purchased for $150." Alfred North Whitehead, too, cautioned against the evil of "bare knowledge" and "inert ideas." He defined education as the art of the use of knowledge, whose importance lies in our active mastery of it—that is to say, it lies in wisdom. "Get your knowledge quickly, and then use it. If you can use it, you will retain it."[16] He wisely noted that "Knowledge does not keep any better than fish."[17]

Lawrence Weed has long objected to our expectation that physicians remember the details in the numerous textbooks they were required to memorize in medical school to pass their examinations. He laments that we further expect them to keep abreast of the newest medical information published and presented at meetings and to apply all this knowledge effectively in their practices. Failure, he believes, is built into those expectations.[18]

Instead of describing methods that rely too heavily on memorizing and learning facts unrelated to current problems, we shall emphasize manual and electronic methods that help physicians access and use information sources efficiently at times when patient problems actually arise. Fortunately, with the explosion of information sources available on the computer, the need for physicians to memorize declines, but they must now concentrate more heavily on seeking and evaluating information and applying the new knowledge prudently.

FRAMING THE RIGHT QUESTIONS

"One learns by asking oneself questions, then finding the answers," said Eugene Stead. The physician must decide what he knows and what he does not know. He must then formulate questions and consult the proper source to answer the questions. With emphasis on methods of organization, storing, and accessing pertinent information, the skill for formulating proper questions becomes essential. "I would be very happy if every student, every resident, and every cardiac fellow felt that it is more important to learn how to ask questions and pursue the answers, themselves, than it is for me to ask questions for them to answer," said Willis Hurst. "I believe that asking questions is what they should do all their lives."

Reading, conferences, and discussions with colleagues alert the physician to knowledge deficits. Associating with other physicians with similar interests helps in formulation of the right questions, and an exchange of information leads to recognition of what needs to be answered. Unanswered questions should stimulate the physician, but one must guard against frustration from failing to find all the answers alone.

KNOWLEDGE IS NOT ENOUGH

The purpose of knowledge and information is to apply them properly in patient care. Proper application of knowledge is not automatic; many advances in patient care are never applied. Physicians who immerse themselves in their practice are likely to learn current developments from their general reading, discussions with peers, attending courses, and browsing an electronic information service. By focused searches for evidence-based information to help them solve diagnostic and therapeutic problems on puzzling patients, they may continually strengthen their knowledge base. How can they assure themselves and their patients that they are applying evidence-based knowledge? (See p. 123)

The classic study by Fox, Mazmanian, and Putnam describes several factors that encourage change,[19] such as curiosity, sense of personal or financial well-being, the desire to be more competent, and stimuli in the clinical environment (opinion of peers, hospital regulations, and community needs).

Most studies have concluded that changes in a physician's delivery of care are due to several factors rather than a single intervention. General practitioners described an average of 3.2 reasons for change and consultants an average of 2.8 reasons. The three most common categories for change were (1) organizational changes, such as regulation by a hospital or health maintenance organization (HMO), (2) an educational activity, such as reading medical journals or attending an educational event, and (3) discussions with a physician or another health professional.[20]

Mazmanian and coauthors found that, after a conference on multiple risk factors in atherosclerotic vascular disease, physicians who indicated on a questionnaire that they planned to change were more likely than those with no commitment to state 45 days later that they made the change.[21]

Evidence indicates that strategies, such as providing feedback reports on practice[22] and the effect of influential peers,[23] are effective in fostering change. Interventions aimed at physicians preparing for change can target the office staff and even patients as well. Reminders and checklists are helpful.[24] Ornstein and coauthors reported that an added benefit of combining patient and physician reminders was an increased adherence of patients receiving preventive services.[25] Patients are a major motivating force to encourage physicians to consider using new knowledge or altering management.[26]

In regularly scheduled meetings with office staff members, dicussions are often helpful to determine problems that are inhibiting delivery of the best care. Writing a plan to effect a change is useful as a commitment as well as a reminder to the physician and office staff. Physicians who systematically study their practice performance have an added advantage of determining what needs to be changed.

START NOW

> The supreme value is not the future but the present.
> The future is a deceitful time that always says to us,
> "Not yet," and thus denies us.
>
> OCTAVIO PAZ[27]

To Roy Behnke, the complaint of some physicians that they are so far behind they can never catch up is merely an excuse. "Many of my colleagues say that the task is so overwhelming, what is the use of trying to catch up? But you must start somewhere. Those who try to make continuing education too formal never get it done: the system beats them. Medicine offers the advantage of informal education. You can pursue it at almost any hour of the day, and five minutes is time enough if you have arranged for the information to be easily accessible." So resist the temptation to procrastinate or defer the task. Remember:

> The Bird of Time has but a little way
> To fly—and Lo! the Bird is on the Wing[28]

REFERENCES

1. Richards RK, Cohen RM. Why physicians attend traditional CME programs. *J Med Educ.* 1980; 55:479–485.

2. Houle CO. *Continuing Learning in the Professions.* San Francisco: Jossey–Bass; 1980:208–209.

3. Osler W. The reserves of life. Address delivered at St. Mary's Hospital, London, 1907 Oct 2. *St. Mary's Hosp Gaz.* 1907;13:97.

4. Shaw GB. *John Bull's Other Island.* In: *Bernard Shaw: Selected Plays with Prefaces.* Vol 2. New York: Dodd, Mead & Co.; 1957:611.

5. Osler W. After twenty-five years. An address at the opening of the session of the medical faculty, McGill University, 1899 Sep 21. *Montreal Med J.* 1899;28:832.

6. Johnson S. *The Rambler.* Vol 5. No. 150, 1751 Aug 24. London: J. Payne and J. Bouquet; 1752:120.

7. Moynihan B. *Abdominal Operations.* Vol 1. Revised, preface to the 4th ed. Philadelphia: W.B. Saunders; 1926:11–12.

8. Osler W. Books and men. In: *Aequanimitas, with Other Addresses to Medical Students, Nurses and Practitioners of Medicine.* 3rd ed. Philadelphia: Blakiston ; 1945:210.

9. Whitehead AF. Technical education and its relation to science and literature. In: *The Aims of Education and Other Essays.* New York: MacMillan; 1959:79.

10. Adler M. Why only adults can be educated. In: Gross R, ed. *Invitation to Lifelong Learning.* Chicago: Follett; 1982:92.

11. Osler W. In: Bean WB, ed. *Sir William Osler: Aphorisms from His Bedside Teachings and Writings.* Springfield, IL: Charles C Thomas; 1968:36.

12. Holmes OW. Scholastic and bedside teaching. In: *Medical Essays; 1842–1882.* Vol 9. Boston: Houghton Mifflin; 1911:273.

13. Maugham WS. *The Summing Up.* Garden City, NY: Doubleday; 1946.

14. Miller GE. Continuing education for what? *J Med Educ.* 1967;42:322.

15. Cohen JJ. Association of American Medical Colleges Memorandum No. 00-32. 2000 Jul 31.

16. Whitehead AN. The rhythmic claims of freedom and discipline. In: *The Aims of Education and Other Essays.* New York: MacMillan; 1959:57.

17. Whitehead AN. Universities and their function. In: *The Aims of Education and Other Essays.* New York: Macmillan; 1959:147.

18. Weed LL. *Your Health and How to Manage It.* Essex Junction, VT: Essex Publishing; 1975:91.

19. Fox RD, Mazmanian PE, Putnam RW. *Changing and Learning in the Lives of Physicians.* New York: Praeger; 1989.

20. Allery LA, Owen PA, Robling MR. Why general practitioners and consultants change their clinical practice: a critical incident study. *BMJ* 1997;314:870–874.

21. Mazmanian PE, Daffron SR, Johnson RE, David DA, Kantrowitz MP. Information about barriers to planned change: a randomized controlled trial involving continuing medical education lectures and commitment to change. *Acad Med.* 1998;73:882–886.

22. Eisenberg JM. *Doctors' Decisions and the Cost of Medical Care.* Ann Arbor, MI: Health Administration Press; 1986.

23. Stross JK, Hiss RG, Watts CM, Davis WK, MacDonald R. Continuing education in pulmonary disease for primary care physicians. *Am Rev Respir Dis.* 1983;127:739–746.

24. McDonald CJ. Protocol-based computer reminders, the quality of care and the non-perfectability of man. *N Engl J Med.* 1976;295:1351–1355.

25. Ornstein SM, Garr DR, Jenkins RG, Rust PF, Arnon A. Computer-generated physician and patient reminders. Tools

to improve population adherence to selected preventive services. *J Fam Pract.* 1991;32:82–90.

26. Towle A. Shifting the culture of continuing medical education: what needs to happen and why is it so difficult? *J Contin Educ Health Prof.* 2000;20:208–218.
27. Paz O. Development and other mirages. In: *The Other Mexico: Critique of the Pyramid.* Kemp L, trans. New York: Grove Press; 1972:68.
28. Khayyam O. *Rubaiyat of Omar Khayyam.* Fitzgerald E, trans. London: John Lane the Bodley Head Ltd; 1922: quatrain 7.

PERSONAL ESSAY

• • •

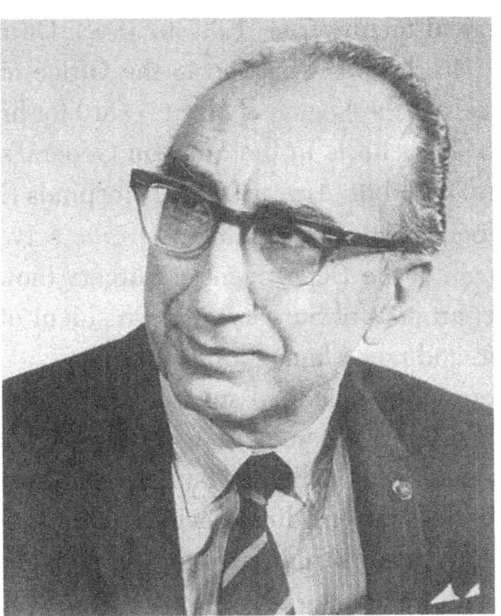

Medicine is an absorbing, even possessive, profession, but the intellectual rewards, humanitarian service, and fulfillment are unsurpassed.

MICHAEL E. DEBAKEY, M.D.

The inscription on the bust of Dr. Michael DeBakey in The Methodist Hospital, Texas Medical Center in Houston, reads "Surgeon, Educator, Medical Statesman. In recognition of one who served so many." Universally recognized as an ingenious medical inventor and researcher, a gifted and dedicated teacher, the premier surgeon of the world, and an international medical statesman, Dr. DeBakey is esteemed and admired by colleagues, students, and the general public for his indefatigable dedication to the service of mankind and is loved by his patients for his skillful and compassionate ministrations.

Dr. DeBakey received his B.S., M.S., and M.D. degrees from Tulane University in New Orleans, served his internship at Charity Hospital in New Orleans, and completed his residency in surgery at Charity Hospital, the University of Strasbourg, France, and the University of Heidelberg, Germany. He served on the Tulane Medical School surgical faculty from 1937 to 1948. On military leave from 1942 to 1946, he was assigned to the Office of the Surgeon General and received the Legion of Merit Award for his outstanding service in 1945. His efforts in the Surgeon General's office led to the development of Mobile Army Surgical Hospitals (MASH units). In 1948, he joined the Baylor faculty, where he served simultaneously as Chairman of the Department of Surgery (now the Michael E. DeBakey Department of Surgery) and President of the College, then Chancellor, and now Chancellor Emeritus.

As an undergraduate medical student, Dr. DeBakey devised a roller pump that later became an essential component of the heart–lung machine and thus helped launch open-heart surgery. He has devised countless new medical devices and operations, as well as more than 50 surgical instruments for the improvement of patient care. In 1939, with his mentor, Dr. Alton Ochsner, he noted an association between smoking tobacco and lung cancer. Best known for his trailblazing efforts in the treatment of cardiovascular diseases, Dr. DeBakey was the first to perform successful excision and graft replacement of aneurysms of the thoracic aorta and obstructive lesions of the major arteries. In 1953, he established the field of surgery for strokes when he performed the first successful carotid endarterectomy. In 1964, he and his associates performed the first successful aortocoronary artery bypass with autogenous vein graft. Four years later, he led a team of surgeons in a historic multiple transplantation procedure in which the heart, kidneys, and one lung of a donor were transplanted to four recipients. A pioneer in artificial heart research, he was the first, in 1966, to use a partial artificial heart successfully—a left ventricular bypass pump, precursor of the current miniaturized DeBakey Left Ventricular Assist Device. It was Dr. DeBakey's testimony before Congress in early 1963 that initiated federal support for artificial heart research.

Dr. DeBakey was a member of the Medical Advisory Committee of the Hoover Commission and was Chairman of President Johnson's Commission on Heart Disease, Cancer, and Stroke. He served an unprecedented three terms on the National Heart, Lung, and Blood Advisory Council of the National Institutes of Health and also served as Chairman of the Board of Regents of the National Library of Medicine, which he was instrumental in establishing.

For his pioneering achievements in cardiovascular surgery and his vast humanitarian endeavors, Dr. DeBakey has received more than 50 honorary degrees from prominent colleges and universities. His countless national and international honors and awards, many from heads-of-state throughout the world, include the Presidential Medal of Freedom with Distinction from President Johnson, the National Medal of Science from President Reagan, the prestigious Albert Lasker Award for Clinical Research, and the Living Legend Award from the Library of Congress. Author of more than 1600 articles and books, many considered landmark publications, he has been the president of various eminent medical organizations, Founding Editor of the *Journal of Vascular Surgery*, Editor of the *Year Book of General Surgery*, and Coeditor of *Christopher's Minor Surgery*.[1] He has also served as editor or editorial board member of many other distinguished surgical journals and as consultant to governmental agencies in the United States and throughout the world. *The New Living Heart*,[2] written for the lay public, was a *New York Times* bestseller. Dr. DeBakey was an early advocate of educating the public about health issues and has long been a frequent guest on network news for this purpose. He has also written widely about medicine and health in the major news media.

As a tribute to his selfless efforts to improve human health, a number of facilities, awards, and scholarships have been named in his honor, including the Michael E. DeBakey Center for Biomedical Education and Research at Baylor College of Medicine, the Metohodist DeBakey Heart Center in Houston; the Michael E. DeBakey High School for Health Professions in Houston; the Texas A&M University Michael E. DeBakey Institute for Cardiovascular Science and Biomedical Devices; the Michael E. DeBakey Heart Institutes in Hays, Kansas, and in Kenosha, Wisconsin; the Michael E. DeBakey International Military Surgery Award and The DeBakey USU Brigade of the Uniformed Services University of the Health Sciences; the Michael E. DeBakey International Surgical Society (formed by his students and residents); the Michael E. DeBakey Award in Journalism of the Foundation for Biomedical Research; and the Michael E. DeBakey Library Services Outreach Award of the Friends of the National Library of Medicine.

As a world-renowned surgeon, he has operated on princes and paupers, providing all with the same dedicated humanitarian service. Known as the "King of Surgeons," Dr. DeBakey has been first and foremost the patient's advocate.

* * * * *

> Dr. DeBakey's total commitment to, and fascination with, medical science and its humanitarian aims have been an inspiration to patients, students, and associates alike. Mike does a tremendous amount of surgery. Many people look upon this as a highly impersonalized, mechanical venture. But you ought to make rounds with Mike about ten o'clock in the evening and watch him go through and touch his people. No one else can do such technical work in a highly personal way as Mike can.
>
> EUGENE A. STEAD, JR., M.D.

> Because of his warmth, compassion, and humanity that symbolize the finest ideals of his profession, he has been beloved by his students, colleagues, and many esteemed friends in every walk of life.
>
> DAVID C. SABISTON, JR., M.D.

REFERENCES

1. Ochsner A, DeBakey ME, eds. *Christopher's Minor Surgery.* Philadelphia: W.B. Saunders; 1955, 1959.
2. DeBakey ME, Gotto AM, Jr. *The New Living Heart.* Holbrook (MA): Adams Media; 1997.

Medicine: Preparing for and Enjoying an Intellectually, Emotionally, and Morally Fulfilling Career

Michael E. DeBakey, M.D.
Chancellor Emeritus
Olga Keith Wiess and Distinguished Service Professor
Michael E. DeBakey Department of Surgery
Director, DeBakey Heart Center
Baylor College of Medicine,
Houston, Texas

EARLY INFLUENCES

Parents

I have often been asked what inspired me to take the path I have pursued in life. The answer lies in my boyhood. My parents, with their keen intellects, natural curiosity, and high standards, were superb models because they sought excellence in everything they did. Anything worth their time was worth doing well. By example, they inspired and encouraged me in that philosophy. They valued education and gave their children every opportunity to learn and to fulfill their potential, not only in school but in music, the arts, and athletics. All of us had music lessons as children; I learned to play several instruments and was a member of the school band. At home, we were surrounded by books, but we were also encouraged to read, in addition to our schoolwork, at least one book a week from the city library. We learned early that books were wonderful companions.

At a very early age, we were also given an opportunity to experience gratification from some special achievement—whether it was mastering a subject in our schoolwork, learning to play a musical composition well, or excelling in sports or gardening. Our parents helped us discover the *delight* of learning, and they often made our new knowledge more significant by relating it to some interesting story in their own lives or to some current or historical event. Although they did not prod or nag us about studying, they did encourage, direct, and support our learning. Almost every family event was a learning experience—whether it was a picnic, where we learned about nature; a hunting trip, where we learned about sportsmanship; or a family meal, where conversations were always stimulating. When we asked questions, our parents satisfied our immediate curiosity with an explanation, but then encouraged us to delve further into the subject by reading about it. If the children had disagreements about certain issues—and children can be extremely opinionated—our parents suggested we could settle the matter by consulting a dictionary, encyclopedia, or other authoritative source. They explained that our opinions would be respected more if we could support them with some evidence, and so we were discouraged from formulating firm opinions without a valid basis or, to express it differently, from developing raw prejudices. Reason and common sense were highly respected in our home.

One incident illustrates how our parents nurtured our education. When I was a very young boy, my Father took me on a hunting trip, and when he set me down in the field, he said, "Now stay right here; I won't be far away." He would go a short distance, glancing back at me often and returning every little while to bring back the ducks that he had shot. On one such occasion, he noticed that I had my hands behind my back, and he said, "What's wrong with your hands?" Eventually, I had to reveal my hands, which were bloody. He was immediately alarmed and asked, "What did you do? Did you cut yourself?" I confessed that I had taken a knife out of the pouch and had opened the ducks. "Why did you do that?" he asked. "I wanted to find out how they fly," I explained. Shortly after that, my Father read me a book about birds flying. He noted my early curiosity, and he encouraged and stimulated it. Throughout my student years, he and my Mother supported my fascination with medicine and surgery.

We hear much today about the disintegration of the American family, and my heart goes out to those who have missed the joys of belonging to a close-knit, loving family. Our parents' affection for us was evident in everything they did, but they also imposed discipline, often in subtle ways. We all had tasks assigned and were expected to exercise personal responsibility and self-reliance in performing them.

I feel fortunate in having received moral and spiritual guidance as a child, because I think it is valuable for everyone, and especially for physicians. Largely by parental example, we learned that honesty, integrity, compassion, and personal and social responsibility enrich life and enhance peace of mind. Intellectual development without these values is compromised, in my view. The family integrity that my parents cherished so deeply gave me a sense of purpose and gave my life direction. It is, perhaps, the greatest legacy anyone can receive, and for a physician, it is indispensable.

Teachers

Having dedicated teachers who reinforced my parents' interest in education encouraged me to do my best in my assignments. I was fortunate to come under the guidance of a number of college professors who took an interest in me, among them my zoology professor. I became so interested in zoology that when I went home on vacation, I set up a large aquarium in my parents' garage and filled it with various kinds of marine life so I could continue my study during the summer. That professor appointed me as a student assistant, and during subsequent summers I continued to work in his department. I taught courses, including graduate courses, and I had to read and study the material thoroughly in order to teach it. My professor of English Literature showed a similar interest in me and invited me to major in that subject. His guidance nurtured my literary bent.

Perhaps the professor who influenced me more than anyone else was Dr. Alton Ochsner, under whose influence I came as a medical student. At that time, I was not sure I wanted to practice surgery, but he and his associate, Dr. Mims Gage, encouraged me to go into surgery and engaged me in laboratory research. I spent a lot of time in the laboratory, and so did Dr. Ochsner. I invented my first medical device when I was still in medical school—a roller pump, which later became an essential component of the heart–lung machine. I think my interest in inventions was whetted by watching my Father constantly improving devices he used and seeking, and usually finding, more efficient ways of accomplishing tasks.

Dr. Ochsner also engaged me in writing papers with him, and, as my early bibliography attests, we wrote a lot of papers together. So I was trained in academic work, and I liked it very much because it permitted continual learning. Dr. Ochsner suggested that I go abroad, where he had received some of his own training and where, in those days, American physicians often studied in prestigious European universities. Although it was around the time of the Great Depression, my parents financed my stay abroad—another indication of how highly they valued education. I worked in the research laboratories of two eminent professors: René Leriche at the University of Strasbourg and Martin Kirschner at the University of Heidelberg. I learned to speak French and German, and I developed valuable associations. It was an extremely rewarding period.

SELF-DISCIPLINE

Next to intellectual curiosity, perhaps self-discipline is most important for continuing education. I see a lot of young students who have not yet developed the self-discipline required for effective organization of their studies and other activities. They flit from one thing to another, allowing themselves to be distracted by matters that are not really helpful. They tend to associate diversion with passive entertainment. Television has probably been responsible, in great measure, for promoting passivity. The enigma is that people can become glued to their television set when the programming is generally so poor. Learning, however, is anything but passive; it is a highly active process that can also be extremely gratifying. Electronic devices represent a remarkable technologic advance, especially because of the speed with which they can provide masses of information, but they are no substitute for human reasoning. And reasoning is at the crux of the physician's daily work.

Reasoning

Few experiences are more enjoyable than reasoning and learning, whether your subject is nature, science, history, or the arts. The exhilaration of solving a difficult problem is hard to match. And when you put your whole heart and soul into whatever you do, your sense of self-worth soars. You gain self-confidence, and you are more at peace with yourself. Today, entrepreneurs make millions selling books and giving courses on "self-actualization" and on finding out "who you are," but if you develop self-discipline and invest your full attention and effort in whatever you do, you will not need a course to tell you who you are. You will know.

Most physicians recognize the need for a good foundation in the sciences, but seem less aware of the importance of the humanities. Since, however, literature deals with all aspects of the human experience—the happy and the tragic, the base and the ennobling—it teaches much about human nature and human life that is useful to the physician. Continuing to read good literature, including history, throughout life is an asset. Our society no longer emphasizes a knowledge or a sense of history, and that is unfortunate. I would urge every young physician to read the major works on medical history. Not only are the lives of the great achievers inspiring, but history puts the present in perspective, and so helps us better understand what is going on now and what the most judicious course might be for the future. In medicine, history also prevents us from duplicating experiments for which the answers are already known.

Philosophy, including ethics and logic, is also an intriguing subject, and those who study it are likely to consider all aspects of an issue, including dissenting views, rather than form dogmatic opinions. Because mathematics enhances reasoning ability, it is useful for physicians. Intellectual and cultural development should go hand in hand with physical development, and all are definite assets for the physician. Athletics improve coordination and physical well-being, in addition to advancing socialization by teaching cooperation and a sense of fair play. A diversity of activities not only affords balance, but provides a stable base for pursuits in adulthood.

Language

And then there is language—the crucial instrument of communication. The whole thinking process is entwined with language—terms and their meanings. Yet I see young people coming out of college today with little understanding of the need for clarity and precision in their speech and writing. Deficiencies in such education can lead to sloppy thinking. Medical students, in presenting a case, will say that a patient had a tumor of the breast without identifying which breast, or pain in the leg without stating which leg. They know that the tumor was in the right breast, but they do not convey that information to their audience. In medicine especially, precision is paramount. To say that a patient has an infarction without precisely defining its site and extent is to withhold information crucial to effective treatment. Simplicity and clarity of expression are as important as precision for the physician, especially in communications with patients. Taking the time to explain a patient's symptoms can relieve anxiety about imagined grave health problems. The compassionate physician will sense a patient's anxiety and will try to assuage it. Moreover, patients who understand their diagnosis and prescribed treatment are likely to be more cooperative in following their physician's advice for remaining well after recovery.

CONTINUING EDUCATION

As every physician knows, the competent practice of medicine requires lifelong learning. I have been able to obtain the kind of information that meets my specific needs by keeping abreast of current publications, by studying topics of special interest more deeply, by arranging regular interdisciplinary discussions, including meetings on research, and by continually analyzing my own surgical results. In The DeBakey Heart Center, we hold weekly meetings at which the staffs in various basic and clinical research disciplines present their current work and bring up complex matters for general discussion. These regular meetings afford a remarkable educational opportunity.

Writing

Writing is also a superb method of continuing education, particularly in medicine, because it requires comprehensive, critical reasoning. Teachers and scientists have an obligation to disseminate new knowledge in this way. Since my early years, when my parents encouraged all of us to write letters and keep journals, I have had an interest in writing. When, as a grammar-school student, I went abroad with my family, I wrote letters to my teachers about our trip and was pleased when the letters were published in the local newspaper. That, of course, further encouraged my literary efforts.

When I began collaborating on manuscripts with my chief, Dr. Alton Ochsner, I would retire to my office or laboratory at the medical school after completion of my routine teaching and clinical duties and would remain there until midnight doing laboratory research, reading published articles, and preparing reports of our results. One long counter in my office was always stacked high with library books, and I spent hours abstracting articles, verifying references, documenting statements, and reverifying statistics. I learned early to take personal responsibility for every step in the preparation of a manuscript for publication or presentation. That self-discipline has been most rewarding.

When I write articles for presentation or publication, I read material that I might not otherwise see in journals I routinely review. At meetings in which I participate throughout the world, I have been able to learn what research is being done and how medicine is practiced in different regions. As a member of various editorial boards over the years, I have also had the opportunity of reviewing manuscripts of research work at the forefront of medicine and have thus been kept informed of the latest scientific developments.

BIBLIOGRAPHIC TECHNOLOGY

When I was a medical student, and until the latter twentieth century, bibliographic searches had to be done manually. This was a tedious, labor-intensive, time-consuming process, involving consulting successive yearly bound volumes of the *Index Medicus*—first selecting articles whose titles suggested pertinence to the subject, then pulling each journal from the library shelves and scanning it for relevance before reading thoroughly those culled for specific information. Today, students cannot conceive of such a laborious process; they search the Internet and find desired sources at the press of a button. As facile as the present process is, you should be aware that current databases usually include references from only the latter twentieth century, so failure to search manually for earlier publications may mean missing historically or otherwise important sources. Research questions you are planning to pursue, for example, may already have been answered, and rare cases may have been described, but missed because they are not entered in current bibliographic databases. You may also inadvertently misattribute priority for certain innovations, discoveries, or advances. My own policy is to make as thorough and as comprehensive a search as possible. One other caveat: do not allow the ease of mechanization to quench your intellectual curiosity or your determination to examine critically, to reason meticulously, and to pursue problems intellectually. Learn to evaluate what you read instead of giving credence to everything that is published. And make sure that the databases you consult are authentic, complete, and current.

Analysis of Clinical Experience

Another excellent method of continuing education for the physician is periodic analysis of personal clinical experience for presentation at meetings or for publication. In my own analyses, I try to determine the factors that affect survival, complications, and mortality. If I am analyzing my clinical results for aortic valve replacement, for example, I do a bibliographic search for articles on a variety of valves and then compare my experience with the results of other surgeons. Such a study may lead me to use a certain valve. After another interval, I will do another comparative analysis of my results with that valve and of results obtained by others. In this way, you can determine whether your techniques are better or worse than those of your peers.

One technique that I use for follow-up is to write the physicians of patients, or the patients themselves, at regular intervals to inquire about their progress and state of health. Not only does this assure patients of my personal interest and concern, but it also provides valuable feedback about treatment or progress of the disease.

In the practice of medicine, you must continually expand your knowledge if you are to give your patients the best available care. When a new surgical technique is introduced, my colleagues and I first study it, and if we decide that it shows promise as a safe and effective procedure, we try it, sometimes modifying and improving it. Continually seeking better ways of treating patients is every physician's obligation, and in my specialty that has sometimes led me to design a new surgical instrument or develop a new operative technique.

From time to time, every physician will have an extraordinarily difficult case about which more information is needed. There are two ways to obtain it. One is to review previous publications to see if anyone has had such a case and, if so, how it was managed. The other is to review your own clinical experience to see if you have had that particular problem before and what the results were. In managing the complex problems referred to me from throughout the world, I have found a continual study of my clinical experience to be invaluable. Reviewing accumulated clinical cases can disclose extremely useful information. The analysis of angiograms of my patients with occlusive arterial disease, for example, allowed me to recognize certain patterns of disease and their segmental nature. Recognition of such patterns led me to devise the surgical treatment for aneurysms before the cause of the underlying disease was fully understood.

We found, also, that the most common cause of death in patients with certain types of vascular disorders was coronary disease. In analyzing that experience, we focused on coronary disease as an important factor contributing to death, and this led us to do specific studies on patients with vascular disease to determine whether they had coronary disease. That analysis showed that in some patients it is important to deal with the coronary disease before you deal with any other vascular disease. We did the same type of study with carotid arterial occlusive disease.

Keeping Current

You can facilitate your continuing medical education by developing a routine for keeping abreast of scientific publications: regularly reviewing selected journals related to your particular practice, and having in your personal medical library or electronic database, for ready reference, books and articles dealing with your own medical discipline. Further, you can attend meetings related to the clinical problems you see in your practice. And if you can set aside several hours a week to participate in hospital or medical school activities, you will not only find them intellectually stimulating, but will also learn of new developments almost as they occur. In most centers such as ours, activities of this kind are well organized. Every hospital, even in small communities, should have a continuing education program, with regular meetings for its medical and allied health staffs. Preparing presentations for such meetings is certainly educational for the speaker, and the information disseminated is useful to the listeners. When such discussions center on patients under consideration at the time, they have a special impact for retention of that knowledge. The interchanges with colleagues and students are mutually stimulating.

In our Surgery Department, we have regular weekly conferences, at which the staff presents analyses of various cases. Clinical data regarding complications and deaths are thoroughly discussed, and interesting cases are presented. Our journal conference is designed largely for residents, who report on designated current journal articles, after which there is a general discussion. When faculty members have been to a medical meeting elsewhere, they summarize the proceedings for the staff, and a discussion follows. For those of us interested in cardiovascular disease, the cardiology and cardiovascular surgery units hold combined conferences, in which basic science personnel engaged in cardiovascular work often participate. When I designed our Cardiovascular Research and Clinical Center, I insisted on having basic scientists and clinicians from all pertinent disciplines housed in the Center, an interdisciplinary arrangement that has been one of its most important and productive features.

My hope is that formal medical education will not become too rigid—that the emphasis will not focus on structure more than on the actual educational process. Continuing education means *active* learning, and whereas guidance, counseling, and direction are helpful, education should not be rigidified. If, for example, the purpose in studying is solely to pass an examination, the student is not going to retain a great deal of knowledge—or gain very much wisdom. The examination should be a means of evaluating one's own state of knowledge, and the emphasis should be on the *knowledge,* not on the test. I would hope that medical education would not be restricted to the absorption of facts, but that it would encourage critical thinking, would include ethical issues, and would foster a humanitarian approach to the care of patients. All learning is useful in expanding the mind and its limits and benefits others when the acquired knowledge is applied for their advantage. In the case of physicians, the application of knowledge often yields dramatic humanitarian results, and we are therefore uniquely motivated, and obligated, to continue our education throughout life. In medicine, helping others while solving complex intellectual puzzles is our special reward.

"MANAGED" CARE

Medicine has undergone dramatic changes over the past few decades, not only because of stunning new discoveries, but also because of proliferating government and managed-care regulations, oppressive administrative burdens, and the enforced ceding of medical decision-making to distant entities.[1–5] Despite the promise that such a plan would control costs, the effort has failed as costs have continued to rise. Not only that, but medical schools and medical centers have had less financial support for medical education, training, and research, all indispensable for optimal healthcare.[6,7]

The advent of managed care has altered medical practice dramatically in ways that few could have anticipated. For those of us who practiced many years before this phenomenon arrived, the transformation imposed by the new system was inconceivable. Who would have believed that a physician—after years of premedical and medical education, followed by three to five or more years of residency training—would be required to submit to managed-care fiats, rendered by distant entities that have never seen the patient? Decisions in medicine have traditionally been made on the basis of the physician's best clinical judgment and scientific evidence, always in the patient's best interests, whereas managed care (more appropriately managed costs) is driven by the desire to control costs and gain maximum profits, directed substantially to the corporate executives. We have all heard and read many heartbreaking stories of patient misadventures with the new healthcare system, including fatal outcomes, and the mounting patient protests may lead to remedial action.

When the time a physician may spend with a patient is severely limited (15 minutes or less in some managed-care organizations), the quality of care may suffer, for the amount of information and conversation is curtailed. The patient, moreover, senses the hastiness and feels shortchanged and less trusting. A system that restricts, rather than facilitates, needed healthcare may be cost-saving but is not cost-effective. Physicians, frustrated by these intrusions into professional care, are opting increasingly for early retirement. Physician shortages are already being predicted.

With the new system came a new lexicon imposed on medicine: physicians became "healthcare providers," and patients became "consumers," terms that encourage the concept of medicine as a trade, not a profession with high ethical standards and noble principles. Such a concept not only lacerates the revered physician–patient relationship, so critical to proper rapport, effective therapy, and the maintenance of good health, but also devalues the time-honored humanitarian code of medicine. Do we want professional physicians to minister to patients or health salesclerks to serve health customers? Of late, the "high cost of healthcare" has been overattributed to the physician's compensation and to the costly technologic procedures patients now expect, less to governmental and managed care restrictions and paperwork. Physicians, like all others, deserve to be compensated fairly for their work. This is not to say that profit should be the primary focus, for I don't believe it should, but it is difficult to understand why physicians, who study longer and at greater personal and financial sacrifice, who work longer hours, and who perform an important public and social service, should receive less remuneration than, for example, attorneys, entertainers, professional athletes, managed-care executives, or a host of other careerists in our society. Physicians today face a choice: If they order the advanced technologic procedures now available, they may be criticized for increasing costs, and if they fail to order them, they may face costly malpractice litigation. Patients expect to receive the latest and best available care, but must understand that increasingly sophisticated and more precise technology carries a higher price tag.

Above all, medicine is a moral profession, with a tradition of humanitarianism and public service. With the intrusion of nonmedical entities into healthercare decision-making, some adverse effects have occurred. Our society must decide whether we want medicine to continue its tradition as a profession, with its code of ethics, or to become a trade, with a compromise in quality. High technology can coexist with humanity. But society must also be realistic; its expectations must be consonant with the realities of the increasing costs of ever more sophisticated technology. No one wants rationing, yet if demands far exceed funds available to pay for them, something has to give. We cannot expect ultrasophisticated healthcare at bargain-basement prices. Medicine's very advances have created thorny ethical and economic problems amid changing social values and an aging population. Physicians today must become informed not only about the scientific aspects of medicine, but also about the economic, ethical, legal, and public policy issues. How can patients become fully informed as partners in their health decisions when a visit of only 12 to 15 minutes is sometimes allowed with their physicians? And how can they become educated in their health maintenance with so little time for communication?

PROFESSIONALISM

Professionalism has intellectual as well as ethical components. Professionalism means being well informed, an expert, in fact, making lifelong learning a *sine qua non* for physicians. In medicine, it means being honest, compassionate, and dedicated—placing the patient's welfare above all other considerations, including personal and financial rewards. The medical professional is *ipso facto* the patient's advocate.

In the words of Oliver Holmes, "The best a physician can give is never too good for the patient."[8] It means sharing your knowledge and experience with colleagues, students, and patients. That educational mission can take various forms: writing, speaking, formal and informal consultations, and educating patients so that they can make informed decisions associated with their diagnosis, treatment, and prevention.[9]

With commercial pressures from managed-care organizations, it is more important than ever for physicians to nurture and maintain professionalism.

PLEASURE IN WORK

Despite the frustrations, strictures, and voluminous, time-consuming paperwork that plague physicians today, if you were attracted to medicine because of a genuine desire to help others and because you enjoy intellectual challenges, you will still find immense satisfaction in your daily work and can preserve the passion for medicine by adopting some of the advice offered in this book by physicians of high achievement. As physicians, we are invited into the most intimate chambers of our patients' lives. We should acknowledge that unfettered trust with dignity, deference, and respect. For a physician, caring for patients is not only a duty; it is a privilege. Alleviating pain and restoring health for another human being induce an exhilaration that few others experience in their careers. That professional gift deserves exquisite care.

Finally, I consider it essential to select a career that greatly appeals to you instead of taking the line of least resistance and indiscriminately or fortuitously entering a path to which you must then commit yourself for life. If your work is not enjoyable, you will look for any diversion or distraction you can find; you will rarely do your best; and you will feel no pride or satisfaction in your performance. If, on the other hand, the career you choose is as enjoyable as mine is to me, you will look forward to going to work each day, and you will feel no desperate need to "escape" periodically. You *will* preserve the passion. Medicine is an absorbing, even possessive, profession, but the intellectual rewards, humanitarian service, and fulfillment are unsurpassed.

REFERENCES

1. DeBakey ME, DeBakey L. The ethics and economics of high-technology medicine. *Compr Ther.* 1983;9(12):6–16.
2. DeBakey ME. The winds of change in medicine [editorial]. *South Med J.* 1993;86:1316–1317.
3. DeBakey ME, DeBakey L. Medicine in the managed care era. *Houston Business Rev.* 1996; Summer: 70–75.
4. DeBakey ME. Rx for the health care system. *The Wall Street Journal.* 1998 Oct 8;CII(70):A18.
5. DeBakey ME, DeBakey L. Should physicians unionize? *The Wall Street Journal.* 1999 Jul 7;CIV(4):A22.
6. DeBakey ME. Medical centers of excellence and health reform. *Science.* 1993;262:523–525.
7. DeBakey ME. Prescription for disaster. *The Wall Street Journal.* 1994 Jun 23; XCIII(122):A14.
8. Holmes OW. *Medical Essays.* Boston: Houghton Mifflin; 1891.
9. DeBakey ME, Gotto AM Jr. *The New Living Heart.* Holbrook, MA: Adams Media; 1997.

REFLECTIONS

• • •

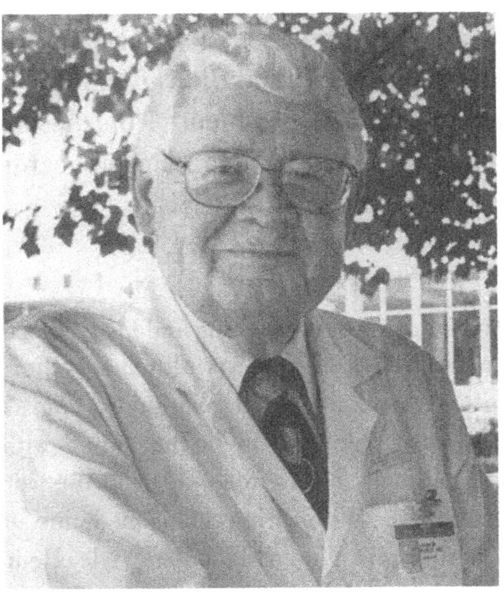

I consider it more important for students, house officers, and fellows to ask questions about their patients and to pursue the answers themselves than it is for me to dispense information to them. For the remainder of their lives, they should ask themselves questions about their patients and seek their own answers. A master teacher guides students in how to learn, so that self-learning becomes a lifelong practice.

J. WILLIS HURST, M.D.

That Dr. Willis Hurst is a master teacher has been validated by his numerous awards, including the Master Teacher Award and the Gifted Teacher Award of the American College of Cardiology, the Distinguished Teacher Award of the American College of Physicians, the prestigious Evangeline Papageorge Teaching Award by former Emory graduates, and numerous other teaching awards. He has also received both the Gold Heart Award and the Herrick Award from the American Heart Association. Author of countless articles on the heart and the teaching process, he published the classic textbook of cardiology, *The Heart*.[1] He was Chairman of the Subspecialty Board of Cardiovascular Diseases, a member of the National Advisory Heart, Lung, and Blood Council, President of the American Heart Association, President of the Association of Professors of Medicine, President Lyndon Johnson's cardiologist for 18 years.

* * * * *

> Willis Hurst's interest in teaching and his genius for instruction are as fresh and powerful today as they were 38 years ago when I graduated from Emory. I have many vivid pictures of Willis striding to the podium with several worn and aged books, ready to read the words of past masters to us. Willis brings to his medicine and his teaching a first-rate mind and a potent style. He has an unerring focus on the fundamentals of medicine. His every action, mannerism, and felicitous phrase are in the service of teaching. He is a striking role model, exemplifying the best qualities to be found in physicians: compassion; clear thinking; and concern for patients, students, and house officers.
>
> KENNETH WALKER, M.D.

REFERENCE

1. Hurst JW. *The Heart.* New York: McGraw-Hill.

A Profession at Risk, but Reasons for Optimism

J. Willis Hurst, M.D.
Consultant to the Division of Cardiology
Former Professor and Chairman
Department of Medicine (1957–1986)
Emory University School of Medicine
Atlanta, Georgia

EARLY INFLUENCES

My father, who was a school superintendent, greatly influenced my interest in, and keen desire for, knowledge and excellence. When I was a child, we lived in a large, dormitory-like house near the school where my Father worked. My aunt, who taught the first three grades at the school, lived in the same building and taught me before I started school. She called on me to read the first day of school, and the entire class laughed; I suppose my class members thought it was a joke on the teacher. Through the third grade, I was exposed to this superb teacher all day long and at night as well. My Father recognized the ability of my next teacher, who lived upstairs in our large two-story house, and transferred her from the fourth to the fifth to the sixth grades as I progressed each year. So, I had only two teachers during the first six grades.

I was also blessed with good high-school teachers, many of whom were an inspiration to me, but my Father's interest in education probably had the greatest influence of all. When I was about 13 years old, he gave up teaching to work for the Federal Savings and Loan Association because he could not support his family on the low salary teachers received during the Depression. But he always loved teaching; he read a great deal and encouraged me to read. I recall my great joy when we purchased our first *Encyclopaedia*. I spent many hours on cold winter days simply turning the pages of the *Encyclopaedia*, and I remember many of the pages until this day.

RESIDENCY AND PAUL DUDLEY WHITE

During my internal medicine house-staff training under Dr. V.P. Sydenstricker at University Hospital in Augusta, Georgia, I was fortunate to meet Dr. Paul Dudley White on a visit to our school. Dr. Harry Harper, the cardiologist at the Medical College of Georgia and a friend of Dr. White's, recommended me to our visitor, who offered me a cardiac fellowship at the Massachusetts General Hospital for 1948, and I quickly accepted. From that point on, Dr. White stimulated me in every conceivable fashion. My friendship with him and Mrs. White continued for many years, and I was honored to give his eulogy at Cambridge.

Paul White used to say that the excitement of medicine had to do with the fact that medicine could link science to humanism. He was a kind, gentle man who did not urge, cajole, or plead with people to perform, but because of his own standard of excellence, he inspired others to achieve. Those who worked with him did their best because he was the recognized authority in cardiology. He had worked with Sir Thomas Lewis and had known Sir James MacKenzie and all the leading cardiologists of the world. He became known as the father of cardiology in this country.

How Paul White Worked and Influenced People

Dr. White recorded the data he collected from his own patients on 4-by-6-inch cards and created what he called a complete cardiac diagnosis. He defined a complete diagnosis as one including the etiology, altered anatomy, altered physiology, and functional cardiac status—a classification later adopted by the New York Heart Association. He took this large collection of cards, along with his bride, Ina, to the Isle of Capri, and wrote his first book, published in 1931. He exemplified the way a scholar works: carefully collecting data on enough patients, interpreting the data, and reporting the results. I think it was that mammoth effort behind the first edition of his book that put cardiology ahead of many other disciplines. That book made the field a recognized specialty in this country, and it remains good reading today. The first edition contained innumerable old references that, regrettably, had to be eliminated in the later editions because of limited space.

Paul White was not only an investigator, superb teacher, excellent physician, writer, and humanitarian, he was also a prophet. He predicted the role of "risk factors" in cases of coronary atherosclerotic disease and taught how to prevent the disease in the late 1940s. Paul White taught me cardiology, but he also taught me what a professional person should strive to be, and he influenced me to teach and write. He used to say that a trainee should see patients one-third of the day, teach one-third of the day, and write one-third of the day.

TEACHING AND LEARNING

I write every day. Writing focuses the mind and, for me at least, is essential for good teaching. Teaching and learning go hand in hand. Physicians should live up to their title, *doctor*, which means teacher. One can always find someone to teach; practicing physicians should teach patients, just as they should interact instructively with colleagues. Instead of dispensing numerous details, the true teacher discusses concepts and approaches to learning. For example, lectures should create interest, stimulate students' curiosity, and motivate them to seek further information. Attending the usual lecture is not the best way to learn. Most often, the information imparted can be read in a fraction of the duration of the lecture. Teachers must also have a good sense of timing and know when to introduce each subject. Success depends in part on personality. The common denominator in the personality of true teachers is their ability to stimulate students to work on problems when the teacher is not present. The true teacher then evaluates the ability of the trainee to think rather than regurgitate facts.

COMPETENCE AS AN IMPORTANT COMPONENT OF COMPASSION

Today, when so much is being said about compassion, we overlook competence as an important sign of the physician's compassion. If the physician cares enough about the patient to ask the necessary questions and is self-disciplined enough to seek the answers, competence becomes a component of compassion. The most competent physicians are usually compassionate. Because they have great concern about being wrong, they make a concerted effort to be right. The most competent, most compassionate physicians have no psychologic problem requesting consultation or admitting that they do not know something.

ASKING THE RIGHT QUESTION AND IDENTIFYING THE PROBLEMS

Most physicians are stimulated to learn as a result of questions arising about the care of their patients. When a question arises about one of my patients, I try to define the problem clearly. In other words, the solution to a problem starts with a clear and simple statement of the problem. I often refer to this process as focusing the mind. The next step is to look up the answer in an authoritative general textbook of medicine and then bring the information up to date by reviewing the index issues of journals published since the latest edition of the textbook. Since the medical library is so close to my office, I use it as my primary information resource. If I were in a different environment, I undoubtedly would rely more on the computer. Finally, I may consult a colleague who knows more about the subject than I do. I learned long ago that experts in a field often know more about individual patients than the information found in a textbook, which presents a generic view of the subject, but not the knowledge honed by valuable clinical experience.

In the hope of initiating a lifelong practice, I encourage students, residents, and fellows to create a problem list on each patient. They are then encouraged to seek the answers to the questions and problems they record. Young children are curious and do not hesitate to ask questions, but as we grow older, the child-like questioning is blocked by external forces, and students are expected only to answer the teachers' questions. I have no objection to testing students by having them answer questions so long as they are also encouraged to *ask* questions of their teachers and, more important, of themselves. If the medical trainee phrases questions properly and has the self-discipline to pursue specific answers in print or electronic textbooks or journals, or in consultations with others, then the teacher has succeeded.

In medicine, as Kipling admonished reporters, we need to ask who, what, when, where, and how.[1] Remember, however, that many obstacles will interfere with asking those simple questions. Medical trainees often have difficulty describing the discomfort of angina pectoris, and they may discuss the irrelevant. Finally, I will say: "*What* does it feel like to the patient? *When* does it occur? *Where* is the discomfort? *How* does it occur?" Not a bad set of guidelines for the description of ischemic coronary atherosclerosis.

When my publisher wanted me to prepare a self-assessment book to help readers test their knowledge of my textbook, *The Heart,* I enlisted the cooperation of second-year cardiac fellows. They had been residents for three years, so they had been out of medical school for five years. I had them formulate questions about each chapter in *The Heart*. I was astounded because the fellows I thought would do a good job did not do well, and vice versa. We had the usual problems with grammar and with clear delineation of the questions—deficiencies that are well known to all teachers. But more than that, some of them wrote questions that had no teaching value, such as: What is the important item on the page? It took about four times longer than I had anticipated to complete this project. I learned that people who are skilled at answering a teacher's questions may not be skilled at asking questions, and vice versa. Those capable of asking themselves important questions, I believe, will be the leaders if they also have the self-discipline to pursue the answers.

EDUCATION OUTSIDE OF SPECIALTY

All specialists should participate at least once a week in discussions in general medicine. Cardiologists need to talk with other cardiologists, but they also need to listen to gastroenterologists, surgeons, ophthalmologists, dermatologists, obstetricians, and other specialists. This is vital to physicians who wish to make good decisions about their patients' problems. We must all concentrate on what *should* be done for a patient rather than what *can* be done. We *can* do many things today, but this does not mean that we *should* do them. The excellent subspecialist must make decisions about patients after reviewing all the problems the patient has. Such decisions, made in that manner, improve the judgment of the physician. Commingling with colleagues outside your own specialty is crucial to enhancing judgment in your own field.

CHAIRING THE DEPARTMENT OF MEDICINE FOR 30 YEARS (1957–1986)

I joined the faculty of Emory University School of Medicine in Atlanta in 1950 when Dr. Paul Beeson was Chairman of the Department of Medicine. I worked with Dr. Bruce Logue to develop Cardiology at Emory University Hospital. In February, 1957, at the age of 36, I became Chairman of the Department of Medicine, a position I held for

30 years. Being Professor and Chairman of the Department of Medicine was exciting and rewarding. I enjoyed the long hours spent in teaching, consulting on private cardiology patients, organizing, writing, developing, and investigating. The full-time faculty grew from 13 to 147 during my tenure. The teaching program attained national recognition, and new research facilities had improved the research thrust of the department. All subspecialties had been developed, and patients came from across the country and abroad. The students, house officers, fellows, and faculty were happy, and the system encouraged learning from one another.

DARK CLOUDS OF UNDESIRABLE CHANGE

I wrote a short paper in 1971, describing the clouds I thought I saw accumulating that would influence the future.[2] I was concerned that the wonderful progress of medicine, which was easily seen, would bring with it new and detracting problems. The cost of medical care would, I feared, create new systems that would displace the physician as the central figure in the care of patients. I believed then that medicine, in general, and medical schools, in particular, would be influenced adversely by changes in the delivery of medical care.

In 1986, as President of the Association of Professors of Medicine, I delivered a short speech, tongue-in-cheek, in which I pointed out that Departments of Medicine in the future would no longer have Divisions of Cardiology, Gastroenterology, Hematology, Oncology, Rheumatology, and the like, but would have Divisions of Legal Affairs, Business, Parking, and Public Relations. The point was that the new approaches to the delivery of healthcare would profoundly influence how a chairman would direct the department.

AFTER CHAIRMANSHIP

I relinquished the chairmanship of Medicine in 1986, but continued as Chief of Medicine and Chief of Cardiology at Emory University

Hospital for several more years. Now, as a Consultant in the Division of Cardiology, I teach nine sessions each week and write the remainder of the time. When asked when I will retire, I answer, "When my memory is not as good as that of the house officers."

I VIEW WITH ALARM

During the past few years, I have written and published, under the title "I View with Alarm,"[3–5] my concerns about certain aspects of medicine that trouble me, including the following:

True teaching has deteriorated, returning many institutions to the simple delivery of information by lecture, assignments in books, or surfing the Internet. Teachers make schedules and give examinations to determine if trainees have, for at least one day, remembered the information. This type of performance is not teaching, and the people doing it should not be called teachers—they are announcers of information.

The true teacher does much more than the announcer. The true teacher understands how people learn. Learning certainly includes information, but the true teacher leads the trainee to use the information thoughtfully. Thinking is the realignment of information into a new perception for the person doing the thinking. The true teacher's goal is to lead the trainee to think. Not to do so implies that the early years in medical school meant nothing to the teacher or trainee. Learning is a step beyond thinking. Learning is successful when trainees practice and practice until they become adept at the skills they are trying to develop, including the skill of thinking.

This discussion is included because it is the basis of the educational process that physicians must use as long as they see patients. True teachers understand that, but announcers do not. I view with alarm the current trend of more and more lectures and less and less true teaching.

The role of the teaching-attending physician has changed for two reasons. First, the managed-care control of medicine diminishes the time true teachers, who are functioning as teaching-attendings, can spend with their patients or with the trainees assigned to them. This is disastrous for the physician, patient, and trainee. Second, teaching-attending physicians must be reminded that true teaching entails more than simply showing trainees abnormalities or how to manage patients. The less time there is to teach, the more true teaching declines. It is through the teaching-attending physicians' efforts that trainees develop their medical thinking, which entails the use of information previously stored in memory.

A PROFESSION AT RISK

What follows here is not written with great pleasure, because I see the profession of medicine at risk. Although it is painful to face the facts, I cannot bury my head in the sand. Admittedly, medical science has advanced with breathtaking speed, additional effective diagnostic and therapeutic procedures becoming available every few months. The downside of this magnificent progress is that the high cost of healthcare makes it inaccessible for many people. In addition, a serious war exists among insurance companies, the government, physicians, patients, and hospitals. The level of happiness of physicians and patients has declined measurably. A more serious problem than the agonizing battle physicians and patients face in the managed-care era is the deterioration of the trust most patients formerly had in physicians.

A number of events suggest that everyone does not understand the attributes of a profession. This confusion is understandable because, for decades, the concept has been popularized that a person who is not paid to perform an act is an amateur and one who is paid to perform the same act is a professional. This superficial thinking has led to such misnomers as professional boxing and wrestling and a number of other "professions" while the finer attributes of a profession are seldom considered.[6]

The November 30, 1999, issue of *The New York Times* contained a two-page article, "When Physicians Double as Businessmen," stating that physicians were working for profit-making companies, or had developed companies themselves, and were creating medical devices for sale. The physicians would perform "research" using the device they created and would then use "educational meetings" to market their new product. Some such medical entrepreneurs made millions of dollars by selling their souls at the marketplace while many dedicated physicians watched their properly earned incomes diminish. On the same day, *The Atlanta Constitution* reported on "Medical Mistakes Are Killers," pointing out that medical mistakes cause an estimated 48,000–98,000 deaths each year in the United States. The National Academy of Sciences reported this devastating news and urged the creation of a new federal agency to protect patients. Both stories undoubtedly had a heavy impact on patients.

In an earlier story in *The New York Times*, reporters discussed their discovery of the "unethical" behavior of physicians who received money from pharmaceutical houses to enroll patients in clinical trials. The trials were often conducted by physicians who had no research training, and many of them had clear-cut conflicts of interest. The story implied that many drugs released during the past few years might not perform as advertised. Many readers undoubtedly concluded that some medical participants in such activity love money more than their patients' welfare.

None of the three scathing reports encourages the public to trust practicing physicians or biomedical researchers. Certainly, with the information in the news reports, the public has a right to question the motives of the physician participants.

At this uneasy juncture, it seems fitting to reemphasize some of the time-honored attributes of a profession.

I have always believed that the medical profession was created to meet the public need for healthcare, not that patients were created to meet physicians' financial needs. I submit that the activities in the news stories mentioned deviate from the professionalism the public expects and deserves. The physicians functioning as businessmen ignored the contribution the public makes to their incomes. The physicians who developed and marketed devices ignored that they used a hospital's equipment and drawing power to perform their work. They forgot that the public gave money to create the facility where they used their products and generously enhanced their incomes. I suspect the physicians would have been highly disturbed if the hospitals had charged them a handsome user fee according to the money they made from marketing the products they created. The public must trust the restaurant staff to serve them clean food, and they must trust the mechanic to repair their cars. Surely, patients should be able to trust their physicians.

The remarkable Mortimer Adler defined "professional" as follows: ". . . in the original and deeper meaning of the term, a professional man is one who does skilled work to achieve a *useful social goal*. . . . In other words, the essential characteristic of a profession is the dedication of its members to the *service* they perform."[7]

Adler noted that the English economist R.H. Tawney defined a profession as "a body of men who carry on their work in accordance with rules designed to enforce certain standards both for the better protection of its members and for the better *service* of the public."[7]

I was just beginning my 30-year stint in 1957 as Chairman of the Department of Medicine at Emory when the brilliant and courageous Judge Elbert Tuttle uttered these unforgettable words (reproduced here with permission) at our graduation exercises: "The professional man is in essence one who provides *service*. But the *service* he renders is something more than that of the laborer, even the skilled laborer. It is a *service* that wells up from the entire complex of his personality. True, some specialized and highly developed techniques may be included, but their mode of expression is given its deepest meaning by the personality of the practitioner. In a very real sense his professional *service* cannot be separate from his personal being. He has no goods to sell, no land to till; his only asset is himself. It turns out that there is no right price for *service*, for what is a share of a man worth? If he does not contain the quality of integrity, he is worthless. If he does, he is priceless. The value is either nothing or it is infinite. So do not try to set a price on yourselves. Do not measure out your professional services on an apothecary's scale and say, 'Only this for so much.' Do not debase yourselves by equating your souls to what they will bring in the market. Do not be a miser, hoarding your talents and abilities and knowledge, either among yourselves or in your dealings with your clients, patients, or flock. Rather be reckless and spendthrift, pouring out your talent to all to whom it can be of *service*! Throw it away, waste it; and in the spending it can be of *service*. Do not keep a watchful eye lest you slip and give away a little bit of what you might have sold. Do not censor your thoughts to gain a wider audience. Like love, talent is useful only in its expenditure, and it is never exhausted. Certain it is that a man must eat, so set what price you must on your *service*. But never confuse the performance, which is great, with the compensation, be it money, power or fame, which is trivial."[8]

Those words became the motto for the department I was developing. Over the years, I have quoted this portion of his speech whenever the opportunity arose. Read it—think about it—read it again—and then pass it on to others to read, because it should be an addendum to the Hippocratic oath.

James Fowler, Charles Howard Candler Professor of Theology and Human Development at Emory University, gave me permission to use the following statements:

- Professionals, and the groups they form, are self-regulating. They set standards for education, apprenticeship, and admission. They administer discipline and have the power and authority to remove colleagues from services for incompetence, malpractice, or character failure.

- The professions carry a public trust. They stand in a fiduciary relationship with those they serve. They must be trustworthy with regard to confidential information, the disclosure of which could be harmful to those they serve. They also have responsibility to exert moral influence on their clients at points where their intents or anticipated actions may do injury to others or to the common good.

- Professionals are, traditionally, expected to provide services—personally or through a collegial network—for persons who have need of professional services, regardless of capacity to pay for their services. Their object is service, not the use of their professional status and skills primarily for personal gain.

While these elements of the traditional understandings of the ethics of the professions may sound quaint to some contemporaries, they offer important windows into the special personal and social responsibilities associated with professional status.

AN OPTIMISTIC NOTE

As I write this, I am optimistic about the future of medicine for the following reasons:

Our knowledge of medicine continues to improve. Despite all the problems, it is better to be sick in 2003 than it was in 1949.

A group of people cannot be persistently repressed. Physicians feel repressed because they cannot always function according to the rules of good medical care. There are definite signs that managed care is failing to satisfy both employees (physicians) and "customers" (formerly called patients). This implies that the managed-care administrators, despite their enormous incomes, are running a bad business, good businesses strive to satisfy their customers. There is light at the end of the tunnel; the current system of health-care delivery is not working, and patients, as well as physicians, will assist in the changes that must be made.

True teaching is making a comeback.[6] Many medical schools and teaching hospitals are beginning to recognize that the future of good medicine lies in the development of true teachers who are supported by funds that are not derived from personal services to patients. There will, in time, be a sufficient number of true teachers serving as teaching-attendings who know how to teach and have the time to do it.

REFERENCES

1. Kipling R. The elephant's child. In: *Just So Stories*. New York: Lancer; 1968:47.
2. Hurst JW. Ten reasons why Lawrence Weed is right. *N Engl J Med.* 1971;284:51–52.
3. Hurst JW. I view with alarm. *Am J Cardiol.* 1995; 75:832–834.
4. Hurst JW. I view with alarm (1997). *Am J Cardiol.* 1997; 80:769.
5. Hurst JW. I view with alarm (1999). *Am J Cardiol.* 1999; 84:1339–1340.
6. Hurst JW. *Teaching Medicine: Process, Habits, and Actions.* Atlanta: Scholars Press; 1999.
7. Adler MJ. *Great Ideas from the Great Books*. New York: Washington Square; 1966:280–282.
8. Tuttle EJ Sr. Heroism in war and peace. *Emory Univ Q.* 1957;13(3):129–130.

2

Reading: Keeping Current

• • •

> All that goes on in medicine is to be the chief matter of interest to you. Hence you must be busy readers; and, as habits form, you will learn to look to medical journals with avidity, and new publications will be examined with keen relish. But to become distinguished, nay, to become even respectable in your profession, you must be something more than readers, you must become active thinkers and sifters of knowledge, learn, as Bacon counsels, to weigh and consider books.
>
> JACOB M. DA COSTA[1]

Reading is the primary source of physicians' medical information. Print is not only the most highly developed and plentiful medium for medical information, but is also relatively economical, convenient, and easily accessible. The electronic media have become competitive with, if they have not surpassed, print media because so much information is readily available at the press of a button. Many physicians are using the Internet to gain easy access to the emerging array of information sources. Almost all the world's recent medical information is readily available to computer-literate physicians. Although this chapter deals primarily with print publications, remember that most recent information is available both electronically and in print.

Beyond new developments in medical care, the need to review fundamental principles necessitates a lifelong plan of reading. In the words of Robert Moser, "Reading is as important a habit for a physician as brushing his teeth and watching his waistline. It becomes a part of his lifestyle, for it is needed to screen useful advances in theory, diagnosis, and therapy and to solve specific clinical problems confronting the practicing physician. If properly engrained, the habit never wanes for the duration of his practice." Just as nonphysicians derive pleasure from reading novels and magazines, many practitioners enjoy reading medical journals. Joseph Van Der Meulen enjoys making new associations with previous knowledge: "The insight that comes with such associations provides the pleasure. I spend leisure time reading practical material in science and medicine that reinforces my medical knowledge."

Physicians who take for granted the accessibility of reading material may find that the words of Shen Jiaqi of Shanghai will give them a better appreciation of their opportunities for enlarging their knowledge. "Throughout his lifetime," Shen stated, "a doctor needs to be informed about new developments in medicine. And there is no shortcut to it beyond reading, but conditions sometimes suppress reading. That the tyrant of the Qin Dynasty burned books and buried intellectuals is a historical fact. During the last disastrous so-called cultural revolution, the 'Gang of Four' spread a fallacy that the more knowledge you have, the more reactionary you are. They duped virtuous people for years into reading little, and the education of a whole generation of youngsters was therefore delayed. Luckily, the horror is over, and the People's Republic of China is now setting off an upsurge of intellectualism. Everyone, old and young, has been moving into the tide of reading to make up for what has been lost in the past.

"With the rehabilitation of Confucius, China's great ancient philosopher and educationist, I would again recommend his famous quotations about reading: 'Reading without thinking is null and void, whereas thinking without reading is critical and riskful.' 'Reviewing old articles yields new ideas.' 'To read constantly is a great happiness.' I think these proverbs are still instructive as guidelines for reading."

GUIDING PRINCIPLES

"Read with two objects," advised Osler, "first, to acquaint yourself with the current knowledge on a subject and the steps by which it has been reached, and secondly, and more important, read to understand and analyse your cases."[2] General undirected reading helps the physician stay current with the state of the art, whereas reading about puzzling individual cases (or a series of cases seen in practice) has an immediate, specific, and practical purpose.

Relating Reading to Experience

Both types of reading, general and specific, will be more valuable if you have an objective in mind or can relate what you read to your clinical experience. Experienced physicians gain the most from general reading because they can associate much of what they read with their clinical observations. As Gerald Plitman noted, "After a certain time practicing medicine, you can hardly pick up a journal without being able to relate an article to some patient you have had. I think all physicians should try to apply the title of each article they read to a patient they have seen."

Screening

John Shaw Billings made an apt observation that illustrates the importance of screening: "There is a vast amount of this effete and worthless material in the literature of medicine. . . . [O]ur preparers of compilations and compendiums, big and little, acknowledged or not, are continually increasing the collection, and for the most part with material which has been characterized as 'superlatively middling, the quintessential extract of mediocrity.' "[3]

The Need. A primary problem has been the proliferation of publications. The 20,000 biomedical journals now published are increasing by six to seven percent a year.[4] To review 10 journals in internal medicine, a physician must read about 200 articles and 70 editorials a month.[5]

Physicians may receive more than 5,000 pages of journal material each month, including advertisements and give-away journals. Much of this contains valuable alternatives and advances in medical practice. Diagnosis is continually being refined by innovations, new drugs provide additional therapeutic options, and newly described diseases also demand attention.

Considerable poorly written or otherwise faulty material infiltrates medical publications. Unfortunately, even peer review in the most prestigious medical journals does not preclude publication of premature, questionably valid, or repetitious scientific reports. DeBakey and DeBakey[6–11] have written extensively on the invalid themes, illogical arguments, inadequate or inaccurate data, and unsupportable conclusions, as well as the ungrammatical prose and generally inferior writing, in some reputable peer-reviewed journals. In a personal communication, John Williamson reported that his extensive study of scientific publications pointed to a "misinformation explosion," in which only 20 percent of published reports today meet even minimal criteria of scientific validity. Sir Thomas Lewis, writing in 1944, emphasized the need for critical reading: ". . . reform, to be useful, must render the student of medicine discriminating in a world where a disquieting proportion of what is offered him in conversation and in the generality of journals and of books is inaccurate, slovenly, or redundant."[12]

"It is important for us to recognize that the reasons for writing clinical articles and the reasons for reading clinical articles may have very little in common," cautioned David Sackett. "We read them to find out how to manage our patients; often, however, authors may write them to obtain tenure. It is our responsibility to determine the validity and applicability of what we read; and we certainly cannot depend on the give-away magazines that provide advice but no data."

Techniques If the busy physician is to avoid unreliable and unintelligible articles, he must read selectively and critically. Observing certain screening techniques can make reading more efficient, whether it is general reading to keep abreast of current medical events or specific reading to solve problems in practice. "Since we recognize that the clinician is never going to have any more time to read than he has now," continued Sackett, "we have formulated specific guides and, perhaps more important to the busy clinician, some screening questions that the physician can apply as he reads scientific articles."

Screening for Relevance All physicians begin by looking at the title and determining whether the article is potentially interesting or useful to them. "Next," advised David Sackett, "review the list of authors; with experience, you will know what their professional reputations are and whether their work has withstood the test of time. Consider the site where the work was carried out, and note whether the patients described are similar to those you see. Turn next to the abstract or summary, which will tell you whether the substance of the article, if true, would be useful to you as a clinician."

Screening for Validity "Readers need to be much more critical than editors, and certainly more so than authors, in determining what is valid and what is going to help their patients," continued Sackett. "Some of the reasons we read, certainly those most pertinent to individual patients, are to understand the cause of a disease, to determine whether a new diagnostic test is worth using, to distinguish useful from useless forms of therapy, and to find out the clinical prognosis of a disorder." If an article concerns etiology, the reader needs to ask basic questions about the integrity of the study (proper selection and prospective follow-up, or simply case reports and undocumented clinical impressions).

"If you want to find whether a diagnostic test is useful," Sackett explained, "you can quickly scan the methods section to see if there is a valid basis for comparison between the proposed diagnostic test and some established standard. Alpha-fetoprotein, for example, is the diagnostic test that has been suggested for hepatocellular carcinoma in patients with preexisting cirrhosis. In this instance, the established standard would not be just the microscopic examination of the liver. The patients with negative biopsies should be followed until they have done well for at least two to three years, so that you can exclude hepatoma. Thus in many conditions, we increasingly use the subsequent clinical course as the standard."

If you are reading to differentiate useful from useless or harmful therapy, the key question, Sackett pointed out, is: "Was the assignment of patients and treatment randomized? That is the only way to be sure that the groups are sufficiently comparable to draw valid conclusions. If the methods section includes terms like 'a table of random numbers,' or 'a computer program of randomization,' you can be reasonably sure that it was a randomized trial. If, on the other hand, you see statements like 'patients were allocated at random,' then you should be skeptical.

"Randomized clinical trials offer the most convincing evidence available today in the study of both therapeutic effectiveness and side effects. We need to compare the incidence of skin rashes, photosensitivity, gastrointestinal upset, headaches, weakness, or dizziness in patients on placebos with those on active drugs. Some side effects occur so infrequently, however, that the usual randomized clinical trial would not be large enough to disclose them. For those, we must rely on a much less powerful design, the case-control study, in which a group of patients with the apparent side effect is assembled and then matched with a control group without the disorder (and that is where we usually get into trouble). Discrepancies between the two groups in the incidence of prior exposure to the drug or other factor would constitute some evidence, although not very strong, that the factor precipitated the disorder.

"If we are reading about the clinical course and prognosis of a disorder, we should find out if the patient group was identified at an early, uniform stage of the disease. If not, a host of biases may interfere. For example, what exactly is the increased risk of colorectal cancer in patients with ulcerative colitis, and does it justify a prophylactic colectomy? When you search the literature to find an answer to that question, you become frustrated because the most 'authoritative' studies of the risk of cancer in ulcerative colitis patients are based on 'grab' samples of patients, many of whom were included because they already had cancer. As a result, the cancer risk associated with ulcerative colitis is vastly overestimated in these studies. The way to answer the question is to collect a group of ulcerative colitis patients at an early, uniform point in the natural history of the disease, such as when they develop the first unambiguous symptoms or receive the first definitive therapy. That is the only way to determine the natural history and clinical course of a disease.

"Critical screening of articles not only substantially increases the validity of the conclusions the reader draws from them, but also increases his efficiency considerably. By applying these basic screening principles, the reader can expeditiously identify which papers to keep and where to file them."

James Young describes how he reads journal articles. "I scan the table of contents of each journal on the day I receive it and quickly read abstracts of papers that pique my interest. I then review the tables, figures, and references cited in these papers. Sometimes I read the entire paper; an in-depth, critical reading is usually reserved for papers I deem particularly relevant, important, controversial, or interesting. I photocopy these articles for files I maintain on subjects I am likely to write or lecture about in the future. Interestingly, I do not leaf page-by-page through my specialty or subspecialty journals. I reserve this practice for general medical journals, particularly *The Lancet* and *The Journal of the American Medical Association,* which contain many newsworthy items, controversies, thought-provoking editorials, helpful book reviews, and moving literature, including poetry and personal perspectives on the humanities as they relate to our profession. Although the scientific content of *The New England Journal of Medicine* may arguably be most laudable, I find an in-depth perusal of *The Lancet* and the *The Journal of the American Medical Association* compelling because of their regular features of poetry, art history, and, in *The Journal of the American Medical Association*, 'A Piece of My Mind.' "

Note-taking and Mental Summaries

Note-taking is a time-honored method of crystallizing what you read. Osler used it to great advantage. According to Cushing, Osler was "a rapid, methodical reader with an exceptionally retentive memory, but in addition he had formed the habit of jotting down the gist of what he had read so that it could be drawn on when needed, and moreover he would often augment the notes with some reflections of his own. It was due to this habit of writing as he read that he finally acquired the charm of style which characterized his later essays."[13]

The late Alton Ochsner, Michael DeBakey's mentor, kept a permanent record of his notes. "Just by looking at those notes," he said, "I can recall relatively easily the thousands of references that I have read." Thomas Callister uses cards for note-taking, and reads them when he is having coffee or has nothing else to do, thereafter filing them at home, where they are easily available. "This system works well for me, even though it has been hard on my coat pockets." Charles Brunicardi recalls that Judah Folkman had a habit of recording five new facts each day, then reviewing those facts at the end of the week. "It is truly amazing what you will remember using this simple technique."

Some physicians use a tape recorder rather than cards or paper for note-keeping. Mentally reviewing and summarizing the important points of an article, in a single sentence if possible, will help fix them in your mind. Richard O'Brien enhances his retention by mentally devising experimental approaches to extend the state of knowledge beyond that reported in the papers that he reads.

A Scheduled Time for Reading

Most physicians agree that learning has to be a daily activity, in which you discipline yourself to read at least one hour a day and adopt a reading schedule that accommodates your lifestyle.

To keep unread journals from piling up, designate a special time to read. Daniel Stone gets up at 4:30 a.m. and reads for one and one-half hours every day except Christmas. "When I get home in the evening, I am too tired to read in an active, aggressive way. I may turn the pages, but I am not really absorbing the information. Furthermore, I prefer spending my evenings with my wife. In the morning, on the other hand, there are no distractions. My mind is fresh, and I can really absorb the material." Richard Field reads from 6:00 to 6:30 a.m., when no phones are ringing and there are no intrusions. "In that short time, I cover about four journals a month."

According to Cushing, Osler read during meals: "During this first year in Philadelphia he usually dined alone at the old Colonnade Hotel, diagonally across the street from his rooms, always it is said with books and manuscript on the table, and he was usually to be seen reading and making notes during the course of the meal."[13]

Allan Ebbin keeps a pile of journals beside his bed to read before retiring: "I know of no better way to fall asleep than to read my journals. Since my wife is also a pediatrician, I can put some of them on her pile, and she doesn't know the difference. Seriously, my best learning has always been at home, alone, with a book or journal. There are only a few things that provide more entertainment for me."

Some physicians prefer to read in brief spurts, at intervals throughout the day—5:30 to 6:30 a.m., at work, after work, and before bedtime. Since a set time for reading is not possible for Lawrence Green, he leaves journals on various tables in his office and home, to be picked up when convenient. Alton Ochsner also used any brief free time to read. "I try to make every moment of my day count, because there is so little time to do things," he said. "I have on my desk journals of all types, and if I have a few spare minutes, I use that time to read." Norton Greenberger reads on several specific subjects in-

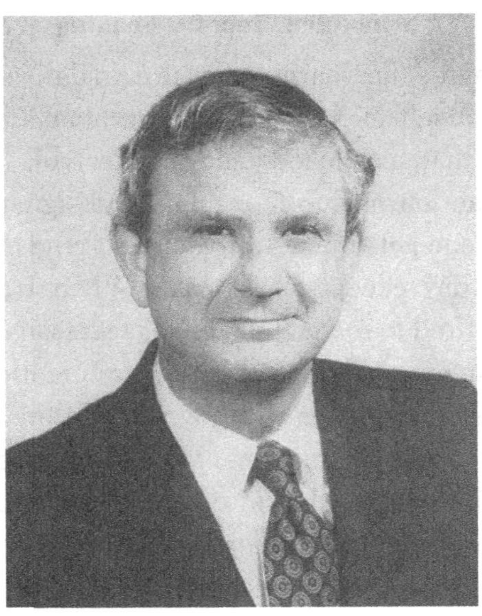

Reading is as important a habit for a physician as brushing his teeth and watching his waistline.

ROBERT H. MOSER. M.D.

Executive Vice President Emeritus
American College of Physicians

stead of concentrating for an hour on one particular topic, which he finds soporific. "When I read, I decide in advance how much I want to accomplish per unit time. I do not read every word; I read for comprehension, recognizing that I have to get through a certain amount at a given time."

Suzanne Knoebel considers her reading time a reward. "Saturday afternoon or Sunday is my 'R and R' time. If I have problems in patient care that I need to read about, I eagerly anticipate this time. But I caution against trying to 'fit' learning into an already tightly scheduled period; pick a convenient 'R and R' time and use it for that."

Some physicians combine reading with other hobbies. David Covell, for example, can be seen every Wednesday afternoon hiking in the

Angeles National Forest above Pasadena reading a current journal, despite the slight risk that engrossing articles can distract attention from tree limbs, snakes, and boulders on the trail.

Reading Retreat Frederick Ludwig and Gerald Plitman use their vacations to catch up on their reading. Plitman created a two-day "reading retreat" for colleagues, which evolved from the practice he and his wife had of going away for a few days every summer, isolating themselves from their usual routine, to read. For each retreat, they invite two professors, who are asked to select topics and to send copies of the selected publications to all others going on the retreat. Everyone reads the material in advance and comes to the retreat ready to discuss these topics. "It is a restful, relaxing event," said Plitman.

Donald Switz and Dan Mohler have initiated similar reading retreats in Virginia. "The format of dual teachers and many papers has worked well for Plitman, but we use a different format," said Switz. "We select three topics per conference and, by rotating the subject, cover all of internal medicine every four years. A single teacher is invited to put together each of the half-day sessions. The teacher selects no more than seven original articles, which he believes are the most important in his field since the last presentations. We ask the registrants to tell us the aspects of each subject they wish to 'catch up' on. We believe physicians learn best when they have a voice in what they will read. Before the reading retreat begins, this information is returned to the teacher, who then has a chance to modify his reading list or to know what to emphasize from his selections. We do not mail the readings in advance, but do distribute a bibliography.

"Like Plitman, we restrict the group to about 25. We retreat to a park-like setting, and families usually come. We make time for walking, loafing, and fishing. The structure of each session is similar to Plitman's. The teacher spends about 30 minutes at the beginning putting the subject of the articles in perspective with respect to current knowledge. We then ask for volunteers to present the pith of each article, after which we retire to read for two hours. When we reassemble, the volunteers present the abstracts, which serve as a basis for discussion by all participants. We spend about 90 minutes discussing the articles in the order the participants desire. There is ample time to ask the teacher for special insights related to clinical cases participants have struggled with.

"Special benefits of the reading retreats are: (1) an opportunity to look critically at original articles, (2) the stimulation of group discussion, and (3) the opportunity to quiz the instructor about clinical matters germane to patients and the articles. We work hard to help participants think about good study design."

Following Specific Investigators

Irvine Page connects facts to people. "I have always been interested in contemporary history; I follow what is going on in the world of medicine largely by associating events with people. History tells me how people make discoveries or observations. My interest in history grows as both the subject and the people grow. A classic example is DNA research. I knew Oswald T. Avery and Colin M. Macleod, both of whom worked on the floor below me at the Rockefeller Institute for Medical Research. I saw the evolution of their work from the beginning, with the accompanying development and skepticism. This is the way I remember things." Donald Seldin also tries to keep abreast of advances by following the work of scientific leaders.

A Historical Perspective

Reading the history of science and medicine provides a good basis for teaching or learning what has happened in the past—how people with keen curiosities were led to important discoveries. Gastone Matioli, however, warns readers: "Validate the historical background upon which the experts base their views. Reviews sometimes distort original intentions or at least phrase them poorly. Americans often ignore history and thus miss the opportunity to identify the source of inherited errors and misunderstanding." Osler advised physicians to "read the original descriptions of the masters who, with crude methods of study, saw so clearly."[14]

GENERAL READING

We use the term "general reading" to refer to that not directed to specific problems in practice or patients under current care. Such reading is enjoyable, useful, and necessary to keep abreast of the general state of medicine. As Paul Wehrle pointed out, "General reading is helpful in following medical progress and disease trends, especially in communicable diseases and new problems." Ian Mackay finds that "General reading provides the opportunity to 'think sideways.' Often, when I have been taxed by a difficult or puzzling clinical problem, or have been startled by an unexpected diagnosis, I am surprised by the number of articles related to that problem that I suddenly encounter; the clinical experience has created an interest in the subject, and I become aware of articles that would otherwise have been overlooked."

Every physician must develop a personal method of selection. Most subscribe to several general journals, such as *The Lancet*, the *British Medical Journal*, *The Journal of the American Medical Association*, and *The New England Journal of Medicine*, as well as one or more journals in their specialties. They usually review the table of contents, checking off the titles that appear interesting. After scanning the abstracts, and sometimes reading an entire article, they file the most significant papers for future use.

Aids to General Reading

Editorials A physician who reads the editorials in two or three major journals can keep fairly well informed about new developments. Of Arthur Rubenstein, Professor of Medicine at the University of Chicago and a specialist in diabetes mellitus, Richard Byyny remarked: "When we went on rounds together, I wondered how he kept up with his busy schedule. One day I asked him how he did it, and he said, 'I am absolutely religious about reading the editorials in *The Lancet* because they are succinct and timely.' "

Letters to the Editor Perusing the letters to the editor in prestigious journals is an enjoyable way to review and gain additional perspective on important medical and related issues of the day. They are not only topical but are often more readable than the more stilted formal articles.

Screening and Abstract Services *The Medical Letter,* a biweekly publication, and the *Yearbook* publications contain excellent information, with expert commentaries. William Waters has made a habit of keeping the *Yearbook of Medicine* at his bedside and reading two or three articles in it every night. "This is the cream of the literature reviewed by the cream of the experts." Some physicians scan abstract journals such as *Excerpta Medica,* whereas others peruse current awareness newsletters, such as *Medical Alert* and *Infectious Disease Alert.*

Self-assessment Programs

Certain specialty societies regularly publish syllabi prepared by experts in the field and containing self-assessment programs, along with objective tests, patient-management problems, and critiques of the questions and answers. Many physicians use the self-assessment programs, such as the Medical Knowledge Self-Assessment Program (MKSAP) or the Surgical Education Self-Assessment Program (SESAP), to keep abreast of new developments or to study for recertification tests. This study combined with the comparison of one's own answers with those of others has proved to be extremely valuable. Between editions, some textbooks offer current awareness volumes, which include self-assessment questions and answers.

Reading in the General Media

The media often release new information in medicine before it is published in the medical journals. Reporters get *The New England Journal of Medicine*, for example, before many physicians receive it. "A patient reads something in *The Wall Street Journal* and calls his physician for an opinion about it," said Alan Gordon. "If the physician hasn't heard of it, he appears not to be keeping up." James Moss pointed out that "Many patients were better informed than their physicians about dimethylsulfoxide (DMSO) after it was featured in a story on 'Sixty Minutes.' " David Sabiston pays attention to medical stories in the public press primarily because he may want to look up such topics in medical publications. "You soon recognize that there are recurring themes in the press. This year it may be obesity, and four years later it may be the surgical treatment of obesity. Cancer, like various new concepts in heart disease, is always there. The subjects repeat themselves in cycles, and it is just a matter of keeping each updated." The *Harvard Medical School Health Letter* and *Mayo Clinic Health Letter* aid physicians in the education of patients about their diseases and general health.

Some physicians post articles on a bulletin board in their offices to convey medical information in the general news to patients. Such a system encourages the physician to assess medical news items as they appear.

READING TO SOLVE SPECIFIC PROBLEMS

Full coverage of medical periodicals is not possible, and even if it were, detailed recall is not. If it is true, as most students of adult education believe, that learning is most effective when a specific problem needs to be solved, overworked physicians can spend their available time most efficiently focusing on information that will help them diagnose and treat the patients under their care. Robert Petersdorf considers patients to be the gateway to new knowledge: "If we direct our reading to conditions we see in our practice, we can keep up reasonably well." Practice-related reading can be classified in two categories: reading about recurring conditions seen in practice, such as hypertension or duodenal ulcer, and reading about puzzling problems in individual patients.

Reading on a Topic of Special Interest

Most physicians develop special interests in certain problems, diseases, drugs, or laboratory studies. A record of the types of problems seen, the drugs prescribed, and the laboratory studies ordered, can direct their reading to their personal experience and can lead to expertise in specific medical topics. (See also Chapter 10.) Donald Seldin explores certain subjects in great depth as they come up. "I try to organize the material in some way, either in the form of notes or in an oral presentation. I prepare not only a catalogue of items but also a synthesis. If I were studying idiopathic edema of women, for example, I would review the literature on that subject fairly thoroughly, and then try to assimilate the material for application to my purposes." Other physicians read on topics they are scheduled to present at medical meetings, in hospital rounds, or informally to colleagues.

Reading About Individual Patients

Eugene Braunwald considers it vital to read about a problem as soon as it arises. "If Mrs. Jones has a mitral valve click and migraine, and you wonder if the two are associated, look the subjects up immediately, not six months later. You will retain the information longer because you will make an association with a specific patient, and this association will help you apply the knowledge you have acquired to similar future problems."

Reading on a particular patient increases retention. "What I remember most," said Edward Shortliffe, "is the information related to specific patients. I may find an interesting article when reading randomly, but it does not stick the same as if I am forced to read because of puzzling questions I have about a patient. Somehow, that becomes better integrated into my memory and helps me deal with similar problems in the future."

When a clinical problem requires additional information, framing the precise applicable question is essential to finding the specific information needed. Rich sources of information, including textbooks, commentaries, and journal articles are now easily accessed electronically. If you are not yet using the Internet, you can consult a recent print edition of a standard textbook or a good review article. If more detailed information is needed, you can consult a medical librarian to obtain pertinent references.

* * * * *

Reading is the most common way for physicians to gain new knowledge and review fundamental concepts. Since there are entirely too many medical publications for physicians to read, they must develop methods of screening journal articles for relevance and validity. As George Sarton said, "The art of reading implies the art of non-reading, and more energy is sometimes needed in order to skip rather than continue useless drifting. Many would-be scholars never learn anything not only because they cannot read, but also because they cannot stop reading: they are like asses turning round and round in a mill with blinkers on their eyes."[15] In addition to reading to remain aware of the state of the art, physicians read about their cases, either about individual puzzling patients or about their aggregate experience with various conditions. Scheduling a daily time for reading and developing related activities such as taking notes, following specific investigators, and relating reading to experience will enhance the value and efficiency of reading. Cultivating a historical perspective about the medical literature and disease entities also enriches understanding and provides a basis for coordinating and integrating new knowledge with old. Editorials in leading journals generally keep one alert to new developments. The physician with limited time can maximize efficiency by concentrating on reading about puzzling individual patients and conditions seen recurrently in practice.

REFERENCES

1. Da Costa JM. Valedictory address to the graduating class of Jefferson Medical College, Philadelphia. Delivered 1874 Mar 11. Philadelphia: P. Madeira, Surgical Instrument Maker; 1874:8.

2. Osler W. The student life: a farewell address to Canadian and American medical students. *The Medical News.* 1905;87:630.

3. Billings JS. Our medical literature. In: Rogers FB, ed. *Selected Papers of John Shaw Billings: Compiled, with a Life of Billings.* Baltimore: Waverly; 1965:128–129.

4. Price DJdeS. The development and structure of biomedical literature. In: Warren KS, ed. *Coping with the Biomedical Literature: A Primer for the Scientist and the Clinician.* New York: Praeger; 1981:3–16.

5. Warren KS. Selective aspects of the biomedical literature. In: Warren KS, ed. *Coping with the Biomedical Literature: A Primer for the Scientist and the Clinician.* New York: Praeger; 1981:17–30.

6. DeBakey L. Critical reasoning: a prerequisite for clear scientific writing. *Int J Cardiol.* 1984;5:629.

7. DeBakey L, DeBakey S. Muddy medical writing: is the culprit "bad grammar," technologic terminology, committee authorship, or undisciplined reading? *South Med J.* 1976;69:1253–1254.

8. DeBakey L. *The Scientific Journal: Editorial Policies and Practices.* St. Louis, MO: C. V. Mosby; 1976.

9. DeBakey L. Releasing literary inhibitions in scientific reporting. *Can Med Assoc J.* 1968;99:360–367.

10. DeBakey L, DeBakey S. Medicant. *Forum on Med.* 1978; 1:38–40, 42–43, 80–81, 83–86.

11. DeBakey L, DeBakey S. The abstract: an abridged scientific report. *Int J Cardiol.* 1983;3:439–445.

12. Lewis T. Reflections upon reform in medical education. *Lancet.* 1944;6298(Pt 1):619.

13. Cushing H. *The Life of Sir William Osler.* London: Oxford Univ. Press; 1940:242.

14. Osler W. In: Bean WB, ed. *Sir William Osler: Aphorisms from His Bedside Teachings and Writings.* Springfield, IL: Charles C Thomas; 1968:79.

15. Sarton G. Notes on the reviewing of learned books. *Science.* 1960;131:1183.

REFLECTIONS

• • •

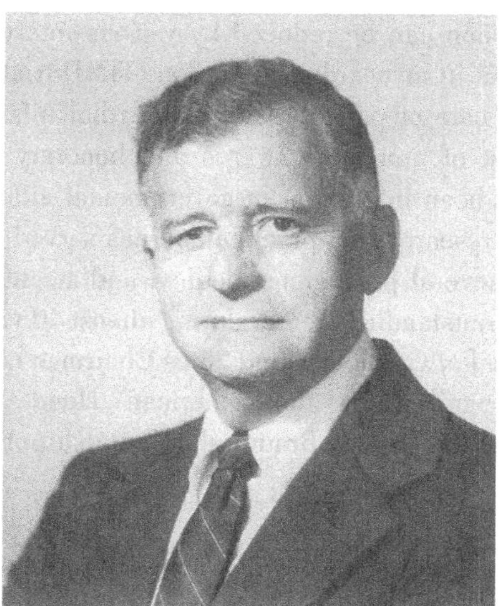

If Mrs. Jones has a mitral valve click and migraine, and you wonder if the two are associated, look the subjects up immediately, not six months later. You will retain the information longer because you will make an association with a specific patient, and this association will help you apply the knowledge you have acquired to similar future problems.

EUGENE BRAUNWALD, M.D.

Dr. Eugene Brauwald's research, reported in more than 1000 publications, has illuminated many aspects of cardiology. He and his colleagues clarified the importance of Starling's Law as a major determinant of human ventricular performance, conducted some of the earliest studies on beta-adrenergic receptor-blocking drugs, and described an important biochemical defect in heart failure—the depletion of norepinephrine in the hearts of patients with this condition. Dr. Braunwald's description of hypertrophic cardiomyopathy and his work on limiting the ultimate size of myocardial infarction have profoundly influenced clinical cardiology. His brilliant animal experiments demonstrated that infarct size after coronary occlusion can be reduced by various interventions, and the thrombolysis in myocardial infarction (TIMI) trials profoundly influenced the care of patients with myocardial infarction worldwide. Recipient of numerous awards and honorary degrees, Dr. Braunwald has been influential in governmental affairs related to cardiovascular research and practice and has served on the editorial boards of several prestigious medical and scientific journals. His work as an outstanding mentor during almost 40 years of teaching—10 as Chief of Cardiology and 28 as Chairman of Medicine—has been recognized by the American Heart Association's establishment of the Eugene Braunwald Mentorship Award.

* * * * *

> Dr. Braunwald is one of the foremost contemporary scholars in the cardiovascular sciences. His contributions are prolific, and his influence is profound in both clinical cardiology and basic research on the heart and circulation. Intense intellectual curiosity and extraordinary analytical abilities are the foundation of Dr. Braunwald's search for knowledge to treat patients afflicted with heart disease. His example has been an inspiration to his students; more than one-sixth of Dr. Braunwald's former trainees are full professors, department heads, or directors of cardiology divisions in major medical schools throughout the world.
>
> WILLIAM F. FRIEDMAN, M.D.

My Three Professional Lives

Eugene Braunwald, M.D.
Distinguished Hersey Professor of Medicine
Harvard Medical School
Chief Academic Officer
Partners HealthCare Systems
Boston, Massachusetts

I lead three professional lives, each with different educational needs. As a Faculty Dean at Harvard Medical School, I must have some basic understanding of the broad aspects of medicine and biomedical sciences in order to deal with recruitment and promotion of senior faculty. My second role is that of author and editor-in-chief of two textbooks: *Harrison's Principles of Internal Medicine* and my own text, *Heart Disease*. We now offer *Harrison's* [textbook] *OnLine*. It was both challenging and exhilarating to prepare the first textbook for this medium. The third component of my professional life is as leader of a clinical trials research group.

I have tried to make all three professional roles support, rather than compete with, one another. As I have observed physicians in academic life whose research is far removed from their clinical work, I have noticed that these two activities are often competitive, not complementary. I am always skeptical about a person who, for example, is a superb molecular biologist but tells me he wants to practice general internal medicine. These two activities do not support each other. If, on the other hand, that person were interested in research on the fundamental mechanisms of cell division and wished to be a clinical oncologist, it would make more sense to me.

For the past 30 years, I have conducted research primarily on the myocardial ischemia. My continuing education in this field derives from the intense association I enjoy with my own research fellows and other colleagues in the field. To keep abreast of the field in which I conduct my research, I must read about 10 hours each week.

THE CASE STUDY

I am becoming more and more convinced that the case-study method, which can be done very readily in a hospital setting, is one that we should be pursuing. Instead of giving a lecture on unstable angina, for example, one can select for discussion six patients who demonstrate different aspects of the problem. Education based on the case-study methods without any didactic lectures is different from the usual grand rounds in which a patient with XYZ diseases is presented and a lecture is given. The case-study method, in which the discussion is about a series of patients, each of whom illustrates different principles, requires much more preparation, but is more effective than traditional educational methods.

MOTIVATION

I have been "programmed" for the work I am doing; my parents expected me to do exactly what I am doing, and that expectation was made clear to me even before I started school. My parents wanted me to do something that they did not have a chance to do, and they saw that I had the capacity to do it, so they encouraged me. I do not regret that. My professional life gives me joy and considerable satisfaction and rewards.

When I began medical school, I intended to practice clinical medicine. Bill Hubbard, then Dean of Students at New York University, introduced the elective system in 1951. When I went to see him, I thought that I wanted a clinical elective—dermatology or orthopedics, as I recall. He said: "I expected that you would do research for your elective," and I said, "No, I do not want to do research. Nothing could be further from my mind." When I sensed that he was becoming angry with this response, I said to myself, "If I fight this, I will get into serious trouble." So I said, "I will be glad to do research." He asked, "What kind of research do you want to do?" I responded, "Oh, no, I am just saying this to please you, and therefore you must make that decision. I really do not want to do any." He called Ludwig Eichna, who at the time was Chief of Cardiology, and said, "I have a man here who is eager to work in your laboratory." "Please send him over," was the reply. I joined Eichna's laboratory, and within days my life was changed forever. Not only did I become enthusiastic about research, but I became fascinated by the cardiovascular system.

As one of the editors of *Harrison's Textbook of Medicine* and *Harrison's OnLine,* I must read all the new material in my field. Thus, my editorial work becomes my continuing education. I also read the major cardiac journals in some detail. This is essential to my position as Faculty Dean, to the preparation of my textbook *Heart Disease,* and to my research program. Thus, my three professional lives are mutually supportive and are built on an infrastructure of continuous updating of my own knowledge base.

REFLECTIONS

• • •

Dr. Philip Tumulty received his M.D. and residency training from Johns Hopkins University. He was twice the recipient of the George J. Stuart Award as Outstanding Clinical Teacher and received an Honorary Doctor of Science Degree from Georgetown University. He published *The Effective Clinician*[1] and wrote extensively on clinical subjects, including the treatment of pneumonia, infectious endocarditis, recurrent malaria, the natural history of systemic lupus, scleroderma, giant-cell arteritis, hepatic hypoglycemia, and functional illness.

In the opinion of Sherman Mellinkoff, Philip Tumulty exemplified what Francis Peabody had in mind when he said, "The secret of the care of the patient is in caring for the patient." Mellinkoff noted that Tumulty, a gifted, lifelong student of medicine, radiated a compassionate concern for all his patients, whatever their backgrounds, their sorrows, and their fates. His devoted care of his patients, even during the search for a diagnosis, is the kind of therapy each of us would like to have and was a lasting inspiration to his students and his colleagues.

REFERENCE

1. Tumulty, PA. *The Effective Clinician. Philadelphia*: W.B. Saunders; 1973.

Preparing for a Fulfilling Career

Philip A. Tumulty, M.D. (1911–1989)
Former David J. Carver Professor Emeritus of Medicine
Johns Hopkins University School of Medicine
Baltimore, Maryland

Students and others have asked me: "Why do you find a career in general internal medicine so completely satisfying?" My answer: Because each day that medicine is practiced properly, I find a full measure of those fulfillments for which we all strive: intellectual enhancement, stimulation, and excitement; an opportunity to increase and expand the best qualities of mind and spirit; a chance to feel the thrill of bringing relief to fellow human beings through the best use of one's intellectual and personal endowments; and finally the daily experience of seeing and understanding more clearly the depths of human nature, with its intense complexities and eccentricities, its good and bad, its sublimity and depravity, its victories and defeats. A clinician is not merely a bystander looking at life as it flows by him; he is an active participant in it, at some of its most crucial stages involving his fellow human beings.

To be effective in such a role, one must, of course, have a number of requisites, including a knowledge of medical science and of the nature of man, both based on the broadest possible clinical experience. One must be stimulated not only by scientific facts and intriguing clinical situations, but by the very simple or exceedingly complex problems arising from patients' human qualities as well. To perform superbly, one must be an eager, persistent, devoted medical scientist whose joy of living comes largely from experiencing the positive effects one's knowledge and talents have on patients' problems, whatever their source may be.

But how does one prepare for such a totally fulfilling yet demanding career, and, once embarked upon it, how does one prevent the practical burdens involved in it from leading to boredom, intellectual and spiritual sterility, and a gradual decline of the stimulus to excellence and of pride in achievement?

Here, we come to the significance of the role of continuing education in our clinical careers. While a proper program of continuing education may keep alive the essential qualities of an effective clinician, it cannot create them. It is therefore the role of the medical schools to select those students with the proper gifts, talents, and abilities of mind, spirit, and character and to create a broad curriculum that fertilizes their growth.

Organized lectures and demonstrations are of undisputed value, but they are not the heart of the matter. The key remains in self-education, and, to my way of thinking, clinical self-education has three essential components:

- Physicians need to have as many and as varied clinical experiences as possible. I see clinical conditions today that I have never seen before, and although they are sometimes insignificant, they may also sometimes be exciting and unusual, as with Takayasu's disease.
- Having had this new experience, the physician must learn more about it. It is important that the clinical experience come first and the reading after.

- Discussion with others of one's new clinical experiences is invaluable, not necessarily by formal consultation but perhaps by informal conversations and exchanges.

A major concern of the clinician is involvement in matters springing from the patient's human nature. Surely the greatest study of mankind is man. A superbly trained scientist who is ignorant of the classics of literature and art and who is naive about social, political, and financial factors is not likely to use these factors positively to ameliorate his patient's illness. How can the physician become more sensitive to these matters? A well-organized schedule, permitting reasonable time for hobbies and interests, social and community activities, and reading, is helpful but is not enough. I recommend a program by the local medical group such as that conceived and developed by George Udvarhelyi of the Johns Hopkins Medical Institutions. In regular informal sessions, often embellished by wine and cheese, those with experiences in widely diverse fields—basic scientists, musicians, actors, clergymen, judges, psychiatrists, social workers, politicans, and others—are invited to talk and to answer questions.

Every physician, whether a specialist or a general internist, should select some clinical condition and begin, at an early date, to develop special knowledge and experience about its natural course and its diagnostic and therapeutic management. Systemic lupus erythematosus, bacterial endocarditis, and giant-cell arteritis, for example, have intrigued me through the years, always as a result of my having seen a patient with the condition. Seeing the patient was followed by a gathering of articles, compilation of a filing index, and slow, methodical collection of case material.

Developing subjects of special interest has several advantages. First, it keeps the clinician intellectually stimulated instead of submerged in the purely routine. Second, in examining the natural history of a disease over time, the physician will acquire a richer knowledge of many other disorders that may simulate it. Third, such clinical studies, if carried out well, may lead to a clinical report, and such a report sometimes leads to an important advance in medicine. Finally, and from a purely practical standpoint, such studies help the young clinician become established as a consultant in the community and as a speaker at medical programs.

Clinicians, then, should be permanent, enthusiastic students of disease and of human beings affected by it, so that they may acquire the ability to cure illness or relieve discomfort and to afford compassion and support to their patients. Without a practical and vital program of continued self-education, these priest-like powers of the superior clinician cannot be fully realized.

REFLECTIONS

• • •

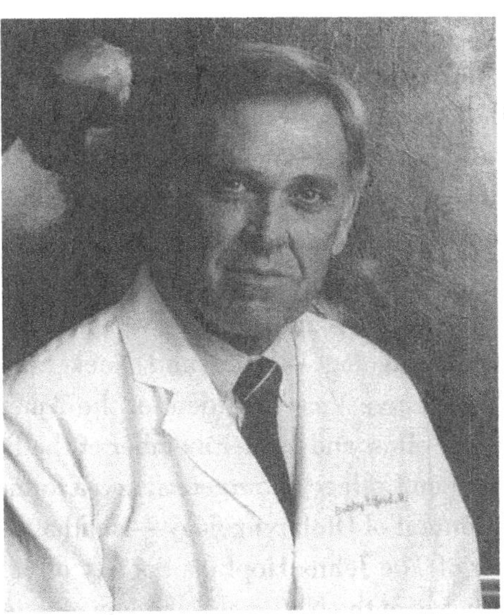

Personal satisfaction and success as a physician depend on an insatiable curiosity, constantly asking "why," then searching for, and finding, the answer.

BOBBY R. ALFORD, M.D.

Dr. Bobby Alford received his M.D. with honors from Baylor University College of Medicine in 1956. After completion of a residency in Otolaryngology—Head and Neck Surgery, he served as a Fellow in Otology at the University of Texas Medical Branch and as a Special NIH Fellow at Johns Hopkins University School of Medicine. He holds the Olga Keith Wiess Chair and is Professor and Chairman of the Department of Otorhinolaryngology and Communicative Sciences, now named in his honor, at Baylor College of Medicine.

Dr. Alford has served on the Advisory Board of Johns Hopkins University School of Medicine and on the National Advisory Council of the National Institute for Neurological and Communicative Disorders and Stroke, the National Advisory Council of the National Institute for Deafness and Other Communication Disorders, the Advisory Council of the Lunar and Planetary Institute, the NASA Headquarters National Advisory Council, the White House "Blue Ribbon" Advisory Committee for the Redesign of the Space Station, and the Aerospace Medicine Advisory Committee (Chairman). He has also served as Consultant to the Surgeon Generals of the United States Army and the United States Navy. He wasCchief Editor of the *Archives of Otolaryngology* for 10 years and has published more than 140 scientific papers.

Dr. Alford is a Fellow and former President of the American Academy of Otolaryngology—Head and Neck Surgery, a former President and Executive Vice President of the American Board of Otolaryngology, a Fellow and former member of the Board of Governors of the American College of Surgeons, and a former President of the American Council of Otolaryngology—Head and Neck Surgery. He is a member of The Johns Hopkins Society of Scholars and the Institute of Medicine of the National Academy of Sciences. As CEO of the newly established and NASA-funded National Space Biomedical Research Institute, he leads a consortium of institutions that includes Baylor College of Medicine as the lead institution.

Dr. Alford was recently awarded the NASA Distinguished Public Service Medal. In 1991, he received the Good Housekeeping Award as one of the "Top 400 Best Doctors in America."

The Prepared Mind

Bobby R. Alford, M.D.
Executive Vice President and Dean of Medicine
Chairman, Department of Otorhinolaryngology
and Communicative Sciences
Baylor College of Medicine
Houston, Texas

"[C]hance only favours the mind which is prepared. . . . "
LOUIS PASTEUR[1]

A lifelong commitment to continual learning, the acquisition of new knowledge, and expanding experience through caring for patients are essential features of a successful physician. Several factors contribute to effective continual learning and the resultant assimilation and application of the latest discoveries for the patient's benefit. An open mind and a learned, disciplined, enlightened approach to the prudent use of new information, technology, and problem-solving are essential. Personal satisfaction and success as a physician depend on an insatiable curiosity, constantly asking "why," then searching for, and finding, the answer. In reflecting on these points, I believe a passage from the Daily Prayer of a Physician, attributed to Maimonides, is as pertinent today as it was when he lived in the twelfth century A.D.: "[N]ever awaken in me the notion that I know enough, but give me strength and leisure and zeal to enlarge my knowledge and to attain ever . . . more. Our art is great, and the mind of man presses forward forever."[2]

There are many well-established ways to advance one's knowledge. For example, access to the latest biomedical information is crucial to a physician's continued development, which, in turn, leads to optimal patient care. Numerous sources are available, but because all are not of comparable reliability, currency, or scientific merit, the physician must select only sources of the highest value, relevance, and credibility. Today, emphasis on evidence-based medicine and the availability of special analytical databases as references provide a wealth of information that helps improve patient outcomes. Traditional sources, such as peer-reviewed journals like *The Journal of the American Medical Association* and *The New England Journal of Medicine,* as well as many specialty journals, are valuable sources of reports of new discoveries in diagnosis and treatment. Textbooks are useful general references, but quickly become outdated as new knowledge emerges. Other valuable sources of timely information that expand overall knowledge are the *Medical Letter* (a nonprofit publication) and the *U.S. Department of Health and Human Services' Morbidity and Mortality Weekly Report* (MMWR), which offer updates regarding drug therapy and public health issues, respectively.

Professional meetings or courses approved by the Accreditation Council for Continuing Medical Education, as well as a variety of clinical and research symposia, also provide updates of the latest developments in the pathophysiology of disease, technology, diagnosis, and treatment. Participation in such activities, which are required to meet specific minimal standards, often requires travel and absence from practice, and the content may not always justify the overall expense. Professional organizations (academies, societies, associations) also offer worthy continuing education materials, some of which are available through printed mailings, audio/video tapes, or electronic media.

In general, biomedical information for physicians should be as broadbased and convenient as possible to expand their knowledge base; a narrow, limited input will not serve their patients well. In recent years, electronic technology, such as the Internet, has provided access to numerous data banks and Web sites, each of which has advantages and disadvantages. The information is extensive, but sometimes lacks peer review and validation. Unless stringent ethical guides are observed, Web sites and e-mail can produce false impressions and border on misrepresentation. The computer-literate public may become confused or be misled by the lack of validity or clarity. Nevertheless, the Internet and e-mail have brought the physician and the public closer to the latest developments in medicine.

An authoritative, critically peer-reviewed, published manuscript continues to be the gold standard in scientific communication and the best source for expanding knowledge. Although electronic versions of such respected scientific communications can shorten the time from submission to accessibility, the technology is often substandard in reproduction of radiographic images and histopathologic materials.

The history of medicine is replete with examples of how learning and the application of knowledge, coupled with astute powers of observation, have resulted in important biomedical discoveries. Sometimes discoveries have resulted from the recognition of something missed by others. A few selected examples bring special meaning to Pasteur's statement that, in the fields of observation, " . . . chance only favours the mind which is prepared. . . .[3] "[1] An experiment in perception conducted by Bruner and Postman[3] asked subjects to identify a series of playing cards that included a few anomalous cards, such as a red six-of-spades and a black four-of-hearts. When these cards were shown briefly, the subjects almost always identified them as normal. The black four-of-hearts, for example, would be seen as either the four-of-hearts or the four-of-spades, without any awareness of anomaly. When the subjects were given gradually increasing increments of time for viewing the cards, most eventually identified the anomalous cards correctly. A few subjects, however, never could identify the anomalies, even when given 40 times the average exposure needed to identify normal cards.

An accidental discovery by the Dutch pathologist Christjaan Eijkman[4] illustrates the importance of recognizing an anomaly. When the supply of rough, unmilled rice ran low, Eijkman fed table scraps of white polished rice to the laboratory fowl, after which he noted that they developed beriberi. When he restored their usual diet of unmilled rice, they recovered. He repeated the experiment several times with the same results, proving that an ingredient of the rice skin—now known as vitamin B—prevents beriberi.

The history of surgery for thyroid disease provides yet another example of how the prepared mind led to a significant advance in medicine. In the late 1800s, the famous surgeon Theodor Kocher[5] observed that one of the young patients on whom he had successfully performed a total thyroidectomy had become extremely tired and cretinoid postoperatively. His astute observation and follow-up of his patient's course led him to describe the clinical picture of hypothyroidism (due to the absence of thyroid hormone) and thereafter to refrain from removing the entire gland. Kocher received the Nobel Prize in 1909 for his outstanding work on the physiology, pathology, and surgery of the thyroid gland. His important observation led to the development of thyroid extract.

One other example of a presumably serendipitous discovery (but more likely the result of a scientist's recognition of the significance of an anomalous occurrence) was that by Alexander Fleming, who noticed that the colonies of mold growing on his contaminated cultures had killed the staphylococci around them.[6] This observation, in combination with much painstaking research, led to the discovery of penicillin.

Each of these discoveries owes much to accident, but each also results from unusually astute powers of observation—the ability first to observe an anomaly, then to recognize its importance, and finally to make productive use of the observation.

Teaching and sharing discoveries or experiences by publishing is another way to learn. Preparing a lecture or a scholarly manuscript is a stimulus for mastering the subject. Invariably, dialogue between teacher and student or author and reader permits a beneficial exchange of ideas, information, and perspectives.

In addition to the formal and traditional ways of keeping abreast of new knowledge and applying it appropriately to patients, other factors add value and success to your medical practice, contribute to new understandings in medicine, and enhance professional growth and development. An open mind that can accommodate an initially radical-appearing idea should be nurtured. In Alexander Pope's words: "Be not the first by whom the new are tried, nor yet the last to lay the old aside."[7] Such an open-minded philosophy is as important in medicine as it is in other endeavors. Regrettably, "instant reporting" must sometimes be retracted as invalid, but that should not close your mind to new knowledge or techniques that, after being carefully reported, prove to have a sound biomedical basis. Indeed, Pasteur's counsel to young physicians (on the celebration of Pasteur's seventieth birthday, December 27, 1892, in Sorbonne) emphasized this very point: "Whatever your career may be, do not let yourselves become tainted by a deprecating and barren skepticism. . . . "[8] Guy de Chauliac (1300–1370), regarded by many as the Father of Surgery, said: "The conditions necessary for the surgeon are four: first, he should be learned; second, he should be expert; third, he must be ingenious, and, fourth, he should be able to adapt himself."[9] Both statements admonish against clinging tenaciously to what you already know as though that knowledge were absolute; have an open mind.

In this past century, one example of narrow-mindedness in surgery stands out as the antithesis of the admonitions of Pasteur and Chauliac: In the late 1930s until the early 1950s, the recommended operation for hearing impairment caused by otosclerosis (fixation of the stapes bone in the middle ear) was the fenestration operation perfected by Julius Lempert. In 1952, Sam Rosen[10] accidentally discovered that mobilization of the fixed stapes would improve hearing in many patients over results from the fenestration operation. Because most ear surgeons of that era did not know how to perform the mobilization operation and because the results in some patients were temporary, there was considerable skepticism about the benefit of the operation, and many surgeons, including Lempert, openly criticized the new procedure. It was, however, Rosen's novel observation that led to the highly successful stapedectomy and stapedotomy procedures still used today to relieve otosclerosis.

Another factor that is important in professional growth and development, and in "preserving the passion," is the pursuit of excellence. In part, it evolves from a personal commitment and discipline. Other special concepts or principles are important to continual learning and the pursuit of excellence:

At Morning Report at many teaching institutions, residents, especially the chief resident, report on the status of patients on a clinical service. When multiple institutions contribute to the training program, such meetings provide not only a review of the diagnosis, plan of treatment, and progress of each patient, but also continuity in care as residents rotate within the affiliated institutions. The Morning Report, which extends the clinical experience of residents beyond their assigned patients, represents shared learning.

Some directors of surgery training programs urge each resident to think of each surgical patient as having three operations: the one the surgeon considers ideal for the patient's diagnosis, carried out mentally before the operation; the actual operation; and a third operation, again performed mentally, that recapitulates the operation performed and changes that may have improved the result.

At several institutions today, it is possible to do a preoperative "virtual operation" with computer-modeling systems. In the future, if not now, it should be feasible to reconstruct the problem or diagnosis encountered during operation and, with virtual systems, reenact the actual operation or design a better one. Such a disciplined approach to surgery, with or without computer systems, adds significantly to the maturity and expertise of a surgeon.

Continual learning and progressive professional development, as described here, may substantially expand the physician's knowledge base and skills for the optimum care of patients. No single learning process can produce "the prepared mind," but two critical elements that assist in that goal are motivation and adaptation to changing times.

REFERENCES

1. Pasteur L. Inaugural lecture, University of Lille, December 7, 1854. In: Vallery-Radot R. *The Life of Pasteur,* Devonshire RL, trans. Garden City, NY: Garden City Publishing; 1923:76.

2. Bogen E. The daily prayer of a physician. *JAMA.* 1929;92:2128.

3. Brunner JS, Postman L. On the perception of incongruity: a paradigm. *J Pers.* 1949;18:206–223. Also discussed in Kuhn T. *The Structure of Scientific Revolutions.* 2nd ed. Chicago: Univ. Chicago Press; 1970:62–64.

4. Kyle RA, Shampo MA. Christjaan Eijkman. *JAMA.* 1980;244:1992.

5. Kocher T. Ueber Kropfextirpation und ihre Folgen. *Arch Klin Chir.* 1883;29:254–337.

6. Maurois A. *The Life of Sir Alexander Fleming, Discoverer of Penicillin.* London: Jonathan Cape; 1959:123–158.

7. Pope A. An essay on criticism: part. 2, line 335. In: Dobree B, ed. *Alexander Pope's Collected Poems.* London: Dent & Sons Ltd, Everyman's Library; 1956:66.

8. Pasteur L. Comments on the occasion of his 70th birthday, Sorbonne, December 27, 1892. In: Vallery-Radot R. *The Life of Pasteur,* Devonshire RL, trans. Garden City, NY: Garden City Publishing; 1923:451.

9. Chauliac Guy de. *On Wounds and Fractures.* Brennan WA, trans. Chicago: W.B. Brennan; 1923:xiii.

10. Rosen S. Palpation of stapes for fixation. *Arch Otolaryngol.* 1952;56:610–615.

REFLECTIONS

• • •

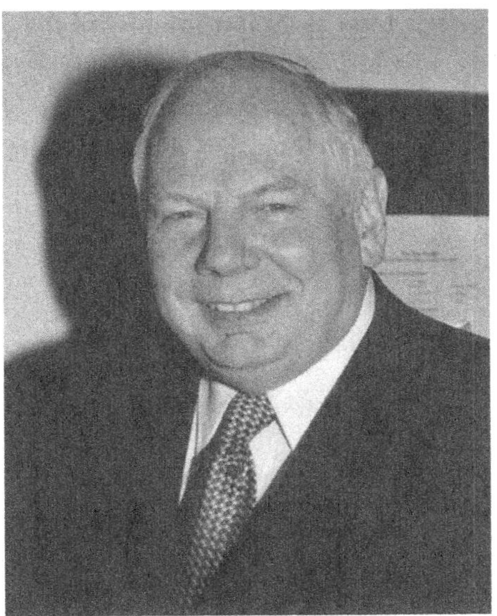

When I encounter a puzzling patient and the available publications do not help, I discuss the patient with my colleagues in the cardiology division, where the combined experience of the group is extremely helpful in reaching a diagnosis, or at least in pointing me in the appropriate direction.

WILLIAM W. PARMLEY, M.D.

Dr. William Parmley received his M.D. degree from Johns Hopkins Medical School and his internal medicine training on the Osler service at Johns Hopkins. He then spent two years in research at the cardiology branch of the National Heart Institute, followed by formal training in cardiology at the Peter Bent Brigham Hospital. He served as Associate Chief of Cardiology at Cedars-Sinai Medical Center in Los Angeles for four years, before becoming Chief of

Cardiology at the University of California at San Francisco (UCSF) for 24 years.

Dr. Parmley has been President of the American College of Cardiology, where he is a Distinguished Fellow and Master. Now completing a 10-year term as Editor-in-chief of the *Journal of the American College of Cardiology,* he is the author or coauthor of more than 350 peer-reviewed publications and 300 abstracts. He has also published four books, 140 book chapters, and 125 editorials.

Keeping Up to Date: Difficult, But Not Impossible

William W. Parmley, M.D.
Professor of Medicine
Araxe Vilensky Professor of Cardiology
University of California, San Francisco
San Francisco, California

I remember an incident as a first-year medical student at Johns Hopkins that greatly impressed me at the time. A lecturer in one of the basic sciences rose one day to advise us that certain material he had presented the previous week had been replaced by new data just published. He carefully reviewed the new data and explained that the old data were partly correct, but had clearly missed some of the major issues. I was impressed by this change in information as a marker of the future changes in "medical truths" that I would experience over a lifetime of learning. At that time, the amount of information one had to absorb and the number of newly published articles were far less than the seemingly endless new information today, especially in cardiovascular disease.

As I have reflected on how I learn information best in this age of high technology, certain patterns have emerged. As third- and fourth-year medical students, and especially during our training years and beyond, we always learned a lot from our patients. No book can adequately describe how each patient with a particular disease is going to present to the physician, and what the course will be. As we gain experience over the years, this information falls into place in our understanding of the variations and long-term course of individual problems. Furthermore, we learn much by seeing individual patients as our focal point and then reading about their problem in textbooks and other available sources. Certainly, the first few patients with diabetes that I saw as an intern provided me with an incentive to study this disease in more detail in textbooks and journals. Somehow, it made more sense to tie my knowledge to individual patients, so that I had a memory bank full of faces that I could link to a given disease. For those who continue the clinical care of patients, I believe that this model will always serve us well. Since the nuances of each patient differ from the one before, we can review the available information on the subject and get a sense of the variety and spectrum of a given disease. The interaction with patients can never be totally replaced by bibliographic searches.

When I encounter a puzzling patient and the available publications do not help, I discuss the patient with my colleagues in the cardiology division, where the combined experience of the group is extremely helpful in reaching a diagnosis, or at least in pointing me in the appropriate direction. The willingness of colleagues in all specialties to share information with one another is a particular advantage in our collective quest for continuing medical education.

There was a time in my training when I was content to confine my learning primarily to the revered textbooks of the day. Although I understood that, at publication, they were almost a year out of date, their authority and the fact that many aspects in medicine do not change gave me comfort that this was the best way to learn about a given disease. This model has served us all well. The reliance on textbooks prompted me to edit a three-volume loose-leaf textbook of cardiology, which, although updated 10 percent each year, was still out of date because of the time lag in publication and the rapid advance in medical knowledge. I no longer buy textbooks, but physicians still flock to "Publisher's Row," and selling books continues to be a brisk business.

Special opportunities to learn about new medical information have come through editing journals. As a previous Associate Editor of the *American Journal of Physiology*, the *Journal of Applied Physiology*, and *Circulation*, and currently as Editor-in-chief of the *Journal of the American College of Cardiology*, I have had a unique opportunity to review the world's latest medical information before it is published. This opportunity is exciting and stimulating because new reports that are going to make a major impact in the cardiovascular community leap out at me in advance. By reading the articles submitted to a journal, including the editorials and review articles, an editor can maintain an excellent perspective on the current state of medical knowledge. For me, this has been an effective form of continuing medical education.

More recently, I have preferentially used an electronic CD-ROM product called UpToDate, which covers internal medicine, including cardiology. The physicians on staff and the editors of UpToDate (including me) scan the world's new publications and important presentations from national and international meetings for those deemed worthy of inclusion on a future UpToDate CD. UpToDate is organized to help the clinician answer specific questions about patients. Each section is written by an expert author, then updated by the full-time physicians employed by UpToDate. Since the CD-ROM is released three times a year, there is a slight lag in information, but this is reduced considerably by the inclusion of items in prepublication form, such as reports that appear on journal Web sites or are presented at medical meetings.

For a scientific search of the world's medical publications, I primarily use PubMed, which quickly sorts out the important articles I need to review and has been extremely helpful for reviews. Although I have occasionally consulted other Web sites for appropriate up-to-date information, the two sources just cited are my current primary supply of information in cardiology. With the continuing explosion of information technology, even better ways of keeping up-to-date may be available in the future. The volume of information, however, is so daunting that we will have to be selective if we are not to drown in an ocean of information when we are really looking for a river of knowledge.

One of the current challenges of journals is the transition to electronic media. Most journals now have full contents of past articles on a Web site usually reserved for subscribers. The NIH proposal for PubMed Central to permit free access will probably be only gradually embraced by publishers of the largest and most popular journals. As one projects forward, however, a large database such as PubMed Central may well be the wave of the future for obtaining data from scientific journals. Concerns remain about the extent of peer review for some submissions and the impact on professional societies.

One of the challenges of the future, of course, will be to determine how continuing medical education (CME) will be offered. Large clinical meetings in cardiology, such as the American Heart Association (AHA) and American College of Cardiology (ACC) meetings, remain popular. The attraction of CME meetings with an outstanding faculty at desirable resort sites (and with family members present) cannot be duplicated on the Internet. It may well be that two types of CME will emerge: traditional CME courses attended for the foregoing reasons, and more specific CME on the Internet, for review of specific topics as well as for collection of appropriate credit hours. As one active in CME over the years, however, I consider the interactive phase of any CME course to be most important. The ability to ask questions of a speaker or a panel and to hear the direct responses is extremely helpful to the practicing clinician. Thus, an attempt must be made to maintain the interactive component of traditional CME if the Internet is to replace it partly or wholly.

Whatever the course of medical education in the future, it will work only if we maintain a passion for learning. Medicine must remain our beloved profession in a way that is stimulating and exciting throughout our professional lives. I remember Dr. John Sampson, past President of the American Heart Association, attending Grand Rounds lectures at the University of California, San Francisco, in his nineties, when he was no longer practicing and after he had sustained a minor stroke. He was still taking notes, reviewing them and asking questions as if he were a new house officer. This insatiable desire to learn is the key ingredient of a lifelong pursuit of medical knowledge and may, in fact, be far more important than the specific method used to satisfy that need. I saw this passion in my father, who had been a physics professor at the University of Utah. At age 99, two days before his death, we had a conversation about advances in astrophysics, based on his journal reading. Fortunately, I believe I have inherited his "desire for learning" genes.

REFLECTIONS

• • •

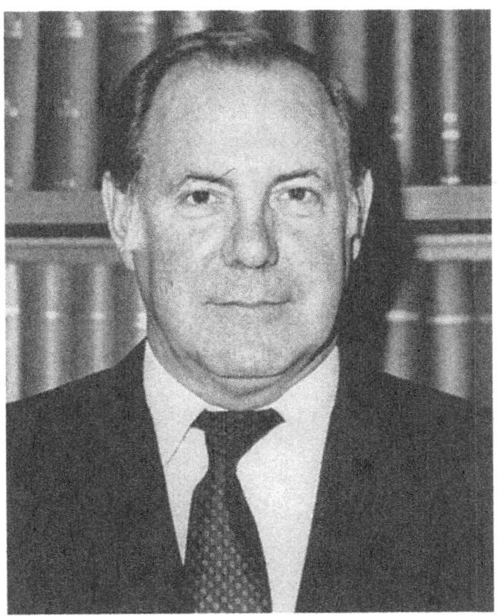

One reason we academicians like our work is that we learn a lot by osmosis. We go to conferences, and we seek out people who have the answers to our questions. So my advice to young physicians is to surround yourself with people who can educate you.

NORTON J. GREENBERGER, M.D.

Dr. Norton Greenberger received his M.D. degree from Case Western Reserve University and his residency training in gastroenterology at University Hospital, Cleveland, Ohio, and Massachusetts General Hospital, Boston. He has served as President of the Central Society for Clinical Research, the American Gastroenterological Association, the Association of Professors of Medicine, and the American College of Physicians, and as Secretary-treasurer of the American Board of Internal Medicine. Past editorships have included *The Journal of Laboratory and Clinical Medicine*, and the *Year Book of Medicine*, and the *Year Book of Digestive Diseases.*

Reading: Finding the Time and Place

Norton J. Greenberger, M.D.
Clinical Professor of Medicine
Harvard Medical School
Senior Physician
Brigham and Women's Hospital
Boston, Massachusetts

Physicians *must* be lifelong learners. When you consider four years of undergraduate education, four years of medical school, three to four years of residency training, three years of fellowship training, and a medical career of 35 years or more, it generally amounts to a 50-year medical experience. With the explosion in new biomedical information, physicians must continually discard irrelevant or obsolete information and assimilate new biomedical knowledge into their daily activities. I am reminded of a statement by C. Sidney Burwell, a noted Harvard cardiologist, who, in addressing the Harvard Medical School graduating class of 1956, said: "My students are dismayed when I say to them, 'Half of what you are taught as medical students will in 10 years have been shown to be wrong. And the trouble is, none of your teachers knows which half.'"[1] This admonition is now quoted each year in many medical schools.

Early in their careers, medical students, residents, and physicians need to develop a method for continued acquisition of reliable information that they can apply in practice. Some physicians are visual learners, some auditory learners, and some learn by both approaches. Many medical students and residents, however, have not learned how to manage their time for reading and studying. In this regard, I distribute my reading rather than concentrate it. With a list of disorders before me that I want to read about and with available textbooks, journal articles, and selected references from my reprint file, as well as other resource material, I will sit down to seek the answers. My extensive reprint collection of more than 40,000 articles organized by disease system has now been largely superseded by computer-generated information, and not a day goes by that I do not use the computer to access information related to subjects I am interested in. I also have about 40 years of bound journals covering the walls of a very large office. I often refer students, house staff, and faculty to classic articles written 20 to 30 years ago and not always readily available from computer sources.

The average student's attention span in the library is about two minutes. I read in my den, where I know I will not be distracted. I read titles, scan abstracts, tables, graphs, and diagrams and read the introduction and first and last paragraphs of the discussion. Then I ask myself what the message is in one sentence. If an article is poorly written and I cannot understand it, I am not going to waste my time with it; it impairs my efficiency.

When I finish reading an article, I often construct mnemonics and try to reproduce the material that I want to remember. Periodically, I also see if I can recall that information, and when I am with students or house staff on rounds, I go through the material for teaching purposes to reinforce my retention. Another trick is to talk about what you have read. At the end of Morning Report, I will ask anyone who may have read something interesting the night before to summarize that reading material.

If we are on rounds and a question comes up that I cannot answer, I will often assign someone to look up the answer and give a five-minute report with references. When we have coffee during rounds, I solicit a list of topics the house staff and students want me to discuss, and when I finish rounds, they generate additional subjects. Such activities stimulate me to read on a given subject and provide me an opportunity to recall information that I may not have used for some time.

REFERENCE

1. Burwell CS. Quoted in Pickering GW. The purpose of medical education. *BMJ*. 1956;2:113–116.

REFLECTIONS

• • •

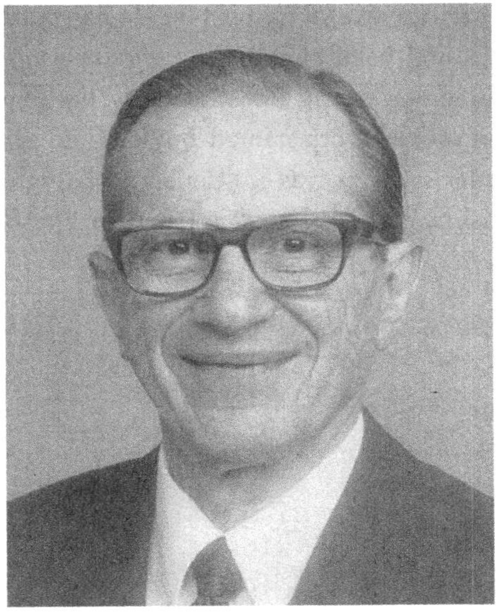

I can think of no avocation that would provide the emotional and intellectual gratification that the practice of medicine does.

ROBERT J. LUCHI, M.D.

The son of a physician, Dr. Robert J. Luchi graduated from the University of Pennsylvania School of Medicine *magna cum laude* and rose to Associate Professor, Associate Director of the Department of Medicine Clinical Research Center, and Professor of Internal Medicine, at the University of Iowa. He arrived at Baylor College of Medicine in Houston in 1970 as Professor and Vice Chairman of Medicine and Chief at the Houston Veterans Affairs (VA) Medical Center. After Dr. Luchi completed a sabbatical with Professor Exton-Smith in London, England, in 1976, he became the Founding Director of a new program in aging at Baylor and the VA

Hospital with exceptional resources for the study of the mechanisms of aging.

Dr. Luchi was the first to discover changes in cardiac myosin in health and disease and the first to describe diastolic dysfunction as a cause of heart failure in elderly people. He has published original research articles and book chapters on geriatric topics. Dr. Luchi has received numerous awards; most recently, the John A. Hartford, Inc. Foundation of New York named Baylor College of Medicine's Huffington Center on Aging as a "Center of Excellence." For his many accomplishments, Dr. Luchi is listed in *The Best Doctors in America.*

Retired Physicians: Preserving the Passion for Medicine

Robert J. Luchi, M.D.
Professor and Chief, Section of Geriatrics, Department of Medicine
Founding Director, Huffington Center on Aging
Baylor College of Medicine
Houston, Texas

Of overriding import in maintaining the passion for medicine is the desire to be useful by contributing to the welfare of others. The passion for excellence is reinforced by my daily practice. As I approach retirement, I must consider how I can sustain the passion for medicine. I can imagine a retirement in which I do not practice medicine in some form or another, but this image is fragmentary and fleeting. I can think of no avocation that would provide the emotional and intellectual gratification that the practice of medicine does.

In full retirement, I will find it harder to keep up. Why keep up if one is not going to practice or teach? One reason is simple: intellectual curiosity. All of our adult lives we have been interested in learning: in school, being taught; in educational institutions, teaching. Learning for the sake of learning becomes part of our being, an ingrained habit hard to break even when the only *raison d'etre* is one's own intellectual stimulation. Being a physician is such an integral part of who we are that it becomes impossible, while health remains, to forgo drinking at the fount of medical knowledge.

But there may be other reasons. Can one fully retire from the practice of medicine? Family and friends, from habit or for more solid reasons, look to the retired physician for advice, direction, second opinions, and the like. What if one were to have only out-of-date information to offer? Most of us value our medical integrity too much to let that happen.

With reduced access to the constant stimulation of challenges arising from daily contact with patients and students, it becomes more difficult to stay on top of things. Certainly, one can attend conferences, chat with colleagues, read the newspapers, and listen to the broadcast media announcing the latest medical news fed to them by medical journals or medical institutions. E-mail and the Internet offer other sources of medical and scientific information. Accessing information is now easy for those with even a modicum of computer literacy; all that is required is some skill in typing, use of the mouse to point and click, and some basic knowledge of how to use a Web browser. Although some information on the Internet is unreliable or unproved, some sources of current medical information, in varying detail, are accurate. Images for slide presentations, difficult to find elsewhere, can be downloaded from some excellent Web sites.

For physicians in retirement, the Internet offers an opportunity to remain productive and current in medical knowledge and practice. New and existing Internet sites continue to seek experts, and the knowledge and skills that physicians in retirement can offer will continue to be in demand, affording the retired physician an opportunity to continue to contribute to the medical and lay communities with the unique perspective long practice offers. And the continuing demand for the retired physician's expertise may well keep the passion for medicine alive when the formal practice of medicine ceases.

REFLECTIONS

• • •

Dr. Andrew Schafer received his M.D. degree from the University of Pennsylvania School of Medicine and his internship and residency in internal medicine at the University of Chicago Hospital and Clinics. He also had clinical and research fellowships in hematology at Harvard Medical School and the Brigham and Women's Hospital in Boston. Dr. Schafer joined the faculty of Harvard Medical School in 1979 and remained there as Associate Professor of Medicine until 1989, when he became Chief of Medicine at the Houston Veterans Affairs (VA) Medical Center.

Dr. Schafer's clinical and research expertise is in thrombosis, hemostasis, coagulation, platelet function, and vascular cell biology. The author of more than 180 original articles, he has edited or coedited five textbooks. He is currently the principal investigator of two National Institutes of Health (NIH) research grants in platelet and vascular cell biology. He has served on NIH and VA research study sections in hematology. A member of the executive committee of the American Heart Association, he is a former Secretary-treasurer of the American Society for Clinical Investigation, is currently Treasurer of the American Society of Hematology, and is a member of the Association of American Physicians. He is on the editorial board of several major journals.

Integrating the Art and Science of Medicine

Andrew I. Schafer, M.D.
The Bob and Vivian Smith Chairman of Medicine
Baylor College of Medicine
Houston, Texas

Twenty-five years after my own graduation from medical school, I now see my son as a first-year medical student. Some colleagues have challenged my unwillingness to discourage him from pursuing this career path during such an unsettling and precarious time. I argue that medicine endures as the most ennobling, spiritually rewarding, and intellectually exhilarating calling imaginable. Yet there is no question that we are now in the midst of perhaps the most turbulent period in the history of American medicine. It is impossible to predict the shape of medicine in general, and academic medicine in particular, that my son will encounter in mid-career. Undoubtedly, it will be radically different and perhaps barely recognizable to those of previous generations.

The recent explosion of new knowledge in molecular biology and genetics poses an intimidating challenge for today's physicians to keep up with the scientific basis of medicine. At the same time, the even more recent dramatic reorganization of medical practice, the chaos of free-market healthcare economics, and the dizzying pace of innovations in information technology have placed enormous new pressures on the already overburdened time of clinicians. Indeed, I have great concern that we are witnessing a rapidly growing schism between clinical practice and basic biomedical research. Practitioners emerging from this generation appear to be abandoning much of the scientific foundation of clinical medicine, and, conversely, physician-investigators are losing sight of the clinical relevance and application of their research. To erect durable bridges between medical practice and medical research and thereby prevent the divergence of these two groups is, I believe, one of the greatest challenges of today's leaders of academic medicine.

There is little opportunity during the workday to acquire any new knowledge except by anecdotal word of mouth. Rigorous organization of my time therefore assumes paramount importance. I continue to set aside about two hours per night to read medical and scientific publications. I try to do this during "prime time" in the evenings and to relegate to the end of the evening, by which time I am virtually decerebrate, the task of sorting through the pile of memos and circulars that invariably accumulate during the day.

My continuing education in the evenings depends on a variety of sources. I subscribe to several journals that are delivered, by intent, to my home; these range from clinical journals, such as *The New England Journal of Medicine* and *The American Journal of Medicine,* to basic science journals, such as *Science* and *Nature.* Articles in these must be reviewed and selectively perused on the day of delivery; once placed on my desk, they almost invariably go unread. During the day, I jot down reminders on an index card of "things to look up" at night; these are triggered by questions that arise in my daily clinical activities, especially those posed by trainees on rounds, as well as problems encountered in my research laboratory, and even challenging issues in healthcare administration. I spend my evening "education time" pursuing these questions and problems. In some cases, I use my home library, but increasingly I rely on computer bibliographic searches, now a more convenient and up-to-date way of surveying publications and sometimes even of reading entire articles. Indeed, I now keep journals only for the past two to three years, and my home library is beginning to suffer serious disuse atrophy.

Although I must ration my commitment to writing scientific or clinical review articles, I continue to volunteer to do these selectively and regularly. I write most of these myself, often as sole author, because they provide me with an unparalleled opportunity for continuing medical education. To the chagrin of my family, writing articles and books is generally assigned to weekends, when I have more uninterrupted time.

Although the revolution in information technology is transforming the instruments of learning and scholarship in astonishing ways, continuing education remains uncompromisingly essential throughout one's career in medicine. I consider it an integral part of my job, not a pastime. The increasing prominence of technology in medicine must continue to be balanced with a deep understanding of its scientific underpinnings. The integration of the art and science of medicine, with its enduring allure, is a legacy I wish my son to inherit.

3

Evidence-based Medicine

• • •

> Evidence-based medicine is patient care based on a synthesis of the most reliable scientific evidence available and the physician's own clinical experience and knowledge of the individual patient under consideration.
>
> PHIL R. MANNING, M.D., AND LOIS DEBAKEY, PH.D.

The basic principles of evidence-based medicine (EBM) link a physician's clinical experience with a systematic appraisal of clinical evidence in medical publications. In the words of Ian Mackay: "The report in 1992 by an Evidence-Based Working Group,[1] in which the McMaster originators were well represented, was a major impetus for evidence-based medicine. The report begins: 'A new paradigm for medical practice is emerging. Evidence-based medicine deemphasizes intuition, unsystematic clinical experience, and pathophysiologic rationale . . . and stresses the examination of evidence from clinical research.' The paradigm was seen as lowering the value of 'authority' (perhaps the authors meant 'authoritarianism'), and the 'final assumption' was that 'physicians whose practice is based on an understanding of the underlying evidence will provide superior patient care.' If a faculty member recommends a therapeutic plan that has been handed down from one generation of physicians to another and the resident assigned to the case questions the basis or effectiveness of that treatment, the resident may wish to perform a computerized bibliographic search, find reliable articles on the subject, discuss them with the faculty member, and proceed to outline an action-plan based on the evidence found.

"What is the contemporary definition of evidence based-medicine? Sackett and colleagues[2] defined it as 'the conscientious, explicit and judicious use of current best evidence in making decisions about the care of individual patients. The practice of evidence-based medicine means integrating individual clinical expertise with the best available external clinical evidence from systematic research.' Sackett emphasized that evidence-based medicine is not restricted to randomized trials and meta-analyses, but also involves the tracking of all the best external evidence with which to answer our clinical questions, whether the accuracy of a diagnostic test or a question about prognosis. The evidence needed may come from the basic sciences, perhaps genetics or immunology. Whatever the case, the idea of evidence-based medicine has proved so appealing that centers have been established to study it, workshops convened to discuss it, and a journal launched to propagate it."

John P. Geyman elaborates: "Evidence-based medicine is neither a substitute for clinical experience and judgment nor a panacea for the clinician's need for knowledge. Many questions, perhaps most, in daily clinical practice can never be studied by randomized clinical trials. Further, as Paul Fischer recently observed, clinical guidelines based on the highest quality evidence still cannot fully answer the clinician's need and responsibility to tailor the best possible care for the individual patient. That process will always require informed partnership decision-making, responsiveness to patient preferences, accommodation for concurrent medical problems, and dealing with ambiguity and uncertainty.[3] Clinical experience remains an essential springboard for clinical decision-making, but is enhanced when combined with judgments based on critical review of the best available evidence." The McMaster group suggests that evidence-based medicine should be merged with excellent skills in history-taking, physical examination, and diagnosis and therapy.[4]

Ian Mackay believes that "Evidence-based medicine has certainly added a new dimension to empirical medical practice, but it should complement, not replace, the conventional skills of the practitioner. Experience-based and intuitive clinical acumen, the art of medicine, is in part the result of a long apprenticeship traditionally used by artisans, navigators, trackers, and others to acquire needed skills. Such skills are required for the care of patients with different stages and features of multiple diseases, with subtleties as infinite as hands of bridge or moves in chess." As an example, Mackay cited a patient under his care, a 78-year-old man with rheumatic mitral stenosis and mild cardiac failure who was being treated with warfarin. In addition, the patient had advanced hemochromatosis and possible autoimmune hepatitis and esophageal varices. Mackay asks: "Should this patient have a liver biopsy? Should long-term venesection be instituted for the hemochromatosis? Should the patient receive immunosuppression?" Since evidence-based medicine cannot answer these questions, Mackay concluded that "Individually acquired experience-based medicine and the developed algorithms of evidence-based medicine should be practiced in unison, at least until we have the clinical equivalents of the IBM 'Deep Blue' program that can match, but not exceed, the skills of the Grand Masters of chess."

David Sackett and his colleagues at McMaster University and Oxford deserve credit for developing systematic approaches to the practice of evidence-based medicine, but intellectuals have long known about levels of quality in the information upon which we base decisions. Sackett and coauthors traced the philosophic origins of evidence-based medicine to the mid-19th century in Paris and earlier.[4]

Spinoza understood the importance of determining the quality of information, cautioning that we must distinguish carefully the various forms of knowledge and accept only the best. In the 17th century, he identified levels of understanding, beginning with *hearsay* information (the date of your birth); *vague experience* (knowing that you are mortal; oil feeds a flame, water extinguishes it); *concluding one thing from another* (after realizing that an object looks smaller as the distance from it increases, we conclude that the moon above is larger than it appears); and *perceiving a thing from its essence alone* (two lines that are parallel to the same line will be parallel to each other).[5] So far as we know, there were no randomized controlled studies in Spinoza's time, but conceptually it is important to understand the limits and advantages of the several kinds of knowledge. No one would contest that the best interest of the patient is served by use of the most reliable evidence available.

"The interesting thing about evidence-based medicine," in the words of Jan Vleck, "is that many physicians think they have been practicing EBM all along, so they either think EBM is nothing new or they oppose it because they do not want to change what they are comfortable with. It is actually easier to rely on local experts or apply traditional treatment forever, even if such actions are not supported, or are even contradicted, by the actual evidence. Many physicians find it difficult to change what they do or to challenge the local experts with evidence. And, of course, convincing patients that the evidence speaks to them is also a challenge. It does not bother me greatly when patients reject the evidence, as long as I have presented it clearly to them. There is always another day, at least in a continuity practice."

Despite some difficulties in the practice of evidence-based medicine, the movement is making practitioners more aware of the need to assess carefully the quality of evidence they use in patient care. Practitioners and medical educators now realize that a systematic approach is necessary.

The classic McMaster approach emphasizes a framework of five steps[4]:

- Convert information needs into answerable questions.

- Track down, with maximum efficiency, the best evidence with which to answer them (from the clinical examination, the diagnostic laboratory, research evidence, or other sources).
- Critically appraise that evidence for its validity (closeness to the truth) and usefulness (clinical applicability). (Also see pp. 121).
- Apply the results of this appraisal in clinical practice.
- Evaluate our performance.

David Slawson outlined his approach to assessing medical information: "When physicians read journals, attend conferences, or consult with colleagues, the goal is to spend the least time and energy finding the best information. We are all busy with important aspects of life besides medicine (family, friends, fun), yet we always want to do the best possible for our patients. Useful information must have three attributes: relevant to everyday practice, correct, and easy to obtain.

"*Relevance* focuses on our ultimate goal: finding information on how to help our patients live long, functional, satisfying, pain- and symptom-free lives. We have a plethora of information about disease: etiology, prevalence, pathophysiology, and pharmacology. These intermediate-level studies are crucial to medicine. We must understand how a disease evolves before we can diagnose, treat, or prevent it. Little of this information, however, tells how to obtain patient-oriented evidence, which provides effective interventions, the ultimate goal of our patients. Only in the past few years has this concept of real-world research surfaced, a concept that focuses on interventions used in clinical practice and their properly tested effects on outcomes.

"For example, an article about prostate cancer screening with the prostate-specific antigen (PSA) assay may report the sensitivity, specificity, and predictive values for identifying men with prostate cancer. Another article may report survival rates for different treatments and stages of prostate cancer. Neither tells us, however, what we and our patients really want to know: whether they will live a longer, healthier, happier life as a result of identifying the cancer. Only a randomized trial evaluating the overall effect of early detection on the mortality and morbidity of prostate cancer will provide that information.

"*Validity* defines to what extent the knowledge gained represents the 'truth.' Well-designed clinical trials that minimize bias are more likely to provide valid conclusions. Validity assessments of research articles are best performed by application of the excellent guides for critical reading published by the Evidence-based Medicine Working Group. Although this task can be delegated to an 'expert,' each of us must accept responsibility for critically assessing validity. We should not accept evidence at face value simply because it is published in a well-known journal or is recommended by a specialist.

"*Work* or time spent is the negative attribute that we must consider when searching for useful information. An inordinate amount of time to establish the validity or relevance of information may be beyond the reach of the overworked physician. On the other hand, a cursory approach may not yield totally valid or relevant information. From the physician's point of view, the best solution is to find highly valuable and pertinent information with minimal effort." A partial solution is to use sources that are based entirely or almost entirely on evidence-based medicine articles, such as the Cochrane Library collection and *Clinical Evidence* (published by the BMJ Publishing Group) and the *ACP Journal Club.* When a physician encounters a difficult search problem, the help of a medical librarian may be essential, both as a time-saver and insurance of a complete search.

Slawson continued: "Using relevance as the primary screen for validity results in the least unnecessary effort. Answering 'yes' to the following three questions will help identify relevant information requiring validation: (1) Is the problem common in my practice? (2) Will this information have a direct bearing on the health of my patients? (3) If valid, will this information require me to change my current practice? When all three answers are 'Yes,' we call the study a POEM because it is *Patient-Oriented Evidence that Matters.* For research articles, the conclusion section of the abstract will usually give all the information necessary to answer these three questions.

"We must also consider our goals for obtaining new information or reviewing previously learned information. Different goals require different approaches. We can (1) *search* for the answer to a question related to a specific patient, (2) *forage* to stay informed about new developments in our field, (3) *keep up* with a specific area of interest, or (4) *retrace* our path by reviewing previously learned information to compare it to new information. But gathering and evaluating patient-oriented information is not enough; the final step is to *incorporate* this new knowledge into medical practice. We may not have all the answers, but we need to find and verify those available. For the rest, we need to start asking the right questions."

David Slawson recommends two specific tools to help physicians efficiently identify information that is highly relevant and valid: "Clinicians need a first-alert method—a POEM bulletin board—for relevant new information as it becomes available. Resources (newsletters, Web sites, continuing education, and others) used by clinicians to update their knowledge should carefully filter out preliminary or unverified information to facilitate keeping-up. Clinicians can purchase POEMs for Primary Care, a database of 20–25 POEMs gleaned from more than 100 primary-care articles and delivered daily in an e-mail update (MedicalInfoPointer: http://www.medicalinforetriever.com) or as a monthly paper supplement to *The Journal of Family Practice, Evidence-Based Practice* (www.jfponline.com). Clinicians also need a way of rapidly retrieving the information to which they have been alerted but that has not yet been cemented into their minds. Computer-based resources, especially handheld portable devices, can provide information in less than 30 seconds. To be lifelong learners, physicians have to use tools that help them forage in the jungle of information."

Ian Mackay described a taxonomy of evidence developed by the National Health and Medical Research Council (NHMRC) of Australia: "Benchmarks for current best practice will vary according to

TABLE 1
Taxonomy of Evidence (Revised 1998)

I	From a systematic review of all relevant randomized controlled trials
II	From at least one properly designed randomized controlled trial
III-1	From well-designed pseudo-randomized controlled trials (alternate allocation or some other method)
III-2	From comparative studies with concurrent controls and allocation not randomized (cohort studies), case-control studies, or interrupted time series with a control group
III-3	From comparative studies with historical control, two or more single-arm studies, or interrupted time series without a parallel control group
IV	From case series, either post-test or pre-test and post-test

Source: National Health and Medical Research Council of Australia.

the circumstances in which evidence-based medicine might be applied. The taxonomy is based on earlier guidelines (Table 1).[6] Thus, when an evidence-based decision is recorded in a medical record, it can be coded according to the quality of the evidence available, as shown in Table 1 (modified from NHMRC's original taxonomy)."[6]

Gary Kelsberg uses his desktop computer to search for answers to clinical problems, such as "Should Type 2 diabetic patients start taking an angiotensin converting enzyme (ACE) inhibitor before there is laboratory evidence of microproteinuria?" or "Are antibiotics likely to benefit a smoker with bronchitis more than the minimal or no-benefit seen in nonsmoking patients?" One of several databases that allow rapid searching is TRIP (Translating Research Into Practice, http://www.tripdatabase. com). Kelsberg explains that "This is a metasite, containing a search engine to comb Patient Oriented Evidence that Matters (POEMs) from numerous sources (*ACP Journal Club, Bandolier, Evidence-Based Practice, The Journal of Family Practice,* POEMs).

More than 10,000 POEMs are available." While he is in clinic, he leaves his computer up and running nearby, so he can usually step out of the room and look something up within two to three minutes.

Kelsberg describes other information sources: "InfoRetriever is proprietary software for the desktop or handheld Windows Pocket PC™ format. It is searchable and has about 800 POEMs, along with drug information and lots of useful clinical calculators, guidelines, and handy tools for prediction. It is updated quarterly. Another is the Cochrane Library, available by subscription on CD ROM and the Internet (or free if you have library privileges at a nearby medical school). It has excellent clinical trials data, analyzed by careful methods. InfoRetriever also contains all of the abstracts from the Cochrane Database, updated quarterly, and allows searching through multiple databases to obtain the highest quality answers to patient care questions. Failing these, several print sources are incorporating evidence in their format, for example, the American College of Obstetrics and Gynecology Guidelines now contain references and ratings about the strength or quality of their recommendations."

Gary Kelsberg and Jan Vleck believe that framing a searchable and answerable question to find the best solution to a medical problem typically requires specifying four elements: population, intervention, comparison intervention, and outcome:

- *Population.* Who is the patient, or how can the patient be described as a member of a group of similar people? Because most research is conducted on groups of subjects, you will be looking for research in which the study groups included people like your individual patient. Example: To research a question involving an asymptomatic, 75-year-old woman with blood pressure of 160/90 mm Hg, you would look for studies examining groups of elderly female hypertensives.

- *Intervention.* What are you or your patient contemplating doing about the clinical situation? Example: What tests or treatments might apply to your elderly female patient with hypertension?

- *Comparison intervention.* There may be a choice of interventions. How does the approach you are considering compare with other intervention choices, or no intervention, in terms of patient outcomes, complications, and costs? You might want to look at outcomes comparing diuretic therapy versus placebo in elderly women with hypertension.

- *Outcomes.* What are the projected outcome differences? The outcomes can be as stark as death, or more subtle like net economic impact. Gary Kelsberg emphasizes: "Remember, if you are going to find evidence, the outcome must be one that can be studied, which in most cases means that it has to be quantifiable. Many quantifiable outcomes are not patient-oriented evidence that matters, so the answers you find may be non-answers. (Does your patient really care about a statistically significant 4 percent improvement in Forced Expiratory Volume 1 [FEV1]?) Be aware also that you and your patient may not value particular outcomes in the same way, so even the best evidence can be thrown out by the court of patient opinion."

At the very least, evidence-based medicine caused most medical schools to incorporate its principles into the medical curriculum, encouraged medical journals to adopt structured formats of abstracts, and heightened the interest of practicing physicians in obtaining the best information available. The definitive basic principles of evidence-based medicine include integrating the best external clinical evidence from systematic research into individual clinical experience.

John Geyman recommends the following concrete steps to physicians desiring to incorporate evidence-based medicine into their own continuing medical education and clinical practice[7]:

- Subscribe to a foraging source of new information as it becomes available, screening for both relevance and validity. Consider

InfoRetriever (http://www.infopoems.com) or *ACP Journal Club* (1-800-523-1546).

- Increase reading of predigested information within your specialty or interest.
- Meet with a librarian at your nearest health sciences library to arrange a tutorial in current search tools, such as PubMed.
- Establish bookmarked Web sites on your office and/or home computer for useful sources of evidence-based abstracts and reports.
- Seek consultants who value and use evidence-based approaches in their practices.
- Reorient your CME to evidence-based courses as they become more available.

David Slawson points out that soon CME will be based on point-of-care learning: "You will obtain CME credit while using handheld portable databases, answering clinical questions as you need the information. This will become possible with embedded files in the software that keep track of usage and can then be sent once a year to specialty organizations to obtain CME credit.

"Gathering and evaluating patient-oriented information is not enough; the final step is to incorporate this new knowledge into medical practice. We may not have all the answers, but we need to find and verify those available. For the rest, we need to start asking the right questions."

Most articles written about evidence-based medicine emphasize selecting the best external information sources. The methods of applying clinical experience, even though extremely important, have received far less attention. All physicians should study and document their clinical experience by knowing their practice mix in order to direct their study, keeping a record of what they learn from puzzling patients and recording outcomes and procedures they perform (see Chapter 10).

REFERENCES

1. Evidence-based Medicine Working Group. Evidence-based medicine. A new approach to teaching the practice of medicine. *JAMA.* 1992;268:2420–2425.

2. Sackett DL, Gray JAM, Haynes RB, Richardson WS. Evidence-based medicine: what it is and what it isn't. *BMJ.* 1996;312:71–72.

3. Fischer PM. Evidentiary medicine lacks humility. *J Fam Pract.* 1999;48:345–346.

4. Sackett DL, Richardson WS, Rosenberg W, Haynes RB. *Evidence-based Medicine: How to Practice and Teach EBM.* London: Churchill Livingstone; 1997.

5. Spinoza, B de. *Spinoza's Ethics and "De Intellectus Emendatione."* Boyle A, trans. New York: E. P. Dutton; 1910: 232–233.

6. National Health and Medical Research Council. *A Guide to the Development, Implementation and Evaluation of Clinical Practice Guidelines.* Canberra, Australia Capitol Territory: NHMRC; 1999:56.

7. Geyman JP. Evidence-based medicine in primary care: an overview. *J Am Board Fam Pract.* 1998;11:46–56.

REFLECTIONS

• • •

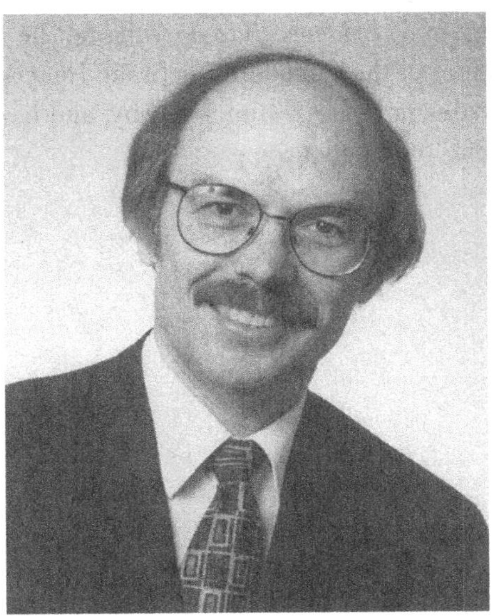

For many health problems, sound evidence from research is still thin or even nonexistent.

R. BRIAN HAYNES, M.D., PH.D.

Dr. Brian Haynes received his M.D. from the University of Alberta, his Ph.D. from McMaster University, and his residency training at Toronto General Hospital, all in Canada. He completed his medical training at St. Thomas Hospital School of Medicine in London. He has had a career-long interest in the methodology of healthcare research and in the validation, distillation, dissemination, and application of healthcare knowledge. Of particular interest are information problems that confront healthcare practitioners and their potential solutions from synoptic writing and information technology. Dr. Haynes led the development of the format for "structured" abstracts, now used by most medical journals. He is a founding member of the Working Group of Evidence-Based Medicine, recognized as one of the most influential ideas of 2001. The Founding Editor for a number of evidence-based journals, including *ACP Journal Club, Evidence-Based Medicine, Evidence-Based Mental Health,* and *Evidence-Based Nursing,* he was also the Founding Director of the Canadian Cochrane Network and Centre. All these activities have been stimulated by, and have contributed to, his passion for lifelong learning.

Learning from Healthcare Research: Evidence-based Medicine

R. Brian Haynes, M.D., Ph.D.
Professor of Clinical Epidemiology and Medicine
Chair, Department of Clinical Epidemiology and Biostatistics
McMaster University Faculty of Health Sciences
Hamilton, Ontario, Canada

Although I was born and reared in Alberta, Canada, I must have had some ancestral roots in Missouri (presumably from United Empire Loyalist times), judging by my compulsion to ask people to show me the evidence on which their pronouncements are based. Such insistence has gotten me into trouble from time to time, notably in my second year of medical school in 1968. My medical school class dubbed that year "trial by lecture," a mind-and-derriere-numbing initiation rite that we had to endure if we were to be found fit for the medical fraternity.

In one lecture on Freud's theories, which mercifully ended before the bell rang, the lecturer asked if there were any questions. I asked what the evidence was that Freud's theories were true. The lecturer broke from his teaching role and admitted that he did not know of any such evidence and did not believe that the theories were valid. He indicated that he had been assigned by the Department of Psychiatry Chairman, a Freudian, to give the lecture. I was dismayed, wondering how much of my medical education to date was similarly based. This revelation and other, if less apocryphal, experiences led me to resolve to combine research with clinical practice. I tried working with a professor in animal research during the summers, but this seemed to be a rather indirect route to learning how human beings and disease interact and what might be done to alter the balance in favor of humans.

I interned at Toronto General Hospital, thinking that the "flagship of the Canadian hospital fleet" might be floating higher in the evidential sea of healthcare. Although there were many good basic scientists there, more than a few would take offense if asked for the evidence supporting their assertions about clinical practice. I realized that I was not going to get what I needed from them and concluded that I would have to study research methods to become a better clinician. Fortuitously, Jack Laidlaw, then Director of the Institute of Clinical Sciences at the University of Toronto (whose favorite question was "What's the evidence for that?"), invited David Sackett from the fledgling McMaster University Faculty of Health Sciences to speak on "Is Healthcare Researchable?" I believe that I was the only house officer attendee, the other attendees having been in epidemiology. I jumped ship at the end of my internship and went to McMaster to study with Sackett and his then small Department of Clinical Epidemiology and Biostatistics. What an experience! In addition to Sackett, I learned at the feet of Alvan Feinstein and met Archie Cochrane—the Canadian, American, and British parents of clinical epidemiology.

I had intended to stay a year at McMaster before returning to clinical training, but stayed three, after which I returned to Toronto, then went to England to complete my training in internal medicine. I found that I could apply much of my training in clinical epidemiology to asking "the right questions" in clinical practice, but the amount of strong research evidence for clinical practice was discouraging. (How times have changed!)

CRITICAL APPRAISAL OF MEDICAL PUBLICATIONS

In 1978, led by Sackett, a group of us organized a series of sessions for residents on how to appraise medical publications. We knew that we were onto something when the attending staff began asking for the sessions (motivated, they said, by the impertinent questions that the house staff was asking on rounds). They wanted their sessions separated from the residents' sessions so as to avoid revealing their ignorance to the residents. To support these sessions, we developed a series of articles that were published in the *Canadian Medical Association Journal* on how to interpret studies on the etiology, diagnosis, prognosis, treatment, and economics of health problems. This led to a textbook on clinical epidemiology, an annual international workshop on how to teach critical appraisal, and invitations to teach elsewhere.

Participants seemed to enjoy the curriculum and indicated that they felt good about mastering the concepts, which they believed would keep them up to date in their clinical work. But we soon realized that even if we could teach these principles and even if some people enjoyed learning them, the volume of publications was far too massive for any practitioner to deal with. It took too much time to determine the best evidence for a given problem. No wonder physicians seemed more inclined to "talk the talk" of critical appraisal than to "walk the walk." Indeed, we ourselves had difficulty making time to find and appraise articles in detail amid the pressure of clinical care.

We felt that we were making the approach too academic. Further, we needed to move the focus from reading and evaluating publications to applying their lessons directly to patient care. We therefore sought to simplify our critical appraisal and to develop resources that facilitated finding sound evidence as it was published and, more ambitiously, resources that provided "current best evidence" for any clinical problem.

To begin the work on resources, we developed a proposal that we took to Ed Huth, then Editor of the *Annals of Internal Medicine* and a devotee of critical appraisal. The proposal called for brief critiques of key articles in the *Annals* so that readers would not have to do the critiques themselves. When the proposal was presented to the *Annals* Editorial Board, the members split along generational lines: the younger Board members were keen, but the older ones feared that no author would submit articles to the *Annals* if they were going to be criticized in public.

This led to a second proposal for authors, themselves, to prepare more informative "structured" abstracts for their articles, providing the key details needed for critical appraisal, including the Objective of the study, Design, Participants, and Setting; the details of any Intervention; the key Results; and only those Conclusions that were directly supported by the data. This proposal was eventually accepted by the *Annals*,[1] supported by Stephen Lock of the *British Medical Journal*, and later adopted by many other clinical journals.

Although structured abstracts provide a means for journal readers to discern studies of relevance and value more readily for their clinical practice, they do not solve the basic problem of medical publications: a small number of important studies (especially from the perspective of any one practitioner) thinly spread among a large number of journals. To overcome this needle-in-a-haystack problem, we developed a proposal for a new breed of derivative journal, to include summaries of articles selected from a large number of full-text medical journals according to explicit principles (an abbreviated set of those developed for critical appraisal of publications), presented in abstracts independently prepared (by research staff and clinical epidemiologists) and critiqued (by a clinical expert with at least a basic understanding of applied clinical research methods). We took this proposal to the American College of Physicians, which accepted it, a decision that led to the bimonthly publication for internists, *ACP Journal Club*. The process of selecting only articles that met criteria for scientific merit and direct clinical relevance clearly demonstrated the myth of information overload: only about one article for every two issues of even the very best journals made the grade. The real problem is "misinformation overload": burying evidence that practitioners need in material inadequately tested for clinical practice but often glittering as if it were relevant.

CRITICAL APPRAISAL OF MEDICAL PUBLICATIONS BECOMES EVIDENCE-BASED MEDICINE DEFINITION

We needed a new term for our ultimate goal, that is, the application of healthcare research evidence at the bedside and in the clinic. Gordon Guyatt coined the term "evidence-based medicine." We discussed this and various alternatives with colleagues, including some rather testy basic scientists who thought the term denigrated their contributions to science (animal and preliminary clinical research being rather low in our hierarchy of "clinically relevant" evidence). The concept was publicized in articles in the *ACP Journal Club*[2] and *The Journal of the American Medical Association.*[3] This term certainly attracted attention, both favorable and unfavorable, and still does. For better or worse, the term has spread around the world, with adaptations for other professions (evidence-based nursing, dentistry, pharmacy), health administration (evidence-based healthcare), and healthy policy (evidence-based policy). In at least some ways, the term is unfortunate. "Evidence," for example, was intended to be used narrowly to mean findings from healthcare research, but those new to the term are rightly confused when they interpret it to mean all kinds of evidence (including that from the patient, the laboratory, and basic research). Further, the term does not translate well into some languages; in French, for example, the term means "self-evident," the opposite of "based on evidence."

To clarify the concept and spread the word, advocates published a new series of articles on applying results of healthcare research to practice in *The Journal of the American Medical Association* beginning in 1993,[4] as well as in numerous books, beginning with one by Sackett and colleagues.[5]

New derivative periodicals have sprung up to help clinicians practicing in various disciplines find sound evidence, including *Evidence-Based Medicine, Evidence-Based Mental Health, Evidence-Based Cardiovascular Medicine,* and *Evidence-Based Nursing*. These journals are based on a systematic review of more than 100 clinical journals, a process that weeds out about 98 percent of medical publications. Further, resources to help clinicians find current best evidence when the need arises have now become available, including *Best Evidence* and the Cochrane Library, which provides electronic access to worldwide, systematic summaries and dissemination of all trials of healthcare interventions. An addition to this panoply of evidence-based resources, with promise of becoming the best, is *Clinical Evidence* from the BMJ Publishing Group. This regularly updated publication summarizes the best evidence for treatment of a widening array of clinical problems.

WHAT'S NEXT?

The interest in evidence-based medicine has probably been premature, raising expectations that healthcare could be readily transformed by this "new paradigm." Perhaps it can, but not so quickly, for a number of reasons. First, for many health problems, sound evidence from research is still thin or even nonexistent. Second, evidence from research can be but one component of a clinical decision, other components being the individual clinical circumstances of the patient, the available resources, and the patient's wishes. Just how these components should be factored in "real time" remains a black box. Continuing education remains a problem—both as to how to practice evidence-based medicine (EBM) and how to adopt the proceeds of the research that it attempts to transfer into practice. We need to become as serious about continuing education as we are about undergraduate and postgraduate education, time and money being the greatest trolls protecting the bridge to learning how to apply new and better healthcare knowledge. Information systems that present evidence in the right way (in a context that fits the problem, patient, and practitioner), in the right place, and at the right time may help, but that remains to be shown in a way that is both powerful and practical.

WHO ARE WE?

The journey described here has been a collegial enterprise. Many people have been involved in addition to those named here, particularly faculty and staff of the McMaster's Department of Clinical Epidemiology and Biostatistics, which has been my academic home for my entire career. I would thank them all, but that would be presumptuous; we're all in this together.

REFERENCES

1. Ad Hoc Working Group for Critical Appraisal of the Medical Literature. A proposal for more informative abstracts of clinical articles. *Ann Intern Med.* 1987;106:598–604.
2. Guyatt GH. Evidence-based medicine. *ACP J Club.* 1991; 114:A-16.
3. Evidence-based Medicine Working Group. Evidence-based medicine: a new approach to teaching the practice of medicine. *JAMA.* 1992;268:2420–2425.
4. Guyatt GH, Rennie D. Users' guides to reading the medical literature [Editorial]. *JAMA.* 1993;270:2096–2097.
5. Sackett DL, Richardson SR, Rosenberg W, Haynes RB. *Evidence-Based Medicine: How to Practice and Teach EBM.* London: Churchill Livingstone; 1997.

4

Medical Information Technology: An Instrument for Learning

• • •

"Knowledge is power,"[1] wrote Francis Bacon. In medical practice, knowledge derives from the critical analysis of the plethora of information now available at the time and place needed. That knowledge, in turn, informs good clinical judgment.

PHIL R. MANNING, M.D., AND LOIS DEBAKEY, PH.D.

The explosive growth of the Internet and the popularity of e-mail have simplified and facilitated physicians' lifelong learning and their communication with colleagues and patients. Continuing medical education courses no longer need to be attended in person, but can be completed on the computer. Medical journals and textbooks are also available online. Daily reports on recent medical advances may be reviewed at the click of a mouse. Authoritative essays on a broad range of current medical concepts are readily accessible. The reality of pertinent information at the point-of-care is approaching. Major changes in medical library services are evolving. Most medical schools (and even high schools and colleges) provide instruction on use of the Internet, ensuring that graduates will be prepared to use this source to enhance their lifelong learning.

With these advances, physicians are able to rely less on memory and more on managing information skillfully by finding, and determining the relevance and validity of, the plethora of available medical information. Advances in electronic information technology, especially information on the Internet, are still rapidly developing. We offer examples of only a few products, realizing that many others exist. With the numerous company mergers and name changes, no one can be certain what will be available in the next few months, let alone the next few years. The only certainty is that access to useful information is becoming easier and faster.

"Where the penetration of managed care has been high, the time available to acquire new information or review old information has diminished," observed Ralph Feigin. "Busy clinicians are allowed less time to pursue academic activities, to expand their knowledge, and to apply new knowledge to the care of their patients. The advent of electronic communications has come at an opportune time in the history of medicine, since the rapid accessibility of information may help offset some of the problems engendered by managed care."

The physician–patient relation is being revised as patients come to the physician's office armed with information gleaned from the Internet, sometimes accurate, sometimes invalid. Physicians need to develop skills in interpreting the information and in guiding patients to the most pertinent sources.

John Wolf cautioned: "The computer-fluent physician will be better prepared than his peers to practice third millennium medicine, but with caveats. First, the Internet, in its infancy, has been replete with erroneous information, a potpourri of poorly edited 'facts' that seem to have taken Mark Twain's facetious advice seriously: 'Get your facts first, and then you can distort them as much as you please.'[2] Furthermore, computers, at least for now, cannot think or teach us how to think. Some insist that computers are of limited value because they can only produce answers. Incisive questions are essential for basic or clinical research in medicine, and only human beings can conceive those questions now."

"At the touch of a button," said Daniel Musher, "I now have access to a plethora of important and unimportant experimental and clinical studies published around the world. Instead of too little information, I now have too much. Moreover, it comes right off my printer in the office, so I no longer have some of the mnemonic clues that helped me remember the text, such as recalling where I sat in the library when reading Beeson and Petersdorf on fever of unknown origin. Culling the current, relevant, and accurate from the mass of unreliable information, much less remembering or being able to cite a reference on rounds, has become a real problem. I have heard colleagues chastise young authors for not being meticulous about bibliographic references, as if that were a new phenomenon. Not so. Some authors have always been meticulous, and others always careless. I have had certain sardonic enjoyment in discovering an article cited out of context or used to support a point that, in fact, it helped refute. I feel confident that my younger colleagues will solve the burden of excessive information, but I cannot, at present, imagine how."

WORLD WIDE WEB

Medical informatician Michael Ackerman pointed out that: "Information, of variable specificity and authenticity, can be found in a few moments whenever and wherever the need arises—the teachable moment. Trips to the library or a CD-ROM purchase may no longer be necessary. The impact that this has on traditional and more formal education remains to be understood. While fingertip opportunities for lifelong learning are endless, the ability of students to recognize reliable sources is problematical. Web access speeds are not fast enough, and Web search engines still do more searching than finding, but these problems will be solved in time. Educational technology will bring credited course material to the physician on demand, a physician's formal progress will be tracked from a distance, and distance learning will be accessed from any site by means of a telephone connection. Educational institutions need to develop the educational and commercial models that will convert these visions to reality."

Technical producer Stephen Nazarian believes that: "Practitioners have traditionally used various print resources (books, journal articles) to keep current. Sources of this information on the Internet are easier to search, accessible around the clock, and almost limitless in quantity. That this information is sometimes valid and sometimes misleading or inaccurate presents new challenges to the physician. By becoming familiar with reliable Web sites, physicians will dramatically reduce the time spent dispelling misleading information for patients."

Yoichi Satomura, President of the Japanese Association of Medical Informatics, believes that formal lecture courses are best suited for medical students, but the best lifelong learning links education to daily practice. Japanese physicians, however, still receive most of their continuing education by conventional means, such as lectures, seminars, and scientific meetings. Most Japanese physicians own computers for accounting or personal use, but accessing information from the Internet is not yet popular. Satomura attributes this to the insufficient time that clinical practice allows to obtain reliable information through the Internet.

As the computerized patient record becomes more prevalent in office practice, physicians will more likely access information from the Internet. The Japanese government has introduced measures to encourage use of the computerized patient record. Satomura believes that, ultimately, information technology will greatly enhance lifelong learning, but conventional methods will continue because of the benefits of social interaction.

Patients: A Driving Force

Stephen Sullivan explained how patients have become a driving force in the use of the Internet: "Today vast clinical knowledge, simple and complex, is available to everyone, and people are increasingly taking advantage of it, as confirmed by the growing medical content sites on the World Wide Web. The number of registered users and page views per month is rising almost exponentially. Patients are reviewing information electronically, joining chat groups or disease-specific forums, and seeking experts, classes, or clinical trials.

"To the surprise of physicians, Personal Health Diaries (PHDs) have gained wide consumer acceptance on the Internet.[3] This patient-controlled clinical repository allows the user to maintain a personal inventory of medical narratives—diagnoses, treatments, events, reminders, and clinical contacts. *The Wall Street Journal*'s weekly 'Health Journal' column features discussions of Internet-available clinical screening-tool questionnaires, such as the one for depression designed by the National Mental Health Association. A San Francisco Bay Area hospital group encourages residents to check their cardiac health by completing similar online screening for coronary artery disease. And on a Web site, http://www.partners.org/healthonline, Internet users can effortlessly find clinical trials related to personal conditions and diseases. Patients not only want more clinical information, but also wish to manage it.

"How are physicians responding? Despite all the new Web-based consumer brands in clinical healthcare, research verifies that patients now believe first and foremost in their local physicians' clinical knowledge and advice. The physician's goal is to use this technology to improve care and enhance the relationship of trust with patients. Besides learning how to respond to patients armed with Web-based general health information and printouts of recent readings, physicians are devising strategies to communicate better with patients. Improved communication between clinicians and patients will be integrated with robust sharing of appropriate, specific clinical information: relevant articles or videos; details about newly prescribed medication from an array of pharmacy databases, textbooks, and even pharmaceutical manufacturers; annotated clinical results linked to personalized explanatory notes; reminders to complete a previously ordered screening or diagnostic study; or even alerts with new genetic information about their condition.

"Patients will be able to review subsets of the clinical information present in their physician's online medical record. This capability will allow patients to submit additions, revisions, and comments for inclusion in their records. This two-way communication should lead to greater efficiency in the physician's office as changes mirror the expectations of Web-literate patients. Routine transactions, like laboratory orders and prescription refills, will become automatic through the Internet, leaving time for more valued communications.

"The clinician will be expected to interpret the complex medical information gathered by the patient as such information continues to explode and patients' unquenchable thirst for it expands. The more medically informed the patients, the healthier they will be as they seek earlier and more effective care.

"The exponential growth of clinical knowledge and of patient expectations for the physicians' mastery of it will lead to more specialization. Routine clinical problems may become the purview of nurse practitioners and physicians' assistants, physicians concentrating on more complex medical issues. The likelihood is real that the patient–physician partnership, based on shared knowledge, will strengthen.

"Yet how can individual physicians manage the knowledge onslaught, even with the best reminder systems? Once a patient's diagnosis has been made, won't the physician insist on consulting an expert to answer the most arcane question that might have arisen during the clinical investigation? Paradoxically, an internist or family physician may have detailed knowledge about an array of maladies, but the patients may be treated by subspecialists, the 'real' experts."

Electronic Services

No longer is there any question about the role of the computer in the physician's daily routine. The Internet offers scores of information resources, but with the frequent mergers and name changes, it is difficult to predict how long services and products will be available in their present state. As more physicians rely on electronic services for current medical information, however, the products will become more sophisticated, efficient, and useful. Two currently popular information resources are Medscape and WebMD. In addition to providing up-to-date information daily, they permit accessing MEDLINE and other databases that are more convenient because they are restricted to key journals. Category 1 continuing medical education (CME) credit is usually available if the physician is willing to take a brief objective test after reviewing written material. Most services also keep records of CME credit earned by the physician.

Medscape (http://www.medscape.com) offers a wide array of information for physicians, other health professionals, and the general public. On the physician's site, each registrant is invited to designate a special area of interest or expertise. Thereafter, the computer will automatically match that registrant with the designated specialty and provide pertinent journal articles.

Once on the personalized home page, the user may choose among many options to obtain desired information. A popular use is to enter a specific search term, upon which nine different databases may be searched without further entry. The usual MEDLINE search produces many citations, sometimes from obscure journals. Medscape Select includes only the 269 journals in MEDLINE chosen as "best" by 77 different criteria. By searching Medscape Select, the user finds fewer articles on any one subject, but all are from the most respected journals, which improves the likelihood of finding reliable and useful information in the shortest time.

Conference summaries are among the most popular Medscape features. Medscape covers many of the best international medical conferences each year. Expert physicians function as medical reporters who create abstracts from the meeting program, decide which presentations to attend, and that evening summarize the presentations, giving full credit to the presenters. After being edited, the reports are posted the next day instead of six to 24 months later, as in standard medical journals.

Medscape provides its own "Medscape Wire" news service. Trained medical reporters scan the best medical journals and write short, readable news stories from them. Medscape publishes *Treatment Updates,* written by experts, based on well-established literature, and couched in language that is easily understood by practicing physicians. This service is free to physicians.

MEDLINE is easily accessed through Ovid. Medical Updates provides 600–800-word summaries of the current understanding of specific diseases, a question-and-answer section, a biographical sketch of the author, and a listing of pertinent guidelines, with hyperlinks to the Web. Quick Facts includes short essays on current topics. Physicians may click onto another version designed for patients. Graphic displays are available to help physicians explain to patients the mechanisms of diseases and how treatments work. Physicians may also access lay medical information by clicking on brief news summaries from such sources as CNN and *The New York Times,* as well as finding tips on wines, travel, and other topics of general interest.

Other Electronic Resources

Standard lecture courses abound on the Internet. Many medical schools are putting lectures and panel discussions online from live CME courses, with speaker and slides, as in traditional CME programs. Each year **World Medical Leaders** (http://www.wml.com) broadcast at least 250 hours of original lectures by highly distinguished medical educators. Detailed information is provided for all drugs mentioned in any lecture, and samples may be ordered directly through the Internet. Other special features include discussion boards that allow physicians to interact with their colleagues regarding lectures or topics of interest, physician-to-physician-only e-mail service for communication with colleagues around the world, and consultation boards to permit physicians to pose difficult diagnostic dilemmas to the medical community.

The ***Encyclopaedia Britannica*** (http://www.britannica.com) offers free general information on medicine, disease, human anatomy, and physiology at its Web site. The comprehensive information will be updated regularly and is written primarily for the lay public. This service will not recommend particular treatments or cures, but should prove useful to physicians by helping patients understand basic information about their diseases and helping build an information partnership among physicians and patients.

Several electronic editions of ***The Merck Manual*** are available for purchase, but the 17th edition (1999) is available free online (http://www.merck.com/pubs/mmanual/). *The Merck Manual of Geriatrics* and part of *The Merck Manual of Medical Information—Home Edition* are also available on the Web site.

Again, the electronic services described are mentioned as examples of what is available. Name changes occur often with mergers, and some services go out of business. Since, therefore, our examples may have changed names or addresses, or may not exist when the reader is ready to investigate them, we recommend that physicians consult a librarian at a medical school or academic hospital to determine what is available. Nevertheless, we are certain that electronic resources will expand and become more valuable each year.

Finding Significant Web Sites

Edward Shortliffe suggested these Web sites and CD services: "The American College of Physicians (ACP) maintains a listing of pertinent Web sites at http://www.acponline.org/computer/ccp/bookmark/index.html?idx. They also maintain a directory of all the Observer articles on computing topics: http://www.acponline.org/journals/news/compmed.htm?idx.

"I consider the best general medical sites for searching the Web to be Cliniweb and Medical Matrix. Cliniweb (http://www.ohsu.edu

/cliniweb/), a resource from Oregon Health Sciences University, is a high quality search interface that helps clinicians find information on the Internet. Medical Matrix (http://www.medmatrix.org/index.asp) offers free registration for physicians and a comprehensive portal for medical topics."

Thomas Lincoln pointed out that many professional societies have their own Web sites and that some Web sites dedicated to particular diseases are run by their nonprofit organizations. These not only offer information for physicians but also organize electronic support groups for patients and their families.

PERSONAL DIGITAL ASSISTANTS

The handheld digital personal assistant (PDA) has enabled physicians to carry large amounts of data in their pockets. According to Oscar Streeter, "The issue for most physicians in practice, at least for the foreseeable future, is not whether you are going to use a personal digital assistant, but whether you are going to use the Palm OS™ or the competing Microsoft Windows CE™ or Pocket PC™ platform. Millions of palm-based devices have been purchased since they appeared on the market in 1996."[4] Many hospitals are providing palm devices for their interns and residents. Wireless palm devices are available and in the future will dominate PDA connectivity with computer networks. They can be connected with a cellular phone or be used as a stand-alone device with a radio antenna. In the August 2000, issue of *Hippocrates* (http://www.hippocrates.com), Leo Burnett listed a compendium of free or inexpensive medical software applications for the Palm™ on the Healthy PalmPilot Web site (http://www.healthypalmpilot.com).[6]

Streeter uses his PDA to get weather reports, stock information, and driving directions using Mapquest™, and to send and receive e-mail anytime, any place. "When I pull the Palm™, out of my pocket and raise the antenna, it connects to an internal transmitter, enabling it to transmit and receive information over the airwaves. To use this feature, however, you must activate the Palm.Net™ wireless communication service, which, like an Internet connection, requires a monthly user fee. Medical software developers, following the lead of physicians, have developed hundreds of medical resources in patient tracking, procedure billing, medical references, and prescription writing for the Palm™.

"Of particular use to physicians is **ePocrates.com™** (http://www.ePocrates.com/), a free drug-database, as opposed to the PDR™ version that you must purchase. The PDR™ version is more complete, but for most of us the ePocrates listing of more than 1,500 prescription drugs is adequate. The Windows version automatically updates itself whenever the Palm™ is HotSynced with your computer. You can search by generic or trade names. **PatientKeeper™** (http://www.patientkeeper.com) is a patient-tracking software program that allows storage of the patient's history, physical examination, laboratory tests completed, and reminders. The information on each patient can be beamed between PDA infrared ports. You can sign out a patient to another physician electronically, with alerts on when to check other laboratory tests or x-rays ordered. This is a boon when you are going out of town and have inpatients or are changing services as a resident. Another patient-tracking software program that serves as a to-do list is **WardWatch™** (http://www.torlesse.com/pilot/wardwatch/). Both of these patient software programs offer a demonstration before you purchase. **Harrison's Principles of Internal Medicine: Companion Handbook™**, which contains the entire companion edition of *Harrison's Principles of Internal Medicine*, and other medical titles are available at http://handheldmed.com. Software is also available for writing accurate, legible prescriptions at the point-of-care."

For those who wish to learn the latest on handheld computers, the magazine *Pen Computing* has excellent reviews and news.

A HOSPITAL DATABASE

Lawrence Cohn described a hospital database that can help in estimating patient outcome: "Brigham has a cardiac surgical database of some

30,000 patients dating from 1972. Such databases are extremely valuable and provide a constant stimulus for faculty and trainees to write of their experience. Analysis of this information allows a better understanding of what we are doing. I may not consult a database at the time I am seeing a patient, but I will have database information at my fingertips about the general disease, procedure, and operation related to the patient. For example, many young candidates for a valve replacement want to know about the results of surgical experience with a homograft or a pulmonary autograft. The constantly updated database allows me to provide patients with numbers and risk/reward ratios, which, in turn, allow the patients to reach an informed decision."

REMINDER SYSTEMS

Many problems that arise in medical care are due not to a lack of medical knowledge but to oversight. The computerized medical record will deliver reminders to physicians while they are seeing patients.

In 1972, Clement McDonald and his collaborators began to construct an electronic medical record system, the Regenstrief Medical Records System (RMRS), which has grown in coverage and scope over the intervening years. At Wishard Hospital, the RMRS now carries coded and computer-readable information about all diagnoses, patient encounters, orders (including prescriptions), and diagnostic studies, as well as all narrative dictations, electrocardiograms, and radiographic images. Some venues, for example, obstetrics, dermatology, and medicine, contain much more clinical detail.[6] The RMRS also includes laboratory and other patient information from four other major Indianapolis hospital systems.[7] The goals of this medical record system have been: (1) to solve the availability and legibility problems of the paper medical record, (2) to facilitate clinical research, for example, the identification of candidate patients for clinical trials and retrieval of patient data for epidemiologic research, and (3) to provide automated guidance to healthcare.

The physician is faced with torrential information flows, random interruptions, and high pressure. Such circumstances are setups for errors due to oversights and omissions.[8] In Samuel Johnson's apt words: "[M]en more frequently require to be reminded than informed,[9]" that is, most errors are due to oversights rather than ignorance. If the computer could check for, and remind the physician about, patient conditions that need attention without requiring the physician to initiate the checking process or (with rare exceptions) feed data into it, the computer could improve patient care. The computer would have to depend on its own content (the electronic medical record) for data needed to generate these reminders.

The computer uses rules to relate patient states to required clinical actions such as treatments or tests. The Regenstrief policy is to implement only rules that are well supported by published scientific evidence and can be sharply defined by computer-stored clinical data. For example, the rule about screening mammograms depends on only three variables: the patient's age (>50), gender (F), and date of previous mammogram (>1 year ago). The rule about the use of angiotensin converting enzyme (ACE) inhibitors depends on echo evidence of left ventricular ejection fraction <40 percent, a normal creatinine clearance, and confirmation that the patient is not yet taking an ACE inhibitor. The computer must have rules with carefully defined criteria if it is to avoid vague and repetitive reminders.

In the 1970s and 1980s, the RMRS rules were delivered to physicians as paper reports. The computer reviewed the patient's electronic medical record for conditions that needed reminders according to pre-defined reminder rules and produced a paper reminder report. The clinic staff delivered the report to the physician by placing it on top of the patient's chart. This method of delivering reminders had powerful positive effects on care, especially preventive care.[10,11]

The paper method continues to be used, but another mechanism has been added that delivers reminders to physicians as they write orders in the hospital, emergency room, and clinics. These reminders are based on a new language called G-care.[12] G-care reminders can deliver simple text reminders or more sophisticated messages that contain preformed orders. The rules can also be used to disagree with certain kinds of physician-written orders before they are completed. Indeed, the computer can suggest an alternative that the ordering physician can accept with one or two keystrokes. Order-related G-care reminders have also had positive effects on patient care.[13] G-care reminders are used for research purposes; for example, physicians can be reminded that a patient with "back pain" might be a candidate for an ongoing clinical trial. If the physician responds online that the patient is an appropriate candidate, the computer will send "e-mail" to the digital pager of the study manager, who can invite the patient to join the study while the patient is still in the clinic.

Physicians receive more than one reminder a day for each hospitalized patient, and an average of two for each outpatient visit. Physicians are free to accept or ignore reminders, as the computer never knows as much about the patient as the physician does. The physician is always the final arbiter.

INFORMATION AT THE POINT-OF-CARE

A long-time dream of physicians has been to ask a specific question and receive a valid and pertinent answer quickly while seeing a patient. Several systems approach this goal.

Systems That Provide Information at the Point-of-Care

MDConsult offers a selection of current textbooks online, a few clicks bringing specific information on a desired topic. Easily accessed are full-text articles from more than 50 clinical journals, as well as MEDLINE. A click or two will access clinical guidelines, information on specific drugs, and written material suitable for patient education. Daily reports of medical news appear with hyperlinks to related current journal articles, along with drug updates and brief discussions of clinical topics.

SKOLAR, M.D. is an integrated information system for learning and decision-making that includes electronic textbooks, drug data, bibliographic information, guidelines, consensus statements, and primary-care teaching modules. Some physicians use the system in the presence of patients. In 1999, in its underdeveloped form, the program could answer, within four minutes, about 80 percent of questions related to patient management that were generated by primary-care physicians. With further development, the percentage of questions answered is increasing.

Scientific American Medicine (SAM), which began as a replaceable text in three-ring binders, is now available on the Internet through WebMD, making it a widely available and frequently updated medical text.

UpToDate is a compact disk product often used for point-of-care information (see page 101).

UPCMD (http://www.upcmd.com), a system developed by the University Pathology Consortium to aid in laboratory diagnosis, is described by Clive Taylor: "This interactive Internet service deals specifically with selection, interpretation, and follow-up of diagnostic and laboratory tests. The Disease Diagnosis section of the site currently contains about 15,000 pages of information designed to assist physicians in selection of diagnostic tests for a wide variety of diseases.

"A physician or other healthcare provider logging onto UPCMD will be able to type in the name of the disease under consideration and within seconds will have a full description of the clinical characteristics of the disease, together with detailed information about test-ordering procedures to explore further the diagnosis. There are also hyperlinks to recent journal articles. In this way, physicians will be able to obtain the most up-to-date information about any disease, even an uncommon disease, encountered in daily practice without leaving their office desk or their handheld wireless PC."

Problem Knowledge Couplers

> A pervasive design flaw in advanced health care systems is their unnecessary dependence on fallible, idiosyncratic inputs from clinical workers. . . . Medical decisions are still based largely on the recall and processing of complex information by highly trained physicians. Yet, their cognitive inputs fall short of what medicine requires, too often producing decisions that are deficient in quality and resistant to organized improvement.
>
> LAWRENCE AND LINCOLN WEED[14]

Lawrence Weed believes that the information retrieval, recall, and synthesis of facts necessary to determine the best care for patients is beyond the unaided mind, even with the help of existing clinical guidelines and computers that deliver knowledge on request. To help solve this problem, he has developed Problem Knowledge Couplers, a computer tool that retrieves and processes information by linking or matching patients' specific data with up-to-date medical knowledge. The Coupler then provides logically organized diagnoses and management options. It is difficult to disagree with Weed's philosophy, but can it work in the real world of clinical practice?

Charles Burger's practice of about 4000 active patients is organized on the Knowledge Coupler concept. The practice consists of one physician, two nurse practitioners, two medical assistants, one registered nurse, and 7.5 full-time-equivalent support staff. Before incorporating the Knowledge Couplers into his practice, Burger conducted an intensive staff-training program in total quality management. For example, medical assistants were trained to gather information from the patient and perform physical examinations. As a first step, Burger employed the triage coupler, which permits the receptionists to perform a triage of the patient's medical complaints to determine if, and how urgently, the patient should be seen by a physician or nurse practitioner, how much time should be allocated for the office visit, and whether any testing should be done before the office visit. Burger found that analyzing a patient's complaint by this method requires 3.9 minutes versus 3.0 minutes for the usual interview by the receptionist, but the results warranted the extra time.

The practice works thus: with the help of the medical assistant, if necessary, patient completes a questionnaire. The completed questionnaire, physical findings, and laboratory findings are keyed into the Coupler system. The paper questionnaire can be replaced by a handheld device that downloads responses directly into the computer. This information, including history, physical findings, and laboratory data, is matched or coupled by the computer with information from current medical publications. The Coupler then provides logically organized diagnoses and management options. Secondary options may suggest further studies to confirm a given diagnosis and comment on the sensitivity, specificity, and costs of the studies. The pros and cons for management options are presented. The clinician's judgment and patient's preferences determine the final management options. The physician or nurse practitioner will spend most of the time clarifying and annotating the history, checking physical findings, and reviewing the results with the patient.

Burger conducted a study indicating that the Coupler-centered practice is successful by measures of patient satisfaction, panel growth (his practice increased from 3554 patients in 1998 to 3991 in mid-1999), provider productivity, satisfaction, and profitability. Burger believes the quality of care has improved without any diminution in empathy or compassion with the use of Couplers. With less time devoted to memorization, he can spend more time developing communication and listening skills. He emphasizes, however, that users should not rely on Couplers or any other single source in making decisions; physicians cannot function competently without their minds actively engaged.

Potential Informatics Approaches

Other systems are being developed in research laboratories. One researcher, Robert Greenes, pointed to the complexity in creating an ideal system: "We need a framework for integrating knowledge and decision support that will provide the physician with access to specific, authoritative, problem-focused information during a patient visit. It should also accommodate the physician's personal notes and observations, as well as offer links to other relevant information that can be pursued more leisurely. Thus, the framework needs to be tailored and updated by both authoritative sources and personal notes and references.

"In seeking ways to provide specific information, we have been pursuing 'Clinical Management State' (CMS), which will address the dual tasks of (1) information access and decision support in the care of specific patients and (2) more general learning needed to stay abreast of medical advances. Each CMS may represent a subclass of patients with a particular disease or problem. Consider, for example, patients with hypertension or diabetes: patients will be in one or another CMS (new onset, workup, treatment, steady-state management, treatment of complications). Knowing a patient's CMS, the physician can predict the kinds of clinical information likely to be needed, decisions to be made, actions to be carried out, and other potentially useful resources relating to that CMS. Questions that arise in practice will be answerable by information resources already linked to the CMS or will be added to the CMS framework. Automatic search tools will use the knowledge model of the CMS, including 'eligibility criteria' for a patient being assigned to a CMS. These criteria will identify appropriate external resources and will update the available information.

"For this approach to succeed, the CMS must be defined for most key problems. We envision that the knowledge models defining a CMS would be reviewed by disease-specific editorial boards. The information will need to be categorized by disease or problem, intended audience, and quality rating, and further categorized by identification of its uses (clinical, biochemical, epidemiologic, diagnostic, therapeutic, or prognostic). The system should also specify the type of information as evidence, opinion, review, clinical guideline, risk assessment, or other decision support tools." While waiting for such a service, physicians can use the principles outlined by Greenes in conceptualizing their approach to medical information.

TOOL TO PROMOTE PRACTICE-BASED LEARNING

An educational program sponsored by the Royal College of Physicians and Surgeons of Canada (RCPSC) encourages physicians to seek information triggered by real problems arising in practice. The Maintenance of Competence Program[15] (MOCOMP) provides a paper diary and computer software (*PCDiary*®) to facilitate practice-based learning. A principle feature provides physicians an opportunity to record a question. John Parboosingh credits the system with assisting physicians in moving efficiently through the learning cycle, beginning with deciding what they need to learn, formulating a question that best describes it (see pp. 164–168), seeking assistance from peers and mentors in the selection of learning resources, and making a commitment to integrate the new learning into their practice. "At a click of the mouse, the diary user may access a searchable Internet database of questions posed by other diary users (the Question Library) and connect anonymously with a physician working on a similar question. The software keeps a record of the learning resources used to complete the task and asks physicians how they intend to use their newly acquired learning. For instance, if the user assigns as the outcome code 'I will modify my practice,' the diary requests a description of how the physician intends to do this.

"*PCDiary*® encourages physicians to focus on the purpose of the learning and to specify its potential impact on their expertise. These two features are reported to increase the likelihood of a change in behavior. Users can search and sort items by topic, stimulus, and assigned outcome. For instance, one may print a list of items for the assigned outcome code 'I will modify my practice' to ensure that necessary changes are made. The search-and-sort capabilities of *PCDiary*® provide feedback, engender ownership, and produce feelings of accomplishment, all of which are reported to motivate independent learners.

"Thus the *PCDiary®*, using the integration of computer and telecommunications technology in the design of personal learning portfolios, will produce a new generation of learning tools that will stimulate learner interaction. Using critical thinking questions, experts will communicate with peers and mentors electronically. *PCDiary®* users contribute entries (the question, the stimulus, the learning resources, and the intended outcome) anonymously by modem transfer of data to the Question Library. It is the first library to house questions rather than answers. As our medical knowledge base rapidly expands and the shelf-life of clinically applicable information falls, answers will inevitably change more often than previously, and the question will likely be the more stable component. Experts will be judged by the quality of the questions they ask and their ability to produce the most accurate and current answers."

The importance of asking circumscribed questions and seeking answers about patients cannot be overemphasized. "In clinical practice, questions always arise that require an evaluation of both the 'old' and the 'new' in published reports," said Stephen Greenberg. "When I am taking care of a puzzling patient, I try to formulate the most critical questions in the case." Of equal importance is the brief recording of results of a search to address the question. If you do not have access to a computer system like MOCOMP, you can keep a paper diary or record your experience on other software.

The Learning Diary

> Physicians [trainees] are ready to leave the fold when they ask searching questions about their patients and vigorously pursue the answers.
>
> EUGENE A. STEAD, JR.[16]

John Toews uses MOCOMP thus: "Although I graduated from medical school three decades ago, only in the past decade have I found a method of lifelong learning that suits my particular style. I enjoy shorter learning activities to solve clearly circumscribed problems, but I thrive on learning in depth. As a psychiatrist, I tend to be more of a conceptual person than one whose first impulse is to fix through action.

"MOCOMP, with its emphasis on lifelong learning, provided a fine avenue to conceptualize and organize my learning through an electronic learning diary (*PCDiary*®). MOCOMP stimulated recording of continuing professional development available to RCPSC Fellows.[17] Two major aspects were participation in group learning activities, such as conferences and rounds, and a diary for recording self-directed learning. Both paper and electronic learning diaries are key features, but it was the electronic diary that facilitated my own learning. Although I have attended my share of conferences and rounds, the *PCDiary*® encouraged me to direct my education to reflect more on my questions and convert them to learning projects. My learning diary now consists of two major types of projects, short ones that arise from immediate practice needs and long-term developmental programs.

"My first step is to frame a question based on the problem I am facing. Framing a question is more effective for me than assigning a title to what I want to learn. Why? Because questions circumscribe the focus more tightly than statements or topics. The questions I ask encourage me to reflect rather than simply describe or list. And my curiosity often keeps me working on the question long after I have adopted an immediate course of action in treating a patient.

"Questions induce a state of tension in the questioner, but the answers provide satisfaction and an enhanced sense of competence. The resulting improved treatment for the patient reinforces the sense of competence, which is a major behavioral motivator.

"Many of my questions are simple: Which antipsychotic medication is safest to use in pregnancy, and what is the evidence for this? I seek and find answers through databases or bibliographic reviews. The questions are duly recorded in my *PCDiary*®. I note the estimated time spent on the problem, the sources used, and the intention, or lack thereof, to change my practice. All this information is forwarded to the RCPSC for my MOCOMP record. I keep the best part, the second electronic page that contains my findings, observations, thoughts, and key references addressing the question, a rich source when I forget something or when I simply page through the questions, remembering fondly past learning experiences.

"When I am not as interested in retrieving specific information as in understanding a more complex process and thus augmenting my knowledge and skill, I select a particular patient as a basis for both a review of knowledge and new learning projects. Such patients become my best teachers as they spur my major learning projects. For example, I had a patient with severe Generalized Anxiety Disorder (GAD). Having had few such patients, I was not sure of the latest medications. I did a MEDLINE search of reviews for the past five years, then framed questions to guide my analysis of the search results: What advances have occurred in the pharmacologic treatment of GAD, and how do they relate to, or change, my previous knowledge? Those questions allowed me to test my previous knowledge against the new information. Since not much had changed, my initial plans for medication were in order. In the process, I also learned about drugs of second and third choice.

"My next questions were: Is there current evidence of advantages from a combination of medication and psychotherapy in GAD? If so, what is the best combination, and what skills do I need to acquire for the psychotherapy? These questions led me to review basic differential therapeutics, a rapidly growing field of psychotherapy research. As I read and attended a workshop on the selected therapy, I constantly reviewed skills, discovering parts in which I was competent and some in which I needed to learn more.

"The final question capped the learning project: What is the evidence for the benefits of combined treatment with antidepressants and cognitive behavioral therapy for GAD, and how will this help my patient? I tied together the symptoms of the patient with a biological and psychological understanding of ways in which this integrative treatment can work. All these questions were recorded and answered as separate, although related, learning projects. This study on GAD required 15 hours over two months. I used a number of sources: published reviews, colleagues, and workshops. What's more, I now have a mental hook; when I think of this patient, I remember my learning and more readily apply it to the next patient. During this project, of course, I saw other patients who presented learning opportunities. I asked initial questions to provide better treatment, but I sought the quickest solution. I recorded in the diary only the questions and solutions that required some time or advanced my knowledge.

"During our experience with MOCOMP, we taught others how to record self-directed learning projects. Many colleagues have difficulty deciding what to enter in learning diaries. Some stated that they were learning so much all the time that they had no time for the diary. A participant in a MOCOMP diary user's focus group found that this system solved this problem. Because he thought he had to know everything, he felt guilty and his learning was diffuse and anxious. With the introduction of the diary, he became more focused in his learning; he entered his projects and systematically worked on them. He saw them as evidence of his continuing learning and resisted chasing every learning impulse. Both the use of the diary and the use of questions gave direction and intention to his learning.

"One further innovation was included in the *PCDiary®:* all the questions submitted electronically became part of a Question Library, which permitted me to see what my colleagues were asking, and to become aware of the leading edge of my field. Further, hot-links were attached to each question, allowing me to be anonymous if I wished and yet have my colleagues interact with me. I received a note from a colleague about one of my question entries, and we had an e-mail exchange about it. This experience illustrated graphically the potential of technology that allows learners to further one another's education. Knowledge is only of half use if it is not shared with a colleague.

"MOCOMP became the official Maintenance of Certification Program of the RCPSC in 2000, and various learning categories are credited. To my great delight, the *PCDiary*® remains, and I continue framing questions because there is no better way for me to learn."

Stephen Sullivan discussed other ways the computer facilitates learning from your practice: "Clinical software will help by inventorying a physician's habits and developing a 'clinical interest profile.' Where does the physician spend most time when resolving a question about a specific disease? Which Web sites or reference sources are used? Which questions are asked? What disease information is sought for a specific patient or in general reading? Based on these cues, the computer will then develop, maintain, and update a personalized library for the clinician. Upon the clinician's request and from that database, the computer will automatically submit questions about material the clinician has read. Continuing medical education will no longer consist primarily of attendance at seminars and random reading, but will be a byproduct of caring for patients and self-teaching about clinical problems."

ELECTRONIC MAIL

The use of electronic mail (e-mail) in the healthcare setting has exploded and continues to expand. Some physicians are using it to communicate with colleagues, to request referrals, to render consultation reports, and to receive laboratory data and follow-up information about their patients.

With practice now increasingly regulated by cost-containment, physicians are becoming ever more pressed for time. Some say time strictures are even jeopardizing their informal consultations with medical colleagues, such as discussions in the doctors' lounge. In such a climate, can e-mail substitute for face-to-face discussions with colleagues about puzzling patients? Can the nuances of a patient's problem be described clearly enough in e-mail to elicit a useful answer? Research is sparse, but physicians will probably need to hone their written communication skills in order to frame questions that will elicit accurate and pertinent responses. E-mail interactions may prove valuable for informal discussions on simple issues of patient care, but they cannot and should not replace personal discussions on more complex issues. An asynchronous method of communicating, e-mail is well suited for some tasks but is not ideal for all.

Stephen Greenberg follows up his e-mail communications with colleagues about patient management issues with a telephone conversation if nuances of a case are difficult to transmit by e-mail. Even so, he considers e-mail more time-efficient and more productive than the telephone or postal mail. Greenberg believes that both written (computer) and oral communication skills will become even more critical for the practicing physician in the future, as teaching and mentoring functions of physicians will be central activities in the 21st century.

A Netherlands study showed that postal mail of admission-discharge reports to general practitioners required a median of two days at one hospital and four days at another. E-mail and electronic data exchange, however, allowed such delivery usually within one hour of being generated. In one hospital, 32 percent of all laboratory reports, and in another 52 percent, were available electronically on the day the samples were collected. Twenty of 27 physicians rated e-mail usefulness as a 4 or 5 (0 = useless, 5 = very useful).[18]

The use of e-mail to communicate with patients is evolving more slowly. (See also pp. 329–331) After an extensive review of publications, Moyer and coauthors[19] concluded that patients between the ages of 20 and 50 years, who represent most subscribers to managed-care organizations, are more likely than older patients to use e-mail to communicate with their physicians. Although the telephone is still their primary means of such communication, they also consider e-mail satisfactory for certain communications, and believe that it increases speed, convenience, and access to medical care. In most cases, a nurse will triage the messages. The medical center staff sees e-mail as competitive with other forms of communication in response rates, value, cost-effectiveness, and communication style, and does not consider reading and responding to patient e-mail to be overly time-consuming. Furthermore, e-mail is ideal for nonurgent problems, such as routine prescription refills, certain laboratory results, and making appointments, and it is well suited to patient follow-up, staff education and training, and patient-care assignments. E-mail prevents interruptions by telephone calls, limits "telephone tag" or long waits on "hold," and thus saves time for physicians, patients, and nurses.

Using e-mail to communicate with patients, however, can get out of hand, and the physician can spend a great deal of uncompensated time answering questions in this way. Methods must be determined to compensate for costs and office staff time required for e-mail. According to Thomas Lincoln, since Frequently Asked Questions (FAQs) comprise almost 90 percent of patients' questions, the physician's investment of time could be reduced by use of a Web site with advice categories or by a list of standard e-mail responses that may be modified to suit specific circumstances.

Other concerns about e-mail communication with patients are the inability to ensure confidentiality, potential medicolegal issues, and the difficulty of authenticating identity (possible impersonation of a patient). These issues are being addressed and should eventually be resolved. Physicians should, of course, not use e-mail to discuss complex issues or to convey negative reports to patients. Face-to-face communication is not only desirable, but is an essential ingredient of the physician–patient relationship.

PRACTICING SKILLS BY SIMULATION

Not only is technology providing information and advancing the study of practice, but it is expanding the use of simulators that permit physicians to learn procedures and other clinical skills. Michael Fordis offered the following observations.

"Information technologies offer opportunities to learn and practice skills in simulated and interactive environments. Future learning and training centers may have simulators and virtual reality stations for such training. The office or home may also have learning sites over the Web, particularly as the bandwidth (or movement of information) increases. Additionally, some such technologies will provide notifications, information, and education at the point of care to enhance learning and patient services.

"Simulation technology for CME can range from interactive case presentations offered on computer networks, CD-ROMs, or the Web to highly sophisticated training with the learner on-site, working with mannequins, haptic devices, and virtual reality.[20–23] Issenberg and colleagues pointed to these advantages of high-fidelity simulations of human conditions: 'Unlike patients, simulators do not become embarrassed or stressed; have predictable behavior; are available at any time to fit curriculum needs; can be programmed to simulate selected findings, conditions, situations, and complications; allow standardized experiences for all trainees; can be used repeatedly with fidelity and reproducibility; and can be used to train both for procedures and difficult management situations.'[24]

"Educators are increasingly applying simulation technology in various medical disciplines, including laparoscopic surgery, anesthesia, cardiology, and emergency medicine, sometimes in continuing medical education.[24] Consider, for example, a sophisticated simulator for endoscopic sinus surgery (ESS) in a virtual reality environment. Because ESS can involve risk to the patient, an effective training tool without patients would be attractive. Furthermore, the relevant anatomic structures lend themselves to a virtual environment. The structures are firm and do not easily become deformed, as soft tissue organs do with contact and pressure. Moreover, imaging datasets are available for creating the virtual environment.

"The ESS simulator uses the head of a mannequin into whose nose surgical instruments can be inserted. The haptic or force-feedback display simulates the resistance that the surgeon experiences in manipulating instruments, such as the endoscope, or in injecting substances into the tissues. The three-dimensional model of human nasal sinus anatomy, developed from the Visible Human Database at the National Library of Medicine,[25] is rendered in real time at

15 to 30 frames per second. The displays are compelling. In addition to the endoscope, the student can use various instruments, including scalpel, injection needle, and forceps. Visualization through the endoscope deteriorates as blood and secretions cloud the tip, requiring the trainee to remove and clean the instrument. When impaling the tissue with the injection needle, the trainee feels the resistance, and the tissue blanches as the injection is made. With inattention to hemostasis, inexperienced surgeons can find their operating field quickly obscured by blood. Different training levels are engineered into the simulator, providing instructional aids to enable the novice and intermediate trainee to accomplish navigation, injection, and dissection. No aids are provided at the advanced level.[26]

"In a formal evaluation of the ESS simulator, non-physicians, non-otolaryngologist physicians, and otolaryngologists with varying levels of experience (second-year residents to senior staff) performed 'clinical' procedures. Participants were evaluated with scoring algorithms based on time, completeness, and accuracy. Performance on the ESS simulator correlated strongly with the degree of prior ESS experience consistent with procedural validity of the simulation model, findings that were supported by subjective evaluations conducted with experienced ESS surgeons.[26,27]

"Whole-body simulators with mannequins have been developed for training in anesthesia and are also being used in continuing education for practitioners; in the training of residents and students in surgery, radiology, obstetrics, and emergency medicine; and in the training of critical care nurses and respiratory technicians.[24,28] The simulation of the cardiovascular and respiratory systems of human subjects allows evaluation of fluid status, acid-base status, pharmacodynamic responses, and temperature.[28]

"Examples of available whole-body simulators include the Eagle Patient Simulator from MEDSIM[29] and the METI simulator from Medical Education Technologies.[30] MEDSIM's vision is 'To create a virtual patient for every medical procedure.'[29] As early as 1999, systems had been developed to simulate problems and treatment in gynecology, obstetrics, vascular disease, cardiology, surgery, and anesthesiology. The METI allows simulation of more than 50 clinical scenarios. The user interacts with a mannequin in which the eyelids open and close; the pupils dilate or constrict in response to light or drugs; the pharynx and tongue can swell; the thumb twitches (the twitches disappear with paralysis); limbs swell to mimic trauma; and urine output can be monitored, as can a variety of pulses and heart and breath sounds. Monitoring also includes electrocardiography, blood pressure, oximetry, Swan–Ganz pressure, central venous pressure, capnography, and inspired and expired concentration of gases. Modeling simulates the injection of drugs, precipitating the appropriate physiologic response for a particular clinical situation. The mannequins can be manipulated and instrumented for intubation, placement of cannulas, cricothyrotomy, chest-tube placement, pericardicentesis, needle decompression for a tension pneumothorax, and defibrillation.[28]

"Whole-body simulators lend themselves most easily to teaching in small groups where participants acclimate to the simulation. Developers of the METI simulator, however, have demonstrated that, with the proper set-up, a large number of persons can participate in such CME during a scientific meeting.[31]

"If the experience of the airline industry and the military is any guide, deployment of whole-body simulators might well expand throughout healthcare training institutions. Some evidence of this already exists.[24,32] Beyond training, whole-body simulators are being considered for assessment and certification of clinical competence. Such considerations invite additional research regarding not only their efficacy in training, but also their validity and predictive power in assessment of performance."[32]

The American Board of Family Practice is revolutionizing physician recertification procedures by developing an online, patient-centered, problem-solving test. A patient simulator provides patient-care scenarios that include multiple questions about the case, employing a branching technique that requires physicians to make clinical decisions at certain points. The patient simulator is designed to ensure that no two cases are identical, removing the possibility that a physician taking a test can use another physician's simulated patients to avoid thinking through a problem himself. An advantage of this program is its focus on clinical decision-making. Instead of taking a single examination every seven years for recertification, the physician can be recertified in steps by completing one or two cases every week or so from the office or home. The program thus serves a dual function as an educational tool, as well as a recertification tool. The test is open-book so that as a physician identifies deficiencies, he may look up appropriate material. Ultimately, the system will provide access to pertinent references and offer educational feedback to the physicians.

SUMMARY

Constant improvement in electronic information is notably changing the way physicians learn and practice. Physicians may communicate with colleagues and patients by e-mail, and they may take courses online. Each morning, their computers may greet them with a summary of breaking medical developments. They may click onto a service that provides a list of published titles suited to their practice, and, with another click, they may be hyperlinked to an abstract or a full-text article. They may also review summaries of major conferences.

Already available are systems that produce prompt, pertinent information at the point-of-care. More rapid, user-friendly, and authoritative sources at the point-of-care are being developed. The recording of specific questions about problems arising in practice is fostering self-directed, practice-related education, and the storage of brief notes on lessons learned on puzzling patients will further enhance learning from experience.

Patients are visiting their physicians with sheets of information from the Internet, valid and invalid, and physicians must acquire special skills to interpret such data. With such easy access to information, memory of detailed facts becomes less important, and the accession and interpretation of pertinent authoritative information becomes paramount.

Since many problems in medical care are due to oversights rather than a lack of knowledge, reminders built into a computerized medical record help physicians avoid errors of omission or memory while they are seeing a patient. The concept of the Knowledge Coupler, which matches information about a specific patient with information in medical publications, is an effort to help physicians retrieve and process information rather than require them to request or process it unaided. The startling scientific advances produced by medical research, coupled with the amazing developments in information technology, make this a challenging and exciting time to practice medicine.

REFERENCES

1. Bacon F. *Meditationes Sacrae. De Haeresibus.* 1597.
2. Kipling R. *From Sea to Sea: Letters of Travel.* New York: Scribners; 1899; letter 37.
3. Katzman MJ, Sullivan SJ. Consumer health informatics: "not your father's electronic medical record." *CPRI-Mail.* 1999;8:9–10.
4. Zucker DF, Barnett S. Enterprise technology for the palm computing platform. *Pen Computing Mag.* 2000; 7:16–30.
5. Burnett L. Pocket computers. Versatile handheld computers are becoming key tools for doctors. *Hippocrates.* 2000;14:18–20.
6. McDonald CJ, Overhage JM, Tierney WM, et al. The Regenstrief Medical Record System: a quarter century experience. *Int J Med Inf.* 1999;54:225–253.
7. Overhage JM, Tierney WM, McDonald CJ. Design and implementation of the Indianapolis Network for Patient Care and Research. *Bull Med Libr Assoc.* 1995;83:48–56.

8. McDonald CJ. Protocol-based computer reminders, the quality of care and the nonperfectability of man. *N Engl J Med.* 1976;295:1351–1355.

9. Johnson S. *The Rambler.* London: Thomas Tegg; Dublin: R. M. Tims;1826:11.

10. McDonald CJ, Hui SL, Smith DM, Tierney WM, Cohen SJ, Weinberger M. Reminders to physicians from an introspective computer medical record. *Ann Intern Med.* 1984;100:130–138.

11. Tierney WM, Miller ME, Hui SL, McDonald CJ. Practice randomization and clinical research. The Indiana experience. *Med Care.* 1991;29:JS57–JS64.

12. Overage JM, Mamlin B, Warvel J, Warvel J, Tierney WM, McDonald CJ. A tool for provider interaction during patient care: G-CARE. In: Gardner RM, ed. *Proceedings of the 19th Annual Symposium on Computer Applications in Medical Care, Oct 28–Nov 1, 1995, New Orleans, LA.* Philadelphia: Hanley & Belfus; 1995 (*JAMIA* Suppl.) 78–182.

13. Overhage TM, Tierney WM, Zhou XH, McDonald CJ. A randomized trial of "corollary orders" to prevent errors of omission. *JAMIA.* 1997;4:364–375.

14. Weed LL, Weed L. Opening the black box of clinical judgment. Part I: A micro perspective on medical decision making. *eBMJ.* 1999 Nov. 13. Available at: http://www.bmj.com/cgi/content/full/319/7220/1279/ DC2/1.

15. Parboosingh JT, Gondocz ST. The Maintenance of Competence Program of the Royal College of Physicians and Surgeons of Canada. *JAMA.* 1993;270:1093.

16. Stead EA Jr. *A Way of Thinking. A Primer on the Art of Being a Doctor.* Haynes BF, ed. Durham, NC: Carolina Academic Press; 1995:1.

17. Parboosingh J. Learning portfolios: potential to assist health professionals with self-directed learning. *J Contin Educ Health Prof.* 1996;16:75–81.

18. Branger PJ, van der Wouden JC, Schudel BR, et al. Electronic communication between providers of primary and secondary care. *BMJ.* 1992;305:1068–1070.

19. Moyer CA, Stern DT, Katz SJ, Fendrick AM. "We got mail": electronic communication between physicians and patients. *Am J Manag Care.* 1999;5:1513–1522.

20. Friedman CP. Anatomy of the clinical simulation. *Acad Med.* 1995;70:205–209.

21. Waugh RA, Mayer JW, Ewy GA, et al. Multimedia computer-assisted instruction in cardiology. *Arch Intern Med.* 1995;155:197–203.

22. Elliott S, Gordon JA. Integration of self-directed computerized patient simulations into the internal medicine ambulatory clerkship. *Acad Med.* 1998;73:611.

23. Human Interface Technology Lab. Surgery simulator evaluations underway. Available at: http://www.hitl.washington.edu/projects/sinus/. Accessed 1999 Oct. 22.

24. Issenberg SB, McGaghie WC, Hart IR, et al. Simulation technology for health care professional skills training and assessment. *JAMA.* 1999;282:861–866.

25. National Library of Medicine. The Visible Human Project. Available at: http://www.nlm.nih.gov/research/visible/visible_human.html. Accessed 1999 Oct. 22.

26. Weghorst S, Airola C, Oppenheimer P, et al. Validation of the Madigan ESS Simulator. In: Westwood JD, Hoffman HM, Stredney D, Weghorst S, eds. *Medicine Meets Virtual Reality. Art, Science, Technology: Healthcare (R)Evolution*™, Proceedings of Medicine Meets Virtual Reality 6, San Diego, CA, 1998 Jan. 28–31. Amsterdam: IOS Press & Ohmsha; 1998:399–405.

27. Weghorst S, Airola C, Oppenheimer P. *Formal Evaluation of the Madigan Endoscopic Sinus Surgery Simulator* (September R-97–34). Seattle: University of Washington, Human Interface Technology Laboratory, 1997.

28. Forrest F, Taylor M. High level simulators in medical education. *Hosp Med.* 1998;59:653–655.

29. MEDSIM. Eagle Patient Simulator Description. Available at:http://www.eaglesim.com/products/patsim/description.html. Accessed 1999 Oct 12.

30. Medical Education Technologies, Inc. METI. Available at: http://www.meti.com. Accessed 1999 Oct. 12.

31. Lampotang S, Good ML, Westhorpe R, Hardcastle J, Carovano RG. Logistics of conducting a large number of individual sessions with a full-scale patient simulator at a scientific meeting. *J Clin Monit Comput.* 1997;13:399–407.

32. Kapur PA, Steadman RH. Patient simulator competency testing: ready for takeoff? *Anaesth Analg.* 1998; 86: 1157–1159.

REFLECTIONS

• • •

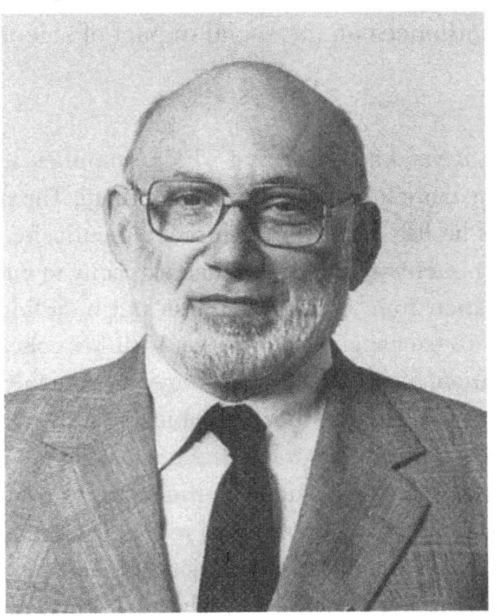

When I approach a problem, I usually immerse myself in it.

JOSHUA LEDERBERG, PH.D.

Dr. Joshua Lederberg received the Nobel Prize in Physiology or Medicine for his work on genetic material in bacteria. His discovery of the mechanism of genetic recombination in bacteria and his career-long work in bacterial genetics provided a principal foundation for contemporary research and biotechnology on gene manipulation in bacteria. Conducting research in artificial intelligence in the 1970s with E. A. Feigenbaum, he spawned one of the first expert systems (DENDRAL), a prototype for practical applications of artificial intelligence. With G. Nossal, he contributed to the conceptual development of monoclonal antibodies by showing that individual immune cells produce single types of antibodies. Dr.

Lederberg played an active role in the National Aeronautics and Space Administration *Mariner* and *Viking* missions to Mars. His interest in improving communications among scientists, the general public, and government policymakers has led him to write extensively for lay audiences on the social impact of scientific progress.

* * * * *

> I have never known anyone who exemplifies lifelong learning more fully than Joshua Lederberg. Throughout his life he has displayed an insatiable curiosity, wide-ranging interests, an extraordinary capacity to integrate information from diverse sources, and unfailing generosity in exchanging information with his colleagues. In addition, he is extremely well organized, highly energetic, and capable of making optimal use of computer technology. One of his trademarks is to send notes with information and ideas highly pertinent to our own interest based on his monitoring of research publications. He is always helpful to his students, friends, and colleagues. Joshua Lederberg is always keenly aware of moving frontiers and is constantly searching for ways to improve the constructive uses of existing knowledge.
>
> DAVID A. HAMBURG, M.D.

The Rapid Changes in Medical Technology

Joshua Lederberg, Ph.D.
Former President and Sackler Foundation Scholar
The Rockefeller University
New York, New York

As the director of a laboratory in molecular genetics and a consultant on infectious diseases for the government, foundations, the National Academy of Sciences, and the biotechnology industry, I have somewhat focused informational needs. All these responsibilities require currency in mechanisms of pathogenesis, innovative approaches to diagnosis and treatment, drug discovery, and interfaces of scientific advance with public policy. The changing informational needs of my various roles have been outpaced by the rapid changes in communication technology. I have been involved with that technology for the past 40 years,[1,2] but in the past decade it has leaped from the academic Arpanet to the now-universal Internet.

We are still in the early stages of that transformation and can but dimly guess its ultimate form. Moore's law,[3] that computer capability will grow at about 60 percent per year, shows no signs of slackening. For example, today's laptop computer far exceeds the mainframe "supercomputer" that powered the entire Stanford University campus 40 years ago. And there is every reason to expect a comparable expansion for the next generation. The entire literary content of the world's libraries can now be stored in an affordable electronic database and can be transported and searched globally within the attention span of human users. It may be some time before the corpus of our technical data and cultural documents is actually converted to electronic bytes; that process would be about as cumbersome as scanning documents through a photocopier. Moreover, many of those documents are on crumbling acidified paper that will demand special preventive measures against disintegration.

Electronic preservation carries certain hazards, the byproduct of rapid technological change. The bytes are not particularly volatile, although perils exist at that level, the more so because of malicious hackers planting computer viruses. More parlous is the rapidly obsolescent hardware for electronic storage. Although everyone was anxious about the Y2K crisis in 1999, few have considered the future problem of reading the 5-inch floppy disks that were the standard a decade ago or the stacks of IBM magtapes that were once the status symbols of electronic sophistication. These concerns, and the question of who will pay for assured sustainability, affect most medical users only indirectly. They become urgent when you are collecting statistics from patient records of a certain vintage, which, if you are fortunate, were protected from deterioration and maintained in a format you can still access.

Of even broader immediate import are the changes in how knowledge is being processed. Starting in the laboratory, bioinformatics plays an indispensable role in the initial generation and processing of laboratory data, most dramatically in the burgeoning of genomics. Every day, new evidence emerges of the association of disease susceptibility with inherited DNA sequences and of the recognition of biodiversification of pathogens like human immunodeficiency virus and *Escherichia coli* O:157. Authors and readers are impatient if they must wait months for new findings to appear in print journals, with further delays in access to index sources. This problem is somewhat mitigated now that MEDLINE appears on the Web only a few weeks after print publications appear. More and more journals are offering near-simultaneous access to their print and Web versions. Print publishers have a natural conservatism toward these alternatives because they jeopardize cost recovery and sometimes substantial profit. The initiative from the National Library of Medicine to make its PubMed Central, PMC (http://www.pubmedcentral.nih.gov/), available as a canonical site to receive Web-based primary papers, opens a new chapter in this challenge. As Chairman of the National Advisory Committee to PMC, I am in the crossfire of publishers' and professional societies' demands to protect their financial stability through copyright monopoly and the scientists' demands for prompt and unencumbered access to any new scientific knowledge.

There are also contentious disputes about the essentiality of peer review, although it is mainly high-energy physicists who consider such a filter dispensable; most biomedical scientists demand such assurance before they expend time and energy reading. The open question is the extent to which immediate access will compromise quality and reliability. We will inevitably see many races for priority—authors rushing onto the Web at the first hint of positive data, hoping that any false starts will be forgotten. Readers will adapt; since they can scan only a tiny fraction of the overall publications, they will rely ever more on their agents—reviewers, interpreters, critical experts—who, themselves, may bear watching. All in all, however, the most important aspect of peer review is critical discourse after publication, which should be enhanced by the Web. Such discussions may be expected to flow from postings on personal Web pages, like http://profiles.nlm.nih.gov/BB. A hazard here is the author's ability to erase yesterday's allegations, confusing everyone and making authorial responsibility a requisite for a reliable archive.

If primary professional publication is just making its way onto the Web, it has been preceded by a tide of didactic material, course outlines, bibliographies, news items, and review material, much of it from reputable academic sources. One of the best of these is the *Encyclopaedia Britannica* (http://www.britannica.com), which does not blink at providing pointers to innumerable Web sites and thus expanding its utility as a first stopping place. Similar resources are being developed in support of clinicians, for example, http://www.Medscape.com and http://www.pdr.com, both of which provide ancillary connections. Professional societies in general medicine (http://www.ama-assn.org), as well as specialties (http://www.geron.org), provide invaluable services with links to many other sites. Users should evaluate these critically, including the reputation of the sponsors. These sites are easily found with the search button on the standard browsers, and journals occasionally publish such lists.

The torrent of commercial peddling (gingko, hypericum, DHEA), is turning more and more patients toward alternative medicine, although verifiable evidence of efficacy remains lacking. An urgent task for the profession is therefore to provide reliable quality control on behalf of the public. To deal with their patients' information and misinformation, primary physicians and specialists will need to familiarize themselves with this cyber-information, encourage critical discourse, and exercise judgment regarding reliability, just as medical societies have done for the flow of print. The volume grows inexorably, but we have powerful tools to separate the valid from the worthless, and it is our responsibility to apply them.

REFERENCES:

1. Lederberg J. Digital communications and the conduct of science: the new literacy. *Proc IEEE.* 1978;66:1314–1319.

2. Lederberg J. Options for the future. *D-Lib Mag.* May 1996. Available at: http://www.dlib.org/delib/may96/05lederberg.html. Accessed 2001 Jul 30.

3. Moore GE. Cramming more components onto integrated circuits. *Electronics.* 1965;38:114–117.

REFLECTIONS

• • •

Dr. George Lundberg received his M.D. degree from the Medical College of Ohio and completed his residency in pathology in San Antonio, Texas. He served 11 years in the U.S. Army during the Vietnam War, after which he was Professor of Pathology and Associate Director of Laboratories at the Los Angeles County/University of Southern California Medical Center, and then Professor and Chairman of Pathology at the University of California–Davis. From 1982 to 1999, Dr. Lundberg was Editor-in-chief, Scientific Information and Multimedia at the American Medical Association. In 1999, he became Editor-in-chief of Medscape on the Internet and in 2002, Editor-in-chief Emeritus. He was founding Editor-in-chief of both *Medscape General Medicine* and CBS Health Watch.com.

Dr. Lundberg's major professional interests are toxicology, violence, communication, physician behavior, strategic management, and health system reform. He is Past President of the American Society of Clinical Pathologists. A frequent lecturer and radio and television guest, and a member of the Institute of Medicine of the National Academy of Sciences, Dr. Lundberg holds professorships at Northwestern and Harvard Universities and has received a number of honorary degrees. In 2000, the Industry Standard dubbed Dr. Lundberg "Online Health Care's Medicine Man."

Computers, the Internet, and Continuing Medical Education

George D. Lundberg, M.D.
Editor-in-Chief Emeritus, Medscape, Inc.
New York, New York
Special Healthcare Advisor
WebMD
Elmwood Park, New Jersey

In 1966, the U.S. Army sent me to the IBM Education Center in Poughkeepsie, New York, for a full-week course called Computing for Physicians. It changed my life. One of my teachers was Donald A. B. Lindberg, M.D., then an Assistant Professor of Pathology at the University of Missouri. We became colleagues and lifelong friends. (Later, when I became Editor of *The Journal of the American Medical Association* [*JAMA*] in 1982, Don became Director of the National Library of Medicine.) In 1968, I began the Laboratory Automation Project at the Los Angeles County–University of Southern California Medical Center, later extended to the entire nine-hospital system of Los Angeles County.

Throughout many of these years, I chaired the Computer Committee of the College of American Pathologists. We held continuing medical education (CME) workshops all over the country, teaching pathologists how to automate the data-processing aspects of their laboratories and, more important, how to organize the systems flow of the operations efficiently, whether or not they installed actual computer equipment.

Today, we speak of electronic medical journalism; some of us even earn our living practicing it. But it is important to remember that the first fully electronic scientific journal was operational at the Massachusetts Institute of Technology in 1967. Sometimes it takes a long time for technology to transfer. In the mid-1980s, the American Medical Association (AMA) contracted with Mead Data Central in Dayton, Ohio, to put all the AMA journals onto its computer system—random access, full-text articles (except for charts, graphs, tables, and color)—as a product called MEDIS, intended to complement the existing and successful products LEXIS and NEXUS. This was highly successful technically, but it failed utterly, as did its competitor, to create a sustaining market. Then around 1990 came CD-ROM, and I thought it was terrific, providing quick, cheap, compact, voluminous, interactive, fully searchable information. We at the AMA put all our best material onto CD-ROM. It was a technical tour de force, but a marketing disaster—already a transitional technology whose time has gone.

The Internet has changed everything in the delivery of information and has opened the door to all types of communication. When the World Wide Web was introduced for medical use in 1994, virtually no U.S. physicians accessed the Internet, according to my personal survey, but by 1995, 3 percent of U.S. physicians did; by 1996, 15 percent; by 1997, 30 percent; by 1998, 60 precent; and by 1999, 80 percent. Computers for physician use have finally arrived. The Internet has been described as an entirely new medium, built on many others, but likely to change all aspects of how we live, just as electricity did. And that includes CME.

We know that physicians change their practice habits over time, but that they are generally skeptical of, and resistant to, change. We know that traditional programmatic CME is popular (even required), but existing data demonstrate no resulting improvement in quality of practice or patient outcomes.[1] Why should it be any different if the CME experience is by way of the Internet? We can only speculate about this, but there is reason to believe that the Internet could become the most effective means of CME. We know that physicians follow recognized physician leaders,[2] and we can take advantage of that leadership on the Internet easily and inexpensively. In addition, the Internet can be accessed from almost anywhere there is a telephone, so physicians can conserve travel time by using the Web for CME. The Internet is interactive; participation produces active involvement, which is a predictor of behavior change. Of course, the Internet knows no geographic, political, or cultural boundaries, so we can teach globally and efficiently. And where certificates of participation or completion are desired, we can generate them instantly and inexpensively for the learner after all proper steps have been met. Now we need studies to see whether positive behavioral change, and even improved patient outcomes, can follow proper Internet CME.

REFERENCES

1. Davis D, O'Brien MA, Freemantle N, Wolf FM, Mazmanian P, Taylor-Vaisey A. Impact of formal continuing medical education: do conferences, workshops, rounds, and other traditional continuing education activities change physician behavior or health care outcomes? *JAMA.* 1999;282: 867–874.

2. Lomas J, Enkin M, Anderson GM, Hannah WJ, Vayda E, Singer J. Opinion leaders vs audit and feedback to implement practice guidelines. Delivery after caeserian section. *JAMA.* 1991;265:2002–2207.

5

The Medical Library

• • •

> The medical library of the 21st century is no longer a structure housing a collection of print books, journals, and multifarious documents, but a resource accessible electronically from distant sites and capable of providing pertinent information at the point of need.
>
> PHIL R. MANNING, M.D., AND LOIS DEBAKEY, PH.D.

"Even more dramatic changes in library services and information management are occurring and will occur in the next decade." This statement concluded the chapter on "The Institutional Medical Library" in the first edition of *Medicine: Preserving the Passion* published in 1987, and its prescience for the revolutionary changes over the past 16 years cannot be disputed. Both availability and ease of access to medical information have dramatically increased during that period, providing clinicians with new and powerful options for continuing the process of lifelong learning and expanding the important role of librarians in healthcare.

Medical librarian William Clintworth explained: "Technology has affected the operation and resources of libraries and is the driving force in transforming the current concept of the library from a centralized physical source of information to a resource for information at any time or place. Technology has made the rapid dissemination of research and clinical data possible, and users demand its accessibility at the point-of-care or where needed most." In the words of Clarence P. Alfrey, "A major event has been the essential transfer of the library into each user's office so that we can rapidly retrieve, from a multitude of sources, a wide variety of information on almost any conceivable medical problem. The Internet offers a remarkable opportunity to look at the interactions of multiple factors, one upon another, since we can so easily search using a variety of different criteria."

Several milestones in information management have contributed to the evolution of the medical library, according to Clintworth: "In the mid-1960s, the National Library of Medicine (NLM) pioneered the development of MEDLINE, one of the world's most sophisticated and comprehensive on-line bibliographic databases. No longer was it necessary for physicians to search the printed *Index Medicus* manually for relevant journal articles on topics of interest. For the following two decades, physicians relied on librarians to act as intermediaries between them and the MEDLINE database. The physician described the information needs, and the medical librarian constructed a search strategy to retrieve the relevant citations and abstracts.

"In the late 1980s and early 1990s, MEDLINE and related biomedical databases became more widely available through a variety of sources, both commercial and academic, and in different formats, including CD-ROM. It became commonplace for physicians to do their own searches by interacting directly with the database. As a result, the role of the medical librarian shifted from a search intermediary to an educator who designed classes, workshops, and tutorials to instruct physicians in retrieval techniques and in understanding the structure and complexity of the databases to be searched.

"The rapid expansion of the Internet and the development of the World Wide Web in the mid-1990s further fueled the physician's interest in online searching. As a result, dozens of search systems were developed to meet the growing need and to provide more user-friendly bibliographic searching strategies. One such effort by the National

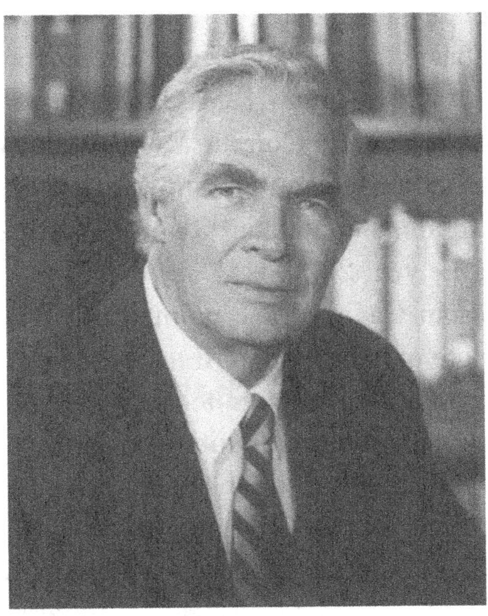

Like everyone else, physicians will need to know where to find the latest information, rather than try to store an avalanche of data in their heads. And they will have to use the computer to find the articles they really need.

DONALD A. B. LINDBERG, M.D.

Director, National Library of Medicine

Library of Medicine was Grateful Med, later developed into the Web version, Internet Grateful Med. The National Center for Biotechnology Information at NLM developed PubMed, employing a different interface and incorporating additional features. It, too, was directed primarily to the novice searcher."

In 1997, the National Library of Medicine's announcement that access to their databases through either PubMed or Internet Grateful Med would be free resulted in an explosion in the number of searches on the NLM system by health professionals, as well as patients and their families. According to National Library of Medicine Director

Donald Lindberg, physicians and librarians, who had primary access to the NLM databases before 1997, conducted about seven million searches a year. In 1998, when NLM's largest database, MEDLINE, could be accessed at no charge on the World Wide Web, the searches rose to 75 million and have continued upward. According to NLM estimates, the public alone conducted 51 million searches of the NLM databases during the year 2000.

Medical librarian David Morse pointed out that some librarians have sounded a note of caution regarding the new accessibility of information: "The availability of more tools is good news, but, like any other form of medical instrumentation, powerful professional tools must be properly used, and even physicians who are relatively confident of their searching skills would do well to consult a librarian occasionally to ensure proper usage or to enlist help designing specific search strategies. It is all too easy to get an apparently satisfying retrieval of information from a database when that may actually represent only a small percentage of the relevant information."

Recognizing the intense public interest in accessing consumer health information, librarians are focusing on the development of collections and Web sites that provide patients and their families with improved methods of accessing relevant, up-to-date information to meet their healthcare needs. Robert Beck believes that physicians may even direct patients to the medical library for help in sifting through the available information. Patients who want to research clinical topics in depth may receive guidance in distinguishing between relatively conclusive and more questionable clinical studies and in finding other patient health information resources. Patient health information, some reliable, some not, is now flooding onto the Internet, presented by specialty organizations, patient advocacy groups, the government (http://www.healthfinder.gov), and a multitude of new business entities.

In Donald Lindberg's words, "Having access to timely and critical health information is important not only to healthcare professionals and faculty, but also to patients, their families, and the public. Libraries need to create that link for all their customers." If patients are to take greater initiative in maintaining their health, access to health information is vital.

William Clintworth believes that perhaps the most significant development in the initiation of remote use of library services was the advent of digital full-text journal content: "Beginning in the mid-1990s, not only could physicians search electronically for relevant citations from medical publications, but they could also link to full-text journal articles, including accompanying tables and graphics. Users began accessing online journals at an astounding rate, and continue to do so primarily because electronic access has now become integral to the daily work of clinicians and academic physicians. This demand will only accelerate. Researchers, clinicians, faculty, and students will expect to access journal articles from any remote site. To keep pace with the demand for, and the proliferation of, information in the next decade, libraries will have to increase electronic access to additional journals. Just as libraries currently pay for and manage institutional print subscriptions, one of their key roles will be to finance and arrange access to electronic resources for their users. In most cases, access is available through the institutional Internet Protocol (IP) address of the computer being used or through authenticated user names and passwords issued and maintained by the institution."

"Even if the library of the future houses fewer print information resources," added David Morse, "the library as an organizational unit will continue to play a critical role in selecting, licensing, organizing, and publicizing resources not necessarily housed in the library. The library's critical mission will be to maximize the benefits of the institution's information resources budget." Although physicians may subscribe individually to commercial electronic resources, they may also have access to their parent institution's library through site license agreements. Licensed resources include not only electronic journals, but also databases and electronic books.

The Internet has also spawned an endless variety of medical Web sites for health professionals. Sponsorship includes professional organizations, medical societies, commercial firms, publishers, foundations, governmental agencies, and nonprofit organizations. "Although these sites focus on the specific needs of the medical community," explained Clintworth, "the content of these sites varies considerably. Many incorporate up-to-the-minute medical news and developments regarding a specific disease condition or medical specialty or simply general information about drugs, treatments, highlights from recent publications, practice management, CME opportunities, medical meetings, and links to other key sites in medicine. Many, such as Medical Matrix (http://www.medmatrix.org) or Medscape (http://www .medscape.com), have editorial boards and on-site peer review. Medical libraries maintain Web sites to publicize the electronic resources licensed for use by their clientele, to provide access to locally developed information, and to link to selected Web sites of interest to their users. They also provide training in the use of the Web and teach Web page development skills to help their institutions create such sites.

"Once again, the introduction of mobile computing within the past two years is quickly changing how physicians obtain and use information in clinical practice and teaching. Already students, residents, and physicians in hospitals and clinics are using portable personal digital assistants (PDAs) to access drug information, electronic books, and medical calculators and to record and organize clinical notes and patient data. Web sites devoted to medical applications of PDAs have proliferated, two of which are pdaMD (http://www.pdamd.com) and Handheldmed (http://www.handheldmed.com). As wireless networks become ubiquitous in the next decade, the use of information tools at the point-of-care will accelerate." Libraries will need to continue expanding the information formats to provide physicians and students with new and efficient technologic applications.

In Clintworth's view, "In addition to disseminating information more widely during the next 10 years, libraries in academic medical centers will also significantly broaden their responsibilities within their parent institutions. Information management will no longer be narrowly restricted to traditional library services, but will extend to organization and management of the plethora of research and clinical data generated within a healthcare enterprise. This invaluable institutional asset, unfortunately, is vastly underused in most complex academic medical environments. Currently, massive amounts of data are created and used through a myriad of independent systems to meet specific clinical and research needs, but because of lack of integration among these systems, data remain isolated in the unit in which they were created and are, therefore, unusable in multiple contexts. Sacrificed are opportunities for collaboration; data mining for research, patient care, and educational applications; and efficiency gained through non-redundant data collection and management. Librarians, as information specialists skilled in database use and design issues, can be effective partners in solving these problems."

Robert Beck thinks that "The rise of powerful computers, an empowered patient population, and Internet technologies are leading to the development of Web-enabled electronic medical records (EMRs) for ambulatory care. The next wave in access to health information will be the integration of electronic information resources with the electronic medical record." Morse added: "Presumably, many of the important links from the EMRs will be to databases of possible drug interactions, normal and pathologic laboratory values, diagnostic algorithms, and the like, which will then be secondarily linked to the pertinent journal articles. The computerized patient-problem list and the list of drugs the patient is taking will link automatically to relevant publications, and searching will be an option on the EMR browser."

Will print collections still be necessary given the proliferation of digital information? "Absolutely," according to Clintworth. "Digital and print formats have different characteristics, each format serving specific functions and critical needs. Digital information offers several key advantages, including rapid access and search capabilities, inherent flexibility of format options, adaptability for integration in different software applications, and instant linkage to other information sources. Digital information is an extremely useful tool, but it cannot in the foreseeable future ensure permanence. Compared to paper, digital information is highly vulnerable to physical degradation and obsolescence as a result of superseded technologies. Paper can be preserved in a usable form for hundreds of years, whereas the lifespan of magnetic data is only of 10 to 30 years. Optical storage formats have a longer physical lifespan but, as with magnetic data, are unreliable for long-term storage and usability because of no accepted standard for guaranteeing continued access. Furthermore, publishers of electronic content often only lease access to the data, such access terminating once the lease terminates. It is crucial for academic libraries not only to provide current access to materials but also to preserve the scholarly record for future users. Until libraries can be assured that digital information can meet the archival standards necessary for continuity, they will need to maintain print, as well as digital, collections."

As Morse pointed out: "Few electronic versions of journals offer backfiles of more than five years, so much clinically relevant information must still be sought in the library stacks. As libraries begin to drop their print subscriptions in favor of strictly electronic ones, archiving will become critical. Publishers may not find it economically advantageous to maintain online files for more than 10 or 15 years, and publishers have a bad habit of going out of business. It is not clear which institution(s) will bear the ultimate responsibility of ensuring the permanence of the electronic record, but academic libraries, national libraries, publishers, and scientific societies should work together closely to avoid catastrophic gaps in the scientific record."

"The next 10 years," Clintworth predicted, "will bring enormous opportunities for health sciences libraries as a result of the unprecedented new technologic tools being spawned and the rapidly changing healthcare environment in which information has a pivotal role. Even the traditional medical school curriculum is currently shifting from lecture-based formats to problem- and case-based approaches to foster analytical and lifelong learning skills. In the coming decade, this shift in emphasis will see the integration of health sciences libraries into the formal curricula for instruction of medical students in the informatics skills needed to use information resources effectively throughout their careers."

Lindberg emphasized the need for physicians to become computer literate in order to keep abreast of the latest medical information: "Like everyone else, physicians will need to know where to find the latest information, rather than try to store an avalanche of data in their heads. And they will have to use the computer to find the articles they really need."

In the words of Morse: "Librarians of the 21st century are no more defined by the physical building in which their offices are housed than physicians are defined by the hospital at which they have privileges. As the role of electronics increases, the walls of the library will gradually become transparent, but the need for information professionals to manage, navigate, and explicate the electronic library will only become more pressing as the universe of available information continues to expand."

6

The Collegial Network

• • •

> To hold him who has taught me this art as equal to my parents and to live my life in partnership with him, and if he is in need of money to give him a share of mine, and to regard his offspring as equal to my brothers in male lineage and to teach them this art—if they desire to learn it—without fee and covenant; to give a share of precepts and oral instruction and all the other learning to my sons and to the sons of him who has instructed me and to pupils who have signed the covenant and have taken an oath according to the medical law, but to no one else.
>
> HIPPOCRATES[1]

When one of us (P. M.) visited Timbuktu, Mali, the native physician, upon learning that a visiting physician was in town, went to the hotel. Although he spoke no English, the conversation, through an interpreter, immediately turned to medicine, lasted six hours, and included discussions of patients, practice, and medical education.

A major advantage of being in the medical profession is the warm spirit of fraternity among physicians the world over. After the introductions, it does not take long for two physicians who have never met to become deeply engaged in conversation about the differences and similarities in their practices. This camaraderie is often most dramatic when physicians are visiting foreign lands, but physicians in offices and hospitals have similar educational discussions daily about patients and practice.

Social interaction can promote intellectual stimulation and satisfaction from learning and can enhance memory. "The current avalanche of information threatens to overwhelm me," confessed Irvine Page. "What to do about it? I learn by associating facts with people. For example, in 1935, at a meeting of the Central Society in Chicago, I had lunch in the Cape Cod Room of the Drake Hotel with Dr. W. W. Herrick. Two things I have never forgotten: first, we had red snapper soup with a small cruet of sherry on the side—a new experience for me; second, Dr. Herrick told me that when he first described coronary thrombosis, the presentation fell like a lead balloon. The result: after nearly 50 years, I have forgotten neither red snapper soup with sherry nor Herrick and his experience in introducing a new idea."

Studies have documented the strength of the information network among physicians, which, although informal, provides mutual support for lifelong learning.[2–5] Physicians are constantly providing information to, and receiving it from, their colleagues to help resolve clinical problems. Thomas Wood believes that his greatest source of learning probably comes from interaction with his colleagues in consultations and informal discussions, as well as in a journal club. "Receiving current medical information from a trusted medical colleague," he finds, "is often as persuasive and useful as the physician's own detailed statistics on a particular subject."

The lifelong student of medicine becomes eligible to join a sophisticated information network by associating with excellent clinicians who are also excellent teachers. You must, of course, uphold your own responsibility in such relations by willingly providing accurate information and contributing your own medical experiences, as well as asking thoughtful questions and listening attentively. It does not pay to be a leech or to try to dominate the relationship. As Francis Moore pointed out, "The more you have to contribute to the education of others, the more welcome you will be in an informal network and the more mutual benefit you and the group will receive."

"As you grow older, it becomes more and more important to associate with young physicians," said Alvin Schultz. "They keep you from withering. They don't accept your answers easily; you have to document what you say. And they have a lot of new ideas." Conversely, young physicians can also profit from the rich experience of older physicians, who are usually anxious to extend a helping hand.

Although you will want to associate with the best informed physicians, you can learn from any colleague. "Even though you may have been the top student at the best medical school and the best resident at the best hospital," counseled James Moss, "every physician you meet will probably know more than you about some aspect of medicine. If you watch him and listen to him, you will discover much that you didn't learn in medical school, and you will then be able to share these new ideas with others."

LEARNING WITH COLLEAGUES

"I really don't begin to think until I am in a situation where there is an exchange of ideas, where my opinion is sought, considered, and perhaps challenged, and where some conclusion is reached," said Jack Tetirick. "The stimulation and the satisfaction of learning come only through social interaction. Maintaining skills in the practice of medicine requires the opportunity to demonstrate those skills to colleagues, with the attendant reinforcement and bolstering of the ego, and then that gentle dangling hook of the fear of losing the circle of approving peers."

Group Practice

Richard Treiman enjoys the advantage of sharing common problems that group practice affords. "It is nice," he finds, "to be able to talk over a clinical problem with an associate who is intimately interested and who will see the patient without a formal consultation or charges. When you run into difficult problems, sharing responsibility relieves the anxiety about whether you are doing the right thing. Every physician should have someone available to share his experiences with." The stimulus of association with a group helps physicians maintain their academic interests and expertise.

Wallace Chambers described the advantages of his group practice thus: "In addition to having discussions almost every hour of the day, we have occasional lunches, and we usually go to breakfast on Fridays, after which we have rounds and see all the group's patients together." Neil Elgee also values the support he receives in group practice: "With 14 of us practicing together, I have an expert on just about everything at my beck and call. I can reach for the phone and pick my colleagues' brains. It is amazing how that takes care of my needs."

Some groups schedule a specific time weekly or biweekly to discuss particular problems of patients under care, an immediately rewarding practice because the discussion is tied to existing problems. In Robert Volpe's clinic, at the end of the day, several patients are kept—provided they are willing—and their problems are discussed with the staff. "The patients have a chance to speak, and seem to appreciate this. It is one of the highlights of our practice." The late Lorin Stephens belonged to a group of eight orthopedists who closed their offices for two and a half hours Monday mornings to discuss their problem patients. When they felt they needed outside help, they called on an expert, usually a faculty member from a nearby medical school, whom they would pay an honorarium. Sadahiro Yamamoto described a practice in Japan: "Groups of private physicians in Japan organize their practice in a way that allows them to invite specialists from the larger hospitals to speak periodically at their offices."

Desmond Julian considers it crucial to go outside a close-knit group from time to time: "The little conferences among members of group practices are sometimes reinforcements for one another's ignorance. One thinks somebody is a specialist in a certain subject whereas, in fact, he may really be a subspecialist who is considered to have a degree of expertise he doesn't possess. In this kind of contact, the specialists must understand their own limitations."

Some practice groups, such as Jean Creek's, have established sabbatical policies similar to those in universities. The younger members of his group have used the sabbatical to finish subspecialty certification, whereas Creek has used it to expand his knowledge of specific diseases. He spent six months of a sabbatical in rheumatology, for example, at Hammersmith Hospital in London and the other six months in the rheumatology service at the University Center in Indianapolis. Although he does not plan to announce himself as a rheumatologist, he found the experience most helpful because there is no rheumatologist in town.

Solo Practice

Although physicians in group practice may have the edge in developing relations with colleagues, the individual practitioner also has ample opportunities to develop collegial relations through his hospital, local medical society, and even medical centers where he has trained or visited.

Academia

Physicians in academia learn by going to conferences and seeking out people who have answers to their questions. Richard Byyny, for example, can walk down the hall and find an oncologist, immunologist, or dermatologist with whom to discuss a problem. Manuel Martinez-Maldonado has established a practice in a Veterans Administration hospital that would also work in group practice and even with nonaffiliated physicians. "Every Friday afternoon I hold a session at which house staff members can present any case they want. I encourage the staff to bring me cases outside my specialty of nephrology. We develop a working list of no more than four or five possibilities according to the history and physical examination of the patient, and then rearrange the list in the most logical, time-saving, and economical way of determining the diagnosis or excluding the one we have entertained. This technique has been extremely effective because it has helped the house staff think about the tests that are essential for diagnosis."

When Lawrence Cohn has puzzling patients, he turns to standard textbooks for a quick survey, to a reprint file, and, most important, to his colleagues on the cardiac surgical service. For a truly unusual case involving something that he and his colleagues have never seen and about which little has been published, he calls a colleague in another city or country.

Curbstone Conferences

Impromptu encounters among colleagues are a useful adjunct to lifelong learning. At such "curbstone" conferences, one physician will question another about a clinical problem or about a new drug or diagnostic procedure. Curbstone consultations offer advantages for both parties. The inquiring physician often receives an answer or is directed to a pertinent reference. The consulting physician, through this opportunity to teach, is required to review personal experience and thus strengthens an understanding of the problem. In addition to practical education, the impromptu encounter provides a brief period of relaxation from the physician's busy routine.

A physician should not hesitate to ask colleagues appropriate questions, but also should not become overly dependent on others. Such dependence is not likely if we organize our thoughts carefully, study the published information on the subject, and then ask appropriate questions. Kenneth Berge recognized this problem: "I work hard at solving problems rather than ask for help prematurely; that is a particular temptation in subspecialty and superspecialty institutions. There is always someone around who knows more about a certain subject than I do. I have found that the best way for me to learn is not to call that person immediately, but to bring the problem to a little better state of resolution in my own mind first, and then ask the questions when I am really backed up to the wall. This procedure establishes whether I really do not know the answer—that after having taken the time to search for it, I have been unable to find it myself."

The Telephone

Francis Moore advocated wider use of the telephone for consultations. "One of the advantages of going to a meeting is that you hear someone talk about a difficult case of intestinal obstruction, for example, and later are able to call him and see how he would handle the patient you now have. Many of us have developed close relations with peers around the country and freely discuss our patient problems with them by telephone."

Frederick Ludwig, the sole surgeon in a rural institution with eight other physicians, calls various consultants around the country when a problem arises in the operating room. "When I am in a tough situation in the operating room, I simply pick up the phone and call a consultant. Using the telephone freely has greatly enhanced my ability to care for my patients." Don't be bashful about calling a colleague for an opinion: most are flattered by such a call. Medical school faculties are almost always willing to answer questions.

R. J. Williamson belongs to a telephone network: "In the communication system of our hospital, we all have telephone lines in our offices tied into the hospital with a three-digit number. Through my extensions in my office and at home, I can dial any extension in the hospital. I can dictate from any one of those extensions into the hospital, or I can do it by long distance."

The University of Alabama has established an excellent telephone consultation service for physicians in the state, Medical Information Service via Telephone (MIST). Using a toll-free number to dial the MIST office, the physician states his problem, which is then immediately referred to the proper faculty member for his advice. Although few medical schools have such a formal telephone consultation service, most faculty members, especially those most highly regarded, receive calls regularly from former students, residents, fellows, and other physicians. Thus, the telephone provides quick access to information and expert clinical judgment.

Correspondence

Some physicians develop teaching/learning associations through correspondence. Andrew Dale, for example, maintains a sizable correspondence. "When I read an article of special interest about which I have questions, I dictate a letter to ask the author about it or state why I disagree with him. Then he will respond with what he thinks. The exchange is always profitable." Correspondence may be especially useful for communicating with fellow physicians in other countries, and today e-mail expedites communication.

SITES OF COLLEGIAL CONVERSATIONS

The Lunch Table

Paul Beeson stated the case clearly: "I have always been impressed by the value of the lunch table, where you can sit down and discuss an interesting case. Our profession, after all, deals partly with guess work; we do not deal in absolutes. A solo practitioner is at a terrible disadvantage because he does not have other people to bounce ideas off, and so the lunch table can be a particularly valuable tool for him. Medical students learn a great deal from other students and from informal conversations and contacts. This is the knowledge that sticks; it is study in connection with a case rather than study in isolation, reading in books."

Too often, however, conversation at lunch drifts to automobiles, the stock market, and golf. With just a little effort, physicians can derive greater benefit and enjoyment through discussion of medical topics. H. Ralph Haymond finds that immediately after reviewing a topic is a good time to start conversations on the subject with your colleagues at lunch or elsewhere. "Not only will they be impressed with your knowledge, but they may fill you in on some aspects of the topic that you have overlooked. Even chance encounters can prove valuable."

The Bedside of Other Physicians' Patients

Gustavo Kuster described the cooperative spirit among the surgeons at his hospital: "Every week the general surgeons make rounds on all the patients we have in the hospital. We do not fully examine every patient unless one of our colleagues needs an opinion. Instead, we are simply overseeing what is happening within our division. An exchange of opinions ensues. If I do a certain operation, I have to justify it to my colleagues."

Ian Mackay advocates inviting specialists, like pathologists and radiologists, on hospital rounds and clinical conferences. "They make excellent contributions. Someone on the service should make sure, however, that they are well briefed on the problem to be discussed. It is unfair to throw a strange laboratory result at them and ask them why the laboratory data do not agree with the clinical impression, with the implication that something went wrong in the laboratory."

Bedside rounds with colleagues are most common in teaching hospitals, but all physicians will find the exercise an opportunity for broadening their clinical outlook.

Study and Discussion Groups

> . . . I had form'd most of my ingenious Acquaintances into a Club for mutual Improvement, which we called the Junto. We met on Friday Evening . . . . Our Debates were to be under the Direction of a President, and to be conducted in the sincere Spirit of Enquiry after Truth, without Fondness for Dispute, or Desire of Victory. . . .
>
> BENJAMIN FRANKLIN[6]

In 1911, because Winston Churchill was denied membership in a dining club originally founded by Sir Joshua Reynolds and Samuel

Johnson, he established, with Mr. F. E. Smith, a club of his own, called "The Other Club." The membership included such prominent men as Generals Kitchener and Montgomery and H. G. Wells. Churchill invited only those whom he considered both estimable and entertaining. "The Other Club" had such significance for Churchill that he insisted on attending even at the height of the Blitz in 1940 and 1941.[7] For this group, politics was the main topic of conversation, but physicians can also profit from medical discussion groups, and, as with Churchill's group, the sessions are most effective when the members are both estimable and entertaining.

Medical colleagues with similar practice problems can profit from discussing individual experiences related to a current clinical problem.

David Covell reflects: "The study group at Huntington Hospital is nearing its twenty-fifth year of 7:30 a.m. Tuesday meetings. Through all this time, from five to nine internists have met weekly to review cases. The continued pleasure we experience is due partly to sharing our individual experiences with similar cases (and noting how diagnosis and treatment of common entities have changed over the long careers of most of us), and partly to the collegiality and lack of one-upmanship the group has fostered. At present, three of the group of seven are retired. Four are in active practice, and one is a young woman in her first year of private practice who brings us a wealth of information about new procedures and devices. Surely the love of learning medicine is the glue that holds the group together.

"We decide what we would like to study, make assignments for each of us to present material, informally discuss the material, and thus learn from one another's experiences. Usually we choose patient-related self-study programs, such as the ACP–ASIM Medical Knowledge Self-Assessment Program (MKSAP) or similar material from major textbooks or medical centers, but the primary value of our group lies in the discussions generated and their relation to our own practice. It is not all serious, however; we enjoy one another's jokes and gripes. Of course, the group would not have lasted so long if we did not all get along. Combining the fun of learning something useful with the fun of a bull session has helped to keep the study group going all this time."

Kunio Okuda of Chiba, Japan, who endorses weekly study sessions to discuss puzzling patients, believes that occasionally inviting young, academically oriented physicians to join the group enhances the discussions.

John Premi and others have developed the Practice Based Small-Group (PBSG) program, which was launched in 1992 as a community-based, peer-led educational program. Groups of physicians are organized in their own communities, and one of their members is a trained educational facilitator. They meet at a time and place of their choosing to discuss PBSG-developed educational modules with or without their own clinical cases. The program has grown rapidly, with a current enrollment of 2700 physician participants organized in more than 400 groups representing all 10 Canadian provinces and both national territories. The concept of practice-based learning is also being adopted by residency programs in family medicine, with 12 to 16 residency programs in Canada participating. (Four peer-led groups and two residency programs in the United States are also involved in the PBSG program at this time.)

A typical module starts with one or more case histories designed to reflect common family-medicine practice problems, each case accompanied by questions to stimulate reflection on the key issues. The second part of the module contains a critically appraised summary of relevant medical publications, followed by an educational commentary outlining application of the published material to the clinical case, specifically addressing issues arising from the questions posed. The commentaries also identify and suggest approaches for the management of barriers to change that may arise when the proposed solutions are applied to practice. Modules are written by practicing family physicians, with support from experienced educators. Educational materials are reviewed by one or more specialists in the relevant field.

Initial evaluation of the program showed an increase in the knowledge of participants as compared to a control group.[8] In the year 2000, a randomized controlled trial involving four cohorts of PBSG groups compared the effectiveness of the PBSG process with that of personal audits on the prescribing behavior of the participants.[9] Of the four possible group interventions (PBSG module alone, PBSG module plus personal prescribing profile, personal prescribing profile alone, and control), all active interventions resulted in statistically significant changes, the combined intervention of prescribing profile and PBSG modules leading to the greatest change.

Visits to Hospital Departments of Pathology and Radiology and the Clinical Laboratory

Pathologists, radiologists, and the clinical laboratory staff are often major teachers in a community hospital. Sir John McMichael, for example, profited greatly from his visits to the pathology department. "Every day I was on duty at Hammersmith, I went to the postmortem room, and never came away without having learned something; often I was a bit humiliated." Ian Mackay confirmed these visits: "Sir John says he visited the postmortem room every day, and he *did*. He never missed. Unfortunately, at our postmortem room the presence of a consultant is a rare event."

The radiologist should be consulted personally to help with the choice of radiologic studies needed in difficult cases. Oscar Balchum stressed the value of personal communication: "I learn a great deal from the radiologist. I personally review with him the results for every patient rather than depend on written reports. Often, the radiologist may suggest pertinent articles to read." Edward Shapiro and his partners start their rounds with a visit to the radiology file room. "We go over the files with the radiologists, an experience that has shown the variation in interpretations and opinions among individuals."

"Forming a close relation with the staff of the hospital clinical laboratory, to discuss the indications and outcomes of certain laboratory studies, new tests, and unusual results, is an easy way to acquire surprisingly useful bits of knowledge," in Joseph Lydon's experience. "From my earliest days I sought out peers whose interests were somewhat different from mine. I made it a practice to 'pick them clean.' I would lunch, lounge, loiter, or take advantage of any contact. As a surgical resident, for example, I would lunch with those who were working in the forefront of hypertension. On slow evenings I would go through the x-ray teaching file with radiology residents who were studying for their Boards. I would hang around the pathology laboratory and look at any specimen that came in. I continued this practice with ophthalmologists, orthopedic surgeons, and cardiologists."

Visits to Other Medical Centers

Will and Charles Mayo made a practice of visiting medical centers in the United States and around the world to learn different surgical techniques and policies. One brother would travel while the other maintained the practice. This arrangement was highly successful for the Mayos, who soon developed a leading medical center that attracted, and welcomed, visiting physicians from all over the world.[10]

Today, many physicians, especially surgeons, visit medical centers regularly. Occasionally, Frederick Ludwig will visit a medical center with a patient he is referring. Frederick O'Dell, who practices in a small community, takes off a week or two every two years to go to Ann Arbor, to Boston, or to Houston, where he observes in the operating room, speaks with the residents, and makes rounds with surgeons. "You can get a lot of useful hints from residents and junior members of the faculty. Not only is the experience enlightening, but it also allows me to form close relationships with many people."

Gustavo Kuster also finds traveling beneficial. "I try to spend one or two weeks every couple of years in centers outside my immediate area—the Midwest or Europe. The instruments and techniques used are considerably different." Additionally, in learning a new surgical technique, he has found it useful to invite a guest surgeon to assist him when he cannot master the technique simply by reading.

A more formal visit may be desired by some physicians. "Unless a physician is in a teaching institution," explained David Sabiston, "he may continue to practice about the same kind of medicine as when he finished his residency. We have mini-residencies at Duke for graduates from outlying areas who can spend two weeks or longer making daily rounds with a particular specialist. These are much better than courses because they allow participation in actual practice, where there is give and take and not just presentations with a stiff question-and-answer period."

Some medical centers are better equipped to receive visitors than others. To avoid inconvenience and disappointment, a prospective physician should have specific goals in mind and make arrangements well in advance of the visit.

Recreational Sites

Fred Turrill likes not only to work with colleagues but to play with them as well—at golf, tennis, fishing, or hunting—and finds that such relaxation with colleagues is a pleasant way to learn. "Not only do you get to know your colleagues better, but you also learn from the medical discussions."

"Perhaps the greatest learning method of all," according to Desmond Julian, "is to be sharing a ski lift with a distinguished colleague who can pass on his expertise to you. He is trapped with you, he is probably in a very good mood, he is preparing for the onslaught of the ski slopes, and he is prepared to speak to you very honestly about what he does. One of the problems about many formal presentations is that we speak in generalities and not about specific problems we encounter or about our shortcomings. We miss physical signs. We misinterpret investigations. Until you talk to someone very frankly, as you can on a ski lift, you really don't find the truth."

LEARNING FROM OTHER HEALTH PROFESSIONALS

A mutually beneficial collegial relationship can also be developed with other members of the health team. Brian Goodell advocates having office staff involved in its own and the physician's continuing education: "If it is a small office staff, you can assign tasks for the collection of relevant information. If someone in our office has read a particularly good article, he will have it copied, distribute it to everyone else who might be interested, and then label and file it for everyone's future reference. Nurses are particularly important resources for this purpose." Desmond Julian thinks he has probably learned more about his patients and practical nursing problems from informal discussions with nurses and other health personnel at coffee and lunch than from the formal sessions.

Joseph Gonnella regrets that physicians do not take full advantage of pharmacists' knowledge: "We still visualize that profession to be the old-time druggist, but in many hospitals there is someone who knows the side effects of drugs better than the doctors, and that is the clinical pharmacist. Some of us, in fact, have graduate students in pharmacy making rounds with us. The director of our pharmacy is a good friend, and since I know he is interested in evaluation of drugs, he and I are always asking each other questions."

* * * * *

This section has highlighted informal learning methods that physicians use each day. These methods may seem self-evident and unsophisticated, but they exemplify the multitude of possibilities available to physicians to profit from the experience of others, to weave education into social and recreational events, and to organize and test thoughts on medical problems. The collegial network in medicine is real and extremely active. It is one of the dividends of being a physician and, if nurtured, will enhance not only the physician's knowledge but his enjoyment of practice.

REFERENCES

1. Edelstein L. The Hippocratic oath: text, translation and interpretation. *Bull Hist Med.* 1943;(Suppl 1):3.
2. Manning PR, Denson TA. How cardiologists learn about echocardiography. *Ann Intern Med.* 1979;91:469–471.
3. Manning PR, Denson TA. How internists learned about cimetidine. *Ann Intern Med.* 1980;92:690–692.
4. Stross JK, Harlan WR. Dissemination of relevant information on hypertension. *JAMA.* 1981;246:360–362.
5. Stross JK, Harlan WR. The dissemination of new medical information. *JAMA.* 1979;241:2622–2624.
6. Franklin B. In Farrand M, ed. *Benjamin Franklin's Memoirs.* Berkeley: Univ California Press; 1949:152.
7. Colville J. *Winston Churchill and His Inner Circle.* New York: Wyndham; 1981.
8. Premi J, Shannon S, Hartwick, et al. Practice-based small-group CME. *Acad Med.* 1994;69:800–802
9. Herbert C, Wright J, Maclure M, Dormuth C, Wakefield J, Premi J, et al. the better "prescribing" project—a randomized controlled trial of an educatkional feedback intervention to support evidence-based practice. *Family Practice Forum 2000*, Ottawa, Ont., Canada, 2000 Oct. 20.
10. Clapesattle H. *The Doctors Mayo.* Minneapolis, MN: Univ Minnesota Press; 1941.

7

Learning from Formal Consultations

• • •

When thou arte callde at anye time,
A patient to see;
And doste perceave the cure to greate,
And ponderous for thee: . . .
Gette one or two of experte men,
To helpe thee in that nede;
And make them partakers wyth thee,
In that worke to procede.

JOHN HALLE, 1565[1]

"Consultation, coupled with a brief bibliographic review on the specific subject, benefits the patient, the referring physician, and the consultant," said Paul Wehrle. "Information is always better retained when associated with specific problems." Consultations also promote interaction among colleagues—the basis for much continuing education in medicine. When a consultation is indicated, it is, of course, necessary for the physician to discuss its purpose with the patient beforehand.

REASONS FOR THE CONSULTATION

Conventionally, referring physicians request consultations because they need assistance in diagnosis or treatment or because the patient requires a special procedure, such as liver biopsy. Occasionally, it is because the patient or the family is unduly anxious or apprehensive. Determining the precise purpose of the consultation before requesting it will expand the knowledge gained and save valuable time.

REQUESTING THE CONSULTATION

Seeking Consultation

George Thorn warned against two extremes in consultations: "At one extreme is the physician who balks at a consultation, as though his own knowledge were being challenged. Patients appreciate the physician who agrees to obtaining a second opinion even when he thinks he knows the answer. Every good clinician realizes this, but some, particularly young physicians, may feel that they are expected to know all the answers. At the other extreme is the physician who gives up too easily, hardly ever solving a problem alone and complicating the situation by involving too many others."

Profiting Most from a Consultation

First Study the Problem Yourself When the referring physician and consultant have a common specialty, the referring physician will usually study the case thoroughly before requesting the consultation. When, however, the consultation is outside the referring physician's specialty, as, for example, when an orthopedist seeks advice from an otolaryngologist, the referring physician may not do a comprehensive study of the condition and may therefore not learn as much as possible for application to future patients, especially since the consultant often proceeds with the patient's treatment.

To obtain the most from a consultation in your field of interest, first look up the subject in a standard textbook or in your personal information file. That will help reduce the scope of the consultation to a few specific questions. Delineation of the problem by one or more explicit questions and a brief review of an authoritative publication on the subject can, in fact, sometimes clarify the problem enough to make a consultation unnecessary.

Summarize the Records All data, including patient records, roentgenograms, and laboratory reports, should be summarized and made accessible to the consultant. While summarizing his data, James Dooley assesses his own performance with the patient, whom he may have observed for 10–20 years, by carefully reviewing all the clinical material accumulated during this time, including his notes.

When the patient is to be seen in the consultant's office, the referring physician may summarize the clinical information in a letter. For hospitalized patients, the summarizing note is made on the chart. Preparation of either summary, when preceded by a careful review, is educational for the referring physician. Regardless of the type of summary used, it is helpful for the referring physician and consultant to discuss the problem in person or by telephone before the consultation.

Ask Specific Questions William Parmley deplores the vagueness of many consultation requests and stresses the importance of informing the consultant of the explicit purpose of the request. The more specific the questions, the more the patient and the referring physician will profit from the consultation.

Example:

> This 23-year-old woman with rheumatoid arthritis continues to have significant symptoms while taking three aspirin tablets four times a day. A dosage of 14 tablets per day produces tinnitus. Should treatment be changed? Are nonsteroidal anti-inflammatory agents indicated? Should we go directly to gold?

Ask the consultant for a listing of the phenomena that should be monitored.

Example:

> What signs, symptoms, and laboratory tests should be monitored and at what intervals? For example, joint symptoms, swelling, fever, and sedimentation rate.

The consultant may also be asked to identify the criteria (signs, symptoms, and laboratory tests) that will require additional consultations.

Warren Williams tests the specificity of his questions by writing his own responses to his consultation requests, outlining diagnostic and therapeutic plans. He then compares his plans with those of the consultant, and they discuss any differences. Consultations thus become a personal and active educational tool.

When R. D. Richards was a young faculty member, he saw a certain patient and decided what he thought should be done. He then asked a senior faculty member to look at the patient and give his recommendation. "To my surprise," said Richards, "he recommended something quite different from my approach, although I still felt my approach was preferable. At that time, I realized that I had not communicated properly with him, and should have specifically stated what I wished to know. Since then, I have never asked for a consultation unless I really wanted it and have always specified precisely what I wished the consultant to do."

Who Is Present During the Consultation?

Some referring physicians like to be present during the consultation. "I call the consultant," said Edward Shapiro, "outline the problem, and make a date to meet with him at the bedside. I watch him examine the patient, I supply additional information if needed, and I interrogate the consultant. In this way, I learn a great deal. One consultant said I cross-examined him, and I don't deny the accusation." Aaron

Feder will not perform a consultation unless the referring physician is there, and will not make such a request himself unless he is present to hear what the consultant has to say.

Most physicians think, however, that the consultant does better without the presence and influence of the referring physician, which may interfere with the consultant's establishing rapport with the patient or may inhibit the patient's responses. Most consultants prefer to have time to organize their thoughts without feeling that they are "on stage."

PROVIDING THE CONSULTATION

"A physician conducts a patient consultation under two different circumstances," said Walter Somerville. "In the teaching hospital, he may be attended by junior staff and students eager to learn and imitate, and by hand-picked senior residents and fellows, critical and watchful for a false move or clinical slip. With such continuous audit, the physician is in the ideal environment to bring out the best in himself as teacher and physician.

"The procedure is different when the physician is alone in his office or face-to-face with the patient in a nonteaching hospital. Two techniques are beneficial to the patient and invaluable to the isolated physician. The first is *patient transposition,* in which the physician imagines the patient's thoughts and feelings: 'I am sensitive and terrified. I am overawed by the doctor, writing down my anxieties, intimate disclosures, and sexual indiscretions, to be read by goodness knows whom? And that tape recorder? No wonder I feel like running away, screaming, from this horrible experience.' Considering the patient's point of view goes a long way toward creating the proper environment for easy doctor–patient communication.

"The second technique is the *invisible audit.* I surround myself with an imaginary audit-jury, drawn from the most constructive critics in my experience. Closest to me, breathing down my neck, is Paul Wood, then Sam Levine, and beside him my most stringent critic, my wife, Jane, whispering emphatically what I'm doing wrong. With my pomposity deflated, affectations minimized, and extempore guesswork challenged, I'm ever aware of my watchful friends. And the patient gets the best service I can give," concludes Somerville.

The Consultant as a Learner

Paul Harvey cited another advantage of consultations: "The consultant has the chance to examine a patient and think over a clinical problem without doing the basic work and with most of the tests completed. This review of the work of others is a unique opportunity to see how others approach problems."

The questions asked by the referring physician may offer a useful perspective. The request may stimulate the consultant to review a recent specialty textbook or personal information file or even do medical library research. If the specific reason for the consultation is not clear, the consultant should ask the referring physician for further information.

Teaching What Not to Order

To promote cost-containment, consultants should point out unnecessary studies that were ordered before they came on the scene, even though such disclosures may be ticklish. In Desmond Julian's opinion, "Consultants don't do enough teaching about when certain tests are *not* needed. Every time you order a test, even an electrocardiogram or roentgenogram, let alone an invasive procedure, you should ask yourself if the information will improve the care of that particular patient. The consultant can often diplomatically point out the limitations of some laboratory work that is ordered."

The Consultant's Report

On completion of the evaluation, the consultant will write a letter or make a consultation report on the hospital chart. Restricting the length of the report forces the consultant to summarize and communicate better. Writing succinctly also reinforces retention. Within 24 hours of the consultation, the consultant should call the referring physician.

Daniel Stone pointed to the instructional value of consultations: "The teaching in my consultation is largely through the letters I write afterwards, in which I review my thinking with the referring physician. I also cite references, and if the physician does not have access to a good medical library, I photocopy relevant articles and append them to the letter."

The inclusion of references must be handled delicately, since some referring physicians may consider such citations to be condescending. On the other hand, many physicians turn to consultants who are known to be outstanding teachers and who often provide useful references in diagnostic workups and treatment.

"The report sent from the consultant to the referring physician upon discharge of the patient," noted Julian "doesn't convey much to the referring physician if the diagnosis or treatment is buried among a mass of data representing the results of tests that he does not understand. I recommend a brief letter, which outlines the diagnosis, the basis for the diagnosis, the treatment selected and its rationale, or, in a complicated case, a more detailed letter further explaining these points." Even the most effective letter does not eliminate the need for a personal discussion after the consultation, whether face-to-face or by telephone.

Discussing the Consultation

Almost all referring physicians arrange for a personal meeting or a telephone conversation with the consultant afterward to discuss details or to ask further questions. Sherman Mellinkoff cautioned: "Physicians sometimes forget the value of conversation. We habitually write notes to consultants in the chart, which is fine—it was prescribed by Hippocrates and remains a good idea today—but I don't think you learn as much or help the patient as much if you rely exclusively on notes in the chart by the attending physician, consultant, or others caring for the patient. If something important develops regarding the patient, it is a good idea to discuss it directly with the consultant. Then both the consultant and referring physician will understand the problem better."

Reporting to the Patient

"The patient often has high expectations of the consultation, and although the consultant may try to withdraw and say he will discuss the case with the patient's doctor, the patient usually wants to hear the consultant's opinion directly," Ian Mackay pointed out. "Consultants should be given an opportunity to express an opinion and perhaps offer a little reassurance to the patient, but this is a delicate issue in the referring physician–consultant relationship."

Desmond Julian added: "The consultant and referring physician should see the patient together after the consultation. It's remarkable how often patients see as major discrepancies the minimal differences in what two physicians tell them. If, for example, I recommend a 1,000-calorie diet and another physician recommends 800 calories, the patient may think: 'These doctors can't agree.' Joint decisions are desirable regarding matters that may seem inconsequential to us but very important to the patient."

The Follow-up

The formal consultation should not end with the consultant's written or verbal communication. When the referring physician remains responsible for the patient's primary care, the consulting physician should be kept posted on the patient's progress. Follow-up telephone calls to review the case or clarify points benefit the patient as well as the referring physician and consultant.

"Whether the consultant should see the patient *again* is," in Ian Mackay's words, "often a touchy matter in hospital practice when a good relationship develops between the consultant and the patient." If the consultant considers it advisable to see the patient again, that should be stated, to avoid disturbing the referring physician–consultant relationship.

THE IDEAL CONSULTATION

To learn the most and ensure the best advice for the patient, the referring physician should delineate the precise reasons for requesting the consultation. Unless the problem is in a totally different specialty, it is desirable to read about the subject in a current textbook or other publication, collect all existing data on the patient, summarize the records in a letter or note on the hospital chart, and formulate specific questions for the consultant.

"In the ideal consultation, the referring physician is present on my arrival, describes the problem he wishes to consult me about, and introduces me to the patient," said Desmond Julian. "That's important because it shows a collaboration of colleagues rather than a physician giving up and having to pass the problem to someone else. After he introduces me to the patient, he leaves while I talk to the patient privately. In this way, the patient is not fearful of telling a different story to one physician from that told to another or of contradicting himself. I take the history and do the physical examination myself. Then I meet the referring physician again and discuss the problem with him. Sometimes something emerges that requires action or further elucidation, or some contradiction in the story may need to be resolved. I like to go back to the patient with the referring physician and explain our joint opinion about diagnosis or treatment."

Even when the patient's problem is discussed in person or by telephone, it is still necessary to write a letter or consultation report. The consultant's report should be clear and concise, providing specific advice on diagnostic and therapeutic plans, along with the rationale on which that advice is based. The consultant should be notified of any significant changes in the patient. Each of these steps offers opportunities for active participation and enlightenment.

REFERENCE

1. Halle J. *An Historiall Expostulation: Against the beastlye Abusers, bothe of Chyrurgerie, and Physyke, in oure tyme: with a goodlye Doctrine and Instruction, necessarye to be marked and folowed, of all true Chirurgiens.* London: Thomas Marshe; 1565. Edited by T.J. Pettigrew, London: Percy Society; 1844:31–32.

8

Formal Courses and Conferences

• • •

> [Lectures] are a temptation to the more contemplative mind to learn diseases by the study of models, rather than of the things themselves. They tend to divorce him from the workshop and the chips and fragments and rude designs that lie about within it, and introduce him into a room swept and garnished and hung round with masterpieces for his contemplation. This may be all very well for gentlemen who patronise the arts; but this is not the way to make the artist.
>
> PETER MERE LATHAM[1]

Formal courses and conferences are the second most popular method of continuing medical education, after reading.[2–4] Numerous studies have shown that physicians learn facts from such formal instruction.[5,6] Courses that focus on physician performance in specific clinical situations, however, can not only transfer facts but can also alter that performance, even though such changes are difficult to measure.

Critics have focused on the limitations of courses and conferences, which are memory based. Because knowledge so acquired may not be used for weeks or months in the care of patients, it may be forgotten by that time. The educational needs of physicians may also vary widely, and yet courses and conferences, which are group enterprises, emphasize common needs, not individual needs. Jesse Rising, who spent decades organizing courses, said: "After retiring as the Associate Dean of Continuing Education, I became a volunteer in the Department of Family Practice at the University of Kansas Medical School, where I have been learning general medicine again. From that experience I am convinced that the critical factor in CME is to take care of patients. Courses are interesting, but learning comes from studying patients."

To Claude Organ, conferences are often simply dull. "To inspire the participants, the course director must create a spirit of learning. This sounds trite, I know, and it is easier said than done."

Despite their limitations, formal courses and conferences can keep physicians aware of current knowledge and new developments, can broaden understanding, and can put the practicing physician in touch with experts and peers. Physicians who gain the most from courses are able to relate course material to their own clinical experience. The fact that these gains are difficult to measure after standard courses or conferences does not vitiate such instruction in a comprehensive lifelong educational program.

REASONS FOR ATTENDING FORMAL COURSES AND CONFERENCES

Physicians are motivated to attend formal courses and conferences by both inner standards and extrinsic forces, such as peer pressure and licensing regulations.[7–12] The motivations varied slightly in different studies conducted, depending on the phrasing of questions, but can be grouped into several broad categories. Physicians frequently cited as motivating factors the opportunity to review and increase medical knowledge by becoming more aware of the general state-of-the-art (with the assumption that the knowledge will make the physician more competent) and by acquiring information pertinent to specific patient problems. Physicians also use courses for self-assessment, to compare their knowledge to that of experts in the field, and to compare their work to accepted standards of practice. Continuing medical education is also seen as an integral part of professionalism by society and the medical community. Professionals are expected to sharpen their knowledge and skills continually. A change of pace from practice and contact with colleagues and faculty are also cited as motivations to attend courses.

Expected Benefits

For Patrick Storey, the single most important benefit of attending a conference or CME short course is a recognition of what the registrant does not know and what he cannot do. As Oliver Wendell Holmes bluntly stated, "The best part of our knowledge is that which teaches us where knowledge leaves off and ignorance begins. Nothing more clearly separates a vulgar from a superior mind, than the confusion in the first between the little that it truly knows, on the one hand, and what it half knows and what it thinks it knows on the other."[13]

Reinforcement of the physician's past knowledge is more valuable to Richard Caplan than the slight new information he may acquire. "Nor must we forget the attitudinal advantages—the re-ignition of languishing fires, the recharging of batteries, the renewal of excitement. Further, a course or conference allows us to place ourselves in the fertile mode of an active learner, free from daily professional responsibilities and interruptions." Even if a physician's knowledge is up-to-date, as Jack Lein said, "attending a course will reinforce the assurance that he is doing his best."

For George Race, the ripple effect is the primary benefit from formal courses. "When physicians hear something new, their interest is piqued, and they will then consult journals, books, or experts to learn more about the subject. Furthermore, the contacts that participants make with course faculty often allow them to identify consultants with whom they can establish ready communication."

"A continuing education course is a wonderful, legitimate excuse to leave behind the responsibilities for children, spouse, and patient care," said Karin Jamison. "The setting is usually some elegant hotel in

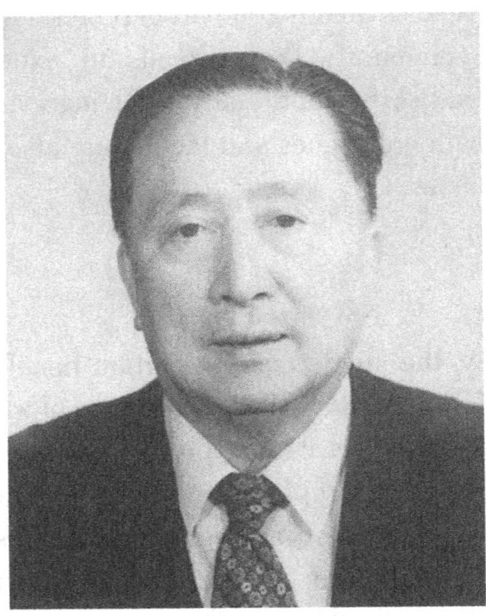

It is important for physicians to summarize and document their clinical experiences, and to remain current with medical progress through reading and attending conferences.

PROFESSOR WU JIEPING
Honorary President
Chinese Academy of Medical Sciences
Beijing, China

a different environment. It is fun to meet people from all over the country and share experiences, joys, and problems, and to discover that what is difficult for one may be difficult for all. Such recognition gives a sense of relief. Even though the meetings are intense, they are still a restful experience. It is an unusual opportunity to laugh at oneself with trusted colleagues who understand. Finally, it is very gratifying to take back home some information that is helpful to one or more patients."

Surveys of registrants in courses given by the University of Southern California illustrate the benefits derived from them:

"It is regenerating to be away from any distractions at home and thus be able to concentrate on the course. I expect to feel more stimulation from the renewal of academic knowledge and to gain more clinical confidence." (Peter Best)

"I want to update my concept of patient care and reassure myself that I am maintaining a high standard of medical practice." (Gerald Farinola)

"Courses give me an opportunity to coordinate the material I read in the literature, and to hear directly from the people in the forefront of their specialties." (Unsigned)

"I expect to get the most advanced knowledge in the field from the course, since I can find the day-to-day knowledge and information in textbooks." (Ragheb Sawires)

"Courses make reading more meaningful, placing the importance of the material in better perspective. Often the writer of an article has spent much of his life doing research on a particular subject and is therefore somewhat biased about the significance of his work." (Wenzel A. Leff)

"I compare what I hear at the course with what is currently in the literature. I expect to come away with a summary of what is new on a subject that will be clinically useful to me." (Daniel Hoffman)

"I want to learn how medicine is practiced in different places and review important developments that I may have missed or do not have in proper perspective." (Unsigned)

"I get the opportunity to compare my method of practice to what is taught in the university hospitals." (Rokay Kamyar)

"I want to increase my medical knowledge and demonstrate to myself how much I don't know, as a stimulus to read." (G.E. Wiebe)

"Courses offer a more provocative approach than sitting at home and reading." (P. B. Jorgensen)

"Attending courses permits me to dilute parochialism a bit—to get views on medical subjects other than those prevalent in my locale." (Donald Jacobs)

SELECTING A COURSE OR CONFERENCE

Content

In deciding whether to take a particular course, Donald Petit suggested that physicians ask themselves: "Do I want a board review? Do I want to find out what's new on a given subject? Do I want to learn something because I think it might be good for me, for example, basic science for clinicians? Courses or conferences for physicians should have a clear statement of content so that the physician will know in advance what to expect." More specifically, Edward Rubenstein advised: "The scope and the level of sophistication should be explicitly stated. For instance, does the program deal in depth with a subject, or does it consist of a number of compressed sessions highlighting the most important or most timely points? Does it emphasize basic science, or does it focus on practical clinical matters? Is it intended for specialists or subspecialists or physicians with other primary interests?"

Lawrence Highman chooses courses that provide current information on problems that arise in practice at his small rural hospital. "I want to find out what changes I can make or what equipment is needed to improve my care of my patients." It is, of course, the physician's responsibility to determine whether the content will make a difference in clinical practice. Richard Caplan suspects that most physicians "respond with a somewhat more visceral than intellectual awareness of what they need. Furthermore, the present methods used by educators to demonstrate needs leave much to be desired. Who is to say that 'visceral wisdom' is not a reasonably good measure of what we need to learn?"

Faculty and Sponsor

The reputation of the sponsor is a fairly reliable index of the competence of the faculty and the value of a medical education conference. "An outstanding course," in Donald Petit's opinion, "depends first on the quality of the faculty—its ability to impart knowledge, its enthusiasm, and its style. Does the faculty stimulate me to learn? Is the experience really enjoyable?"

Course Design

A program that promotes active participation is most beneficial, with ample opportunity for questions or concerns of the participating physicians through direct question-and-answer periods or discussion forums. Programs are enriched by multiple formats such as lectures, panel discussions, and problem-solving sessions. Informal periods at lunch and coffee breaks are useful for discussion among participants.

Facilities and Site

Are the chairs comfortable, and are the tables convenient for writing? Is the lighting good? Are the audiovisual facilities adequate? Is the temperature comfortable? These may seem like minor factors before one attends a conference, but once the sessions are under way, their absence can become a major detriment.

National or regional courses or conferences are held at medical schools, hospitals, hotels, convention centers, or popular vacation sites. "With tuition, air travel, and the practice of conducting courses in posh resort areas, not to mention the expense of maintaining the office and staff while the physician is away, cost is becoming a tremendous factor," noted Wenzel Leff.

On the other hand, a relaxed setting is important because it removes physicians from the tensions and distractions of practice and thus allows better concentration. A relaxed setting may also lower the barriers between faculty and participants and permit interaction to continue at the beach, poolside, or dinner table. Because a vacation setting is also pleasant for the faculty, it may attract superior teachers. In our view, a combined course and vacation will enhance educational activities rather than detract from them, provided that the sponsor plans a superior course that leaves no question that the prime purpose is learning. Recreational activities should be scheduled outside of course hours. Courses that appear to be simple tax dodges, with little or no educational value, are deplorable. That such courses exist does not argue against the superior programs set in vacation surroundings. Participants must be particularly alert in assessing the quality of the faculty and suitability of topics to ensure the legitimacy of the program and the applicability to their needs.

Fruitful and Worthless Courses

Some interviewees gave examples of fruitful as well as worthless courses. Cited most often as worthwhile were courses with information for practical clinical application, with opportunity for interaction with an outstanding faculty, and with emphasis on new information and skills rather than overviews. The most useful courses, in Robert Palmer's view, are those that apply directly to the physician's own practice, whereas the most worthless are those that suggest that the only proper care of patients is given in a large medical center or "Ivory Tower" setting. In J. Young's opinion, controversy and discussion are crucial components of a good course. "Passive didactic instruction does not really encourage intellectual growth. A great number of panel discussions are worthless, the 'professors' merely scratching one another's backs."

ENSURING OPTIMAL BENEFIT

Preparing for a Course or Conference

When Frederick Ludwig goes to a meeting, he has a specific goal in mind. "A day or two in advance of the meeting, I will study what I am going to be dealing with. Then at the meeting, I take notes, and when I get home, I organize my thoughts and dictate a summary for my secretary to transcribe so that I have a record of it. Later I can go back and consult those notes." Donald Feinstein also reads the abstracts the night before. "It is extremely inefficient if I do not prepare." Trying to think in advance of something worthwhile to contribute makes Kenneth Berge much more attentive to the content.

Being Active During the Course

Most interviewees take notes during the sessions, and some rewrite them the same evening to reinforce the concepts. Summarizing your notes while the presentation is still fresh in your mind gives "double exposure" to important ideas. Some physicians corral the speaker after the presentation to ask questions not answered during the sessions; others discuss particular cases with other participants. A good course syllabus is a great help but, unfortunately, is rare.

Follow-up Study

After a course, some physicians summarize their notes or the provided syllabus and file the material under the appropriate heading in their files. New information can be condensed into a few basic statements, written on one sheet of paper, and reviewed periodically over the next few days. To disseminate new information, as well as to help retain it, the physician can dictate and distribute to interested colleagues a summary of the meeting. Also, a presentation based on the subject can be given to the hospital staff. Many physicians probe further into subjects that engage their interest or that they do not fully understand, looking for articles to compare, refute, or reinforce what was covered at a conference.

Daniel Bird uses his active learning participation in courses to improve patient understanding. "As an aid in patient education, I have typed short summaries of lectures I've attended and have placed them in a special corner of my waiting room or occasionally mailed them to certain patients. This ensures the wide dissemination of accurate and timely medical information and strongly underlines the concern of physicians for the welfare of their patients. Patients take these sheets of information home, discuss them with family and friends, and thus introduce the physician to many persons as one who both knows and cares."

CONFERENCES OFFERED BY HOSPITALS AND SPECIALTY SOCIETIES

The general principles discussed under formal courses and conferences are applicable to all such programs, although hospital conferences and annual sessions sponsored by specialty groups may present a different orientation from courses offered by medical schools.

HOSPITAL CONFERENCES

All hospitals have staff meetings, many have section or departmental meetings, and some have general educational meetings. Hospital conferences are convenient for physicians and can be designed to solve specific medical problems in the hospital. They also promote interaction with peers and may enhance the physician's visibility while improving cooperation among physicians, nurses, pharmacists, and other health professionals.

In place of medical grand rounds consisting only of a clinical lecture, Samuel Rapaport prefers a case presentation to serve as the springboard for more generalized comments on mechanisms or treatment. Paul Beeson favors morbidity and mortality rounds, along with case reviews and medical pathology reviews. "These sessions permit physicians to review frankly what happened and where the treatment went wrong. Nothing sticks with you like a mistake. Having someone looking over your shoulder and saying 'No, it is not what you think it is, but it is this,' gives you a healthy humility. I have had just enough experience in private practice to know that no matter what you do, 90 percent of your patients are going to get well, and unless someone points this out to you, you may begin to feel that what you are doing is responsible."

Hugh Lawrence also lauded the review of morbidity data, with open discussion of cases, followed by an audit. "The audit report suggests a plan of action, and a later audit indicates if there has been any progress. When I came to our hospital about seven years ago, several different bowel preparations were used by the 20 surgeons. We discussed this and found the infection rate in intestinal surgery to be about 18 percent. We narrowed the protocols to four, and the infection rate dropped to 5.8 percent. The new practice was presented at a morbidity and mortality conference, which led other surgeons to refine the protocol, with a further reduction in infection rate to 1.8 percent. We found, however, that some surgeons were having a higher infection rate than this. At first we thought that the nurses were not carrying out the procedures, but an audit showed that certain doctors had not been writing orders satisfactorily."

Analysis of hospital patient care data can be used beyond conference planning, extending into direct conversation about quality assurance. If a physician is having a high complication rate for a given disorder, Hugh Lawrence will approach the physician privately. "I will not communicate with him by memorandum or letter, but will go to him personally, solicit his help with the problem, and ask him how he would approach it. I will pick the physician with the next worse complication rate and say, 'You are one of two people here who are having a problem, and I just wonder how we can eliminate it.' In this way, I encourage him to produce the action himself."

Death conferences and clinicopathologic conferences, which have been important educational tools in the past, have declined in popularity because they focus on exotic diseases and rare diagnoses. James Moss would like to see these conferences directed toward patients with avoidable deaths. Unfortunately, the litigious atmosphere today makes discussions of this kind very difficult.

Morbidity and mortality rounds can be inordinately dull, "a slow unfolding of the inevitable, ending with a pathology demonstration," according to Ian Mackay. "In addition, although an outcome may be unfavorable and the criticism severe, there may have been, in retrospect, no other course to follow, or the course followed may not have been at all unreasonable at the time."

Francis Moore encouraged the staffs of small hospitals to review their own experiences. "The average surgeon or internist or pediatrician probably does not analyze his practice data. The purpose of staff committees and staff review groups in small hospitals should be to encourage that kind of review of one's own work."

Desmond Julian advocates a switch from mortality to morbidity. "Whereas the postmortem room used to be the main learning area, with all the tests we have today on living patients, the biopsies and the radiologic investigations, we learn more from morbidity conferences than mortality conferences, that is, from what goes wrong in patients who survive."

Discussions of medical care in which the physician should have acted differently are essential, but some physicians may have a tendency to cover up their actions, as Paul Wehrle explained: "Facilitating discussions with medical colleagues is an interesting art and requires a certain amount of understanding. Some practicing physicians in small rural private hospitals are unwilling to discuss candidly patients who have been mismanaged. Each staff member knows precisely which physician treated which patient and must use special tact to make constructive criticisms and suggest alternate diagnostic or therapeutic approaches. Unless the discussion leader is experienced and diplomatic, the atmosphere can become tense and painful for those responsible for the medical decisions under scrutiny." It is best to relate these meetings to educational activities, lest overly harsh punitive measures drive the errors underground.

Claude Organ considers the best hospital meetings to be those directed at deficiencies disclosed by a properly designed audit. He advises physicians to resist wasting time at hospital staff meetings about administrative and statistical reports that lead to no conclusions. The primary purpose, after all, is to improve patient care through education. Charles Brunicardi agrees: "If you take an active approach, conferences can help you remain current. I choose several conferences relevant to my needs and attend them weekly. Taking notes at these conferences requires discipline, but is well worth the effort, since it helps me to concentrate and process information."

Annual Sessions

Annual sessions of specialty and state societies and associations can provide excellent opportunities for learning and reviewing the state of knowledge. As in any other educational event, preparation and participation make attendance more productive.

Advantages Programs sponsored by a subspecialty society, which usually give an in-depth view of the latest research and clinical information, differ from the formal course given by a medical school, which is often a review of a topic. The formal course or conference generally entails broad coverage, whereas annual sessions often spotlight recognized authorities on given subjects.

Because of its many concurrent sessions, an annual meeting may have a wider appeal than a three- or four-day postgraduate course and may provide better opportunities for division of groups by special interest. Unlike most postgraduate courses, it usually also has commercial and scientific exhibits, which may include teaching media, such as computer-based or audiovisual programs. The commercial exhibits usually alert the practitioner to new drugs and devices.

Discussions with fellow physicians from different areas of the country are enlightening. As William Davis has found, "You learn as much or more in the halls between sessions as you do from listening to the presentations." The "Meet the Professor" sessions with informal discussion of clinical problems provide divergent views.

Limitations Not only do annual out-of-town sessions require a protracted absence from one's practice, but large meetings do not always offer the best opportunities for fellowship and may be dominated by political rather than professional issues. The large audience can also be an obstacle to learning, with less opportunity for face-to-face interchanges. There may also be housing problems, and less choice of scheduling. On the other hand, the physician can choose the month and general location desired for a postgraduate course.

Of little value are prolonged discussions of rare diseases and syndromes that few physicians will ever see, as well as presentations of new diagnostic procedures or therapeutic measures that have not been studied adequately and that may subsequently prove to be of no benefit. For Marsha Wallace, it is a mistake to design information for everyone from country doctors to those in urban centers, each with vastly different needs. "By the time basics are rehashed, there is often little time left for what is new."

* * * * *

Courses and conferences are traditional and remain popular. When most physicians think of continuing education, they think of a classroom presentation. Courses and conferences may define to the physician directions for further study, reinforce past knowledge, acquaint the physician with experts in the field, and provide opportunities for informal discussions with peers, as well as present new information and developments. Such group teaching and learning help keep the profession aware of the current state of knowledge and of contemporary standards, but cannot provide all the detail a physician needs for daily practice. Courses are therefore no substitute for reading or for colleague consultations on specific problems. Physicians who have developed methods for reviewing their practice according to problems seen, drugs prescribed, and studies ordered may profit most from courses and conferences because they can compare their experience and performance with those of the instructors.

REFERENCES

1. Latham PM. A word or two on medical education. In: Martin R, ed. *The Collected Works of Dr. P. M. Latham.* London: New Sydenham Society; 1878:562.
2. Manning PR, Denson TA. How cardiologists learn about echocardiography. *Ann Intern Med.* 1979;91:469–471.

3. Manning PR, Denson TA. How internists learned about cimetidine. *Ann Intern Med.* 1980;92:690–692.

4. Vollan DD. Scope and extent of postgraduate medical education in the United States. *JAMA.* 1955;157:703–708.

5. Manning PR, Abrahamson S, Dennis DA. Comparison of four teaching techniques: programmed text, textbook, lecture-demonstration, and lecture workshop. *J Med Educ.* 1968;43:356–359.

6. Manning PR. Pre- and post-course testing as a teaching aid. *The Mayo Alumnus.* 1966;2:18–20.

7. Stein LS. The effectiveness of continuing medical education: eight research reports. *J Med Educ.* 1981;56:103–110.

8. Richards RK, Cohen RM. The value and limitations of physician participation in traditional forms of continuing medical education, Part II. Kalamazoo, MI: Educational Service Department, Upjohn; 1983.

9. Houle CO. *Continuing Learning in the Professions.* San Francisco: Jossey–Bass; 1980.

10. Schuknecht HF. The risks and limitations of the course as providing competent training. *Trans Am Acad Ophthal Otolaryngol.* 1976;82:640–641.

11. Meighan SS. Continuing medical education: philosophy in search of a plan. *Northwest Med.* 1966;65:925–929.

12. Cervero RM. A factor analytic study of physicians' reasons for participating in continuing education. *J Med Educ.* 1981;56:29–34.

13. Holmes OW. Border lines of knowledge in some provinces of medical science. In: *Medical Essays: 1842–1882.* Boston: Houghton Mifflin; 1911:211.

REFLECTIONS

• • •

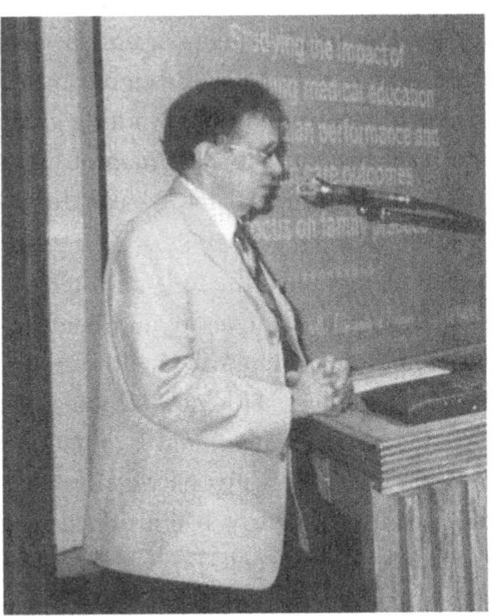

Persuasive evidence suggests that the learning phase in formal CME begins not with the course, but with the identification of clinical needs or deficits.

DAVID A. DAVIS, M.D.

After completing his medical training at the University of Western Ontario and the University of Toronto in 1969, Dr. David Davis entered private family practice in Burlington, Ontario, and began a lifelong interest in continuing medical education (CME), culminating in the development of a community hospital-based continuing education program at Burlington's Joseph Brant Hospital. In 1977, he became Director of CME at the new Faculty of Health Sciences, McMaster University in Hamilton.

Dr. Davis's efforts at McMaster led to a number of academic CME developments: the concept of a CME Society, the application of problem-based learning principles to CME, a comprehensive competency assessment program supported by the provincial licensing body, a Ministry of Health-funded national audioconferencing network, the use of innovative needs-assessment and evaluative techniques, including standardized patients, a unique database of CME research (Research and Development Resource Base in CME), and the evolution of an evidence-based CME working group.

In 1986, Dr. Davis became the Chairman of Continuing Health Sciences Education and Clinical Professor in the Department of Family Medicine at McMaster University. Three years later, leaving his Burlington practice, he joined the full-time staff of the Faculty of Health Sciences of McMaster University and became a staff physician at the North Hamilton Community Health Center, an inner-city primary-care teaching practice. He is now a Professor in the Departments of Health Policy, Management, and Evaluation and of Family and Community Medicine at the University of Toronto.

Dr. Davis has published nearly 100 articles, monographs, and chapters and coedited a textbook on CME, *The Physician as Learner.*[1] A speaker, workshop leader, and consultant on four continents, he has served as Chairman of the CME Committee of the Ontario Council of the Faculties of Medicine, President of the Standing Committee on CME for the Association of Canadian Medical Colleges, President of the Alliance for CME, and President of the Society of Medical College Directors of CME (now the Society for Academic CME).

REFERENCE

1. Davis DA, Fox RD, eds. *The Physician as Learner. Linking Research to Practice.* Chicago, IL: American Medical Association; 1994.

Lifelong Learning: A Physician's Perspective

David A. Davis, M.D.
Associate Dean, Continuing Education, Faculty of Medicine
University of Toronto
Toronto, Ontario, Canada

Formal continuing medical education (CME) has traditionally comprised planned educational activities, usually didactic, with stated objectives and accreditation standards. In the current professional environment, its effectiveness is being increasingly examined. First, the rising number of accredited activities[1] presents an often bewildering choice for the practicing physician. Second, each course involves costs, including registration fees and travel. Third, most short courses produce little change in physician performance.[2] Finally, perhaps most surprisingly, because many physicians have difficulty determining their own learning needs, they do not select programs of greatest value to them. In the 1980s, Sibley and colleagues[3] reported that family physicians often chose course subjects in which they were already competent, ignoring, or ranking lower, topics in which they were less proficient. Similar findings have been obtained in other specialties.

PRECOURSE: THE DETERMINATION OF LEARNING NEEDS

Persuasive evidence suggests that the learning phase in formal CME begins not with the course, but with identification of clinical needs or deficits. What steps can the physician take to gain the most from current educational opportunities? A recent review of 14 randomized controlled trials of CME activities showed that in four of five trials in which needs were assessed in advance, the change in physicians' clinical competence was greater than when no formal preliminary needs assessment was done.[4] Physicians can, of course, do their own needs assessment. Reading and attending courses help uncover knowledge deficits, but better still is a log or list of clinical questions arising in individual practice, with steps to address those questions. The ultimate test of any physician's performance lies in the patient outcomes, useful measures of which are infection rates, length of hospitalization, blood pressure, and laboratory tests.

EVIDENCE FROM RANDOMIZED CONTROLLED TRIALS

In our previously mentioned review of 14 randomized controlled trials (RCTs) of formal CME,[4] physicians' performance did not change when instruction was didactic and little time was available for questions or interaction. Interactive conferences and workshops, on the other hand, or a mix of didactic and interactive sessions (hands-on workshops, skills-building sessions, role play, animal labs, case discussion conferences) improved physician performance or healthcare outcomes more.[5] In addition, one-day events were less likely to change performance than those held on two or more occasions over time. We theorized that repeated exposure at intervals allows the learner to reflect on the new knowledge, incorporate it into practice, and then return to the next learning session to reinforce the new practice, acquiring and incorporating new skills in the process.[4]

We also concluded that group size was not important to outcomes, perhaps because even with large audiences, small-group learning activities are possible. Also helpful was sending reminders to registrants after the course. Three of four trials incorporating patient educational material, or physician reminders and protocols, improved healthcare outcomes.[4]

SOFTER EVIDENCE OF THE EFFECTIVENESS OF COURSES

Educational theories and common sense have dictated a number of other questions that enhance learning and provide a fairly reliable checklist for choosing formal CME (Table 1).[6] First, what are the major *themes* or broader *goals* of the conference? Do these, and the learning objective listed in precourse materials, match the physician's specific needs identified by subjective or objective means? The more precise the answer, the better. In general, attending a course with a clear and articulated vision of what you wish to accomplish is better than a vague set of objectives ("I want an update in cardiology"). Second, there may be impediments to the *credibility* of a program. It is wise to inquire about sponsorship, industry involvement, and the specific use of critically appraised material or publications.

AFTER THE COURSE: MAKING THE CONNECTION TO PRACTICE, CLOSING THE LOOP

Follow-up after the course is as important as the course itself. Study of materials distributed during the course or provided later (examples of patient contracts,[7] reminders, and flow charts) can encourage changes in practice. Anecdotal evidence suggests that many attendees do refer to course handouts to refresh their memory. Postcourse reminders generated from the CME director, a Web site at which registrants can find support materials, and updated mailed information are helpful in reinforcing lessons learned.

The astute CME participant will complete the cycle that began with needs assessment. With sufficient attention to the knowledge deficits and related data sources, it should be relatively simple to satisfy the learning need. If subjective data were used for the needs assessment (reviewing a learning log, reflecting on practice patterns and outcomes),

TABLE 1
Choosing a CME Course: Factors to Weigh

Factor	Related Questions	Evidence Base[a]
Precourse activity	Have I done a needs-assessment on my own practice?	A
	Are there specific and well-described objectives? Do they match my own objectives and goals?	D
	The planning committee: have physicians with similar backgrounds planned this course?	D
Format	Does the format allow for interactivity?	A
	Is there sufficient time for questions and answers? For interaction with the faculty?	B
	Are there learning resources provided (protocols, reminders, patient education materials)?	A
Credibility	Is the major sponsor of the event a credible institution or group?	D
	Is there a corporate or other sponsor? If so, are the fees reduced or social activities provided that might produce bias?	D
	In general, am I satisfied that sufficient safeguards are in place to prevent or identify bias?	D
Logistics	Are the conference site, timing, and other considerations convenient?	D
	Is the conference locale suitable for interaction and comfortable learning?	D
Postcourse activity	Is there a Web site or other resource for ongoing materials and support after the course? If so, is it acceptable and accessible for me?	D

[a]Level A evidence: from reviews of publications, meta-analysis of randomized clinical trials (RCTs); level B evidence: from one or more RCTs; level C evidence: from descriptive studies; level D evidence: common sense.

simple postcourse reflection may be sufficient to close the loop: Did I meet my objectives? What questions were left unanswered? If more objective data were used (practice-based Continuous Quality Improvement [CQI] data sources), reviewing them within three to six months may determine the effectiveness of the course.

ALTERNATIVES TO THE SHORT COURSE

For almost two decades, directors of continuing medical education have been wrestling with alternatives to formal courses. Distributed CME consists of such print materials as practice guidelines generated by specialty societies and others or audiotapes, videotapes, monographs, and newsletters. If unsolicited and unlinked to needs, they generally have little effect.[2] Other alternatives are visiting speakers and academic detailers. Visiting lectureships usually have little impact, especially if the subject is unrelated to local needs. Evidence suggests, however, that academic medical educators who focus on some aspect of clinical practice, such as prescribing practices, are effective.[8,9] Community-based interventions, generally sponsored by a disease-related organization (diabetes, HIV–AIDS, smoking cessation), include media, public and patient education, and sessions with local physician leaders. Practice-based interventions are increasingly used by cost- and quality-conscious organizations. These may include a combination of lectures, reminder systems (print or electronic), audit and feedback, and other methods borrowed from CQI publications.[10] Finally, interventions that target the patient directly, for example, patient reminders about preventive practices (flu shots in the elderly or mammography) and more comprehensive practices, including patient education, as in diabetes, have optimized physicians' clinical performance.

REFERENCES

1. Accreditation Council for Continuing Medical Education (ACCME) homepage. Available at www.accme.org/sec_acc_fl.html. Accessed 2001 May 14.

2. Davis DA, Thomson MA, Oxman AD, Haynes RB. Changing physician performance. A systematic review of the effect of continuing medical education strategies. *JAMA.* 1995; 274:700–705.

3. Sibley JC, Sacket DL, Neufeld V, Gerrard B, Rudnick KV, Fraser WA. Randomized trial of continuing medical education. *N Engl J Med.* 1982;306:511–515.

4. Davis D, Thomson O'Brien MA, Freemantle N, Wolf EM, Mazmanian P, Taylor-Vaisey A. Impact of formal continuing medical education: do conferences, workshops, rounds, and other traditional continuing education activities change physician behavior or health care outcomes? *JAMA.* 1999;282:867–874.

5. Steinert Y, Snell L. Interactive learning: strategies for increasing participation in large group presentations. *Med Teach.* 1999;21:37–42.

6. Davis DA, Thomson MA. Continuing medical education as a means of lifelong learning. In: Silagy C, Haines A, eds. *Evidence Based Practice in Primary Care.* London: BMJ Publishing Group; 1998:129–143.

7. Wilson DM, Taylor DW, Gilbert JR, et al. A randomized trial of a family physician intervention for smoking cessation. *JAMA.* 1988;260:1570–1574.

8. Thomson O'Brien MA, Oxman AD, Davis DA, Haynes RB, Freemantle N, Harvey EL. Educational outreach visits: effects on professional practice and health care outcomes. Cochrane Database and Systematic Reviews (2):CD000409, 2000.

9. Soumerai SB. Principles and uses of academic detailing to improve the management of psychiatric disorders. *Int J Psychiatry Med.* 1998;28:81–96.

10. Laffel G, Berwick DM. Quality in health care. *JAMA.* 1992;268:407–409.

REFLECTIONS

• • •

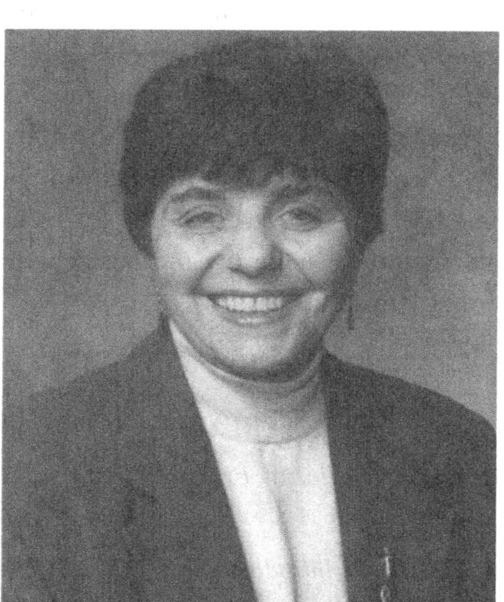

The medical profession has been forced to function in a business mode when providing clinical services. It is imperative that our educational mission not be compromised by the for-profit concept.

CATHERINE D. DEANGELIS, M.D.

Dr. Catherine DeAngelis received her M.D. degree from the University of Pittsburgh School of Medicine and her M.P.H. from the Harvard Graduate School of Public Health (Health Services Administration). As Editor-in-chief she oversees *The Journal of the American Medical Association* (*JAMA*) as well as the *Archives* publications and the *JAMA*-related Web site content. Before this appointment, she was Vice Dean for Academic Affairs and Faculty at Johns Hopkins University School of Medicine, where she is still Professor of Pediatrics. From 1994 to 2000, she was Editor of the

Archives of Pediatrics and Adolescent Medicine. She has been a member of numerous other medical journal editorial boards.

Dr. DeAngelis has written or edited 10 books, including *Pediatric Primary Care*[1] and *An Introduction to Clinical Research*[2], and has published more than 150 original articles, chapters, editorials, and abstracts. Several of her recent publications have focused on conflicts of interest in medicine, women in medicine, and medical education. A member of the National Academy of Science, Institute of Medicine, she has also served as an officer in a number of national academic societies, including the past chairmanship of the American Board of Pediatrics.

REFERENCES

1. DeAngelis CD *Pediatric Primary Care*, 3rd ed. Boston: Little, Brown; 1984.
2. DeAngelis CD *An Introduction to Clinical Research.* New York: Oxford Univ Pres; 1990.

Physician Education and Conflict of Interest

Catherine D. DeAngelis, M.D.
Editor-in-Chief, Scientific Publications and Multimedia Publications
American Medical Association
Chicago, Illinois

The programs sponsored by medical schools and medical societies are often supported in part by unrestricted educational grants from pharmaceutical and technology companies. One major concern is the potential misuse of the CME venue to sell or promote a product rather than to educate. Such financial support is acceptable so long as the rules promulgated by the Accreditation Council for Continuing Medical Education (ACCME) are followed, that is, disclosure of potential conflicts of interest and assurance that the accredited activity is unbiased and scientifically sound. The result: better continuing education of physicians and, ultimately, better patient care.

Editors of medical journals, which provide a great deal of CME with or without CME credits, are aware that subscription income alone cannot sustain their publications. The real income is generated by advertisements, reprint sales, and some licensing fees. Pharmaceutical and technology firms purchase most advertisements, and some pay licensing fees. Again, the potential for conflict of interest weighs in heavily. Editors, authors, and reviewers must disclose personal or financial interest in any pharmaceutical company that has a role in a manuscript accepted for publication. Many studies, especially clinical trials, are funded, at least in part, by pharmaceutical companies that seek testing of drugs and publication of results. This is acceptable if journals rigidly adhere to appropriate rules regarding conflict of interest and if the companies' grants are unrestricted, so that results may be published, whether favorable or unfavorable.

Drug and technology companies spend hundreds of millions of dollars and play a vital role in developing new products and evaluating their efficacy beyond the requirements of the Food and Drug Administration's rules and regulations. In 1999, the top five pharmaceutical firms spent more than $20 billion on research, while the National Institutes of Health spent $18 billion. The firms have a right to profit from their investments and to make clinicians aware of their products, but strict ethical principles are mandatory.

The medical profession has been forced to function in a business mode when providing clinical services, but it is imperative that our educational mission not be compromised by the for-profit concept. Profits from the provision of educational services should be reinvested in educational enterprises to ensure that physicians will receive the most effective, current, and unbiased information for ministering to patients. To mask the promulgation of biased information as education rather than as promotion is to endanger the health of the public. We simply cannot allow this to happen.

9

Learning by Teaching

• • •

Men learn while they teach.
[H]omines, dum docent discunt.

SENECA[1]

The word "doctor" is from the Latin *docere,* meaning to teach. The title of "doctor" became associated with the medical profession after the 15th century, probably because only the medical doctors, of all the members of faculties, went out among the people. "Doctor," by common usage, thus became associated with medicine. Physicians often find themselves teaching patients, colleagues, other associates, and the general public. Academic physicians have primary responsibilities for teaching, but all practicing physicians have such opportunities. In our interviews, we have explored teaching as a method of learning for the physician, have elicited ways of ensuring self-education as a by-product of teaching, have reviewed the attributes of master teachers, and have discovered how practicing physicians create opportunities to teach clinical medicine.

BENEFITS OF TEACHING

"The safest thing for a patient," Charles Mayo was quoted as saying, "was to be in the hands of a man engaged in teaching medicine. In order to be a teacher of medicine the doctor must always be a student."[2] Leigh Thompson identified three ways teaching helps him to learn: "First, it stimulates me to search published material, learn new facts, and update my knowledge. Second, it forces me to organize my knowledge for my presentation. Third, it provides the opportunity for feedback from the audience." Stephen Greenberg added: "I regularly teach someone—a student, resident, fellow, or colleague—about the latest information on a given topic. Having to communicate this information requires continuously updating my own databases on various topics." Garret T. Lynch agreed: "Academicians have the advantage of learning while teaching. Questions from students compel teachers to expand their knowledge base. Teachers also learn from students who, at the bedside or during conferences, share information from their own extensive reading."

Attributes of Effective Teachers

In the words of Ralph Feigin, "The common thread through all of academic life is teaching, and although academicians may develop individual styles, anyone can learn to be an effective teacher if the desire to impart knowledge is sincere and if sufficient time and effort are invested. The motivating forces for clinical teaching are caring for and respecting trainees and being committed to their success. Caring for trainees implies being a good listener and focusing adequate effort and attention on them. An effective teacher cares about students as people beyond their training. This does not necessarily imply acceptance of all the trainees' qualities, but the teacher should encourage positive behavior and point out how certain behavior can be improved. The ideal teacher is enthusiastic, has a good sense of humor, sets standards that motivate students to do their best, and has a broad knowledge base organized in a way that the trainee readily understands.

"Respecting the trainee requires willingness to communicate by explanation as well as demonstration. Every effort should be made to answer questions satisfactorily without making the trainee feel inferior for having posed the question. Ensuring the success of the trainee requires the teacher to have a clear and explicit expectation that is communicated to the trainee. Teaching is important to me because it stimulates me to pursue new knowledge continually and to grow professionally. I generally learn something from every new teaching experience."

In addition to knowledge of one's discipline, Joseph Van Der Meulen listed the following attributes of outstanding teachers: "They must be able to abstract the essentials from a subject and present them in an organized and interesting way. They should be able to accommodate their pacing to the complexity of the subject. They should be receptive to constructive criticism, be adaptable to change, and remain current. They must be sensitive to the needs of the audience and to its receptivity. Sensitivity is probably innate; I doubt that it can be acquired, but the other attributes can be acquired by experience and constructive feedback."

"An outstanding clinical teacher," said Clifton Cleaveland, "shows a profound regard and empathy for each patient seen on teaching rounds. A second attribute is a dedication to upgrading and renewing one's own fund of clinical information. A third is the ability to stimulate open, frank, nonthreatening communication with house staff and students."

For William Waters, the compulsion to share new learning, insights, and revelations is the competent teacher's primary attribute. "Other qualifications include verbalism, enthusiasm, intellectualism, warm feelings for students, and—not by any means least—brains. Most of these can be developed by example and experience."

Edwin Overholt emphasized "intellectual honesty, high intelligence, enthusiasm, attention to detail, and a joy in interacting with one's colleagues. A teacher must respect his colleagues. The help that an outstanding teacher can give his colleagues and his house staff is the ultimate reward. Teachers should encourage young physicians with a potential for teaching to pursue such a career. Exposure to an outstanding teacher is a great motivator." The opportunity to give case presentations and literature reviews, with constructive comments from their teachers, is extremely valuable to house officers.

A good teacher should possess enthusiasm, self-discipline, and the ability to transmit ideas with clarity, humor, and intelligence. The teacher must show respect and sympathy for students without pandering to sloppiness of thought or performance.

Teachers must know the subject from all standpoints, according to Leigh Thompson, including personal involvement in research and practice. "They must present the right amount of information in the right sequence with the right timing and the right graphics."

One phenomenon that is clearly a handicap, according to Thomas Burns, is a large information differential between teacher and audience. "We all know people with a great fund of knowledge who are barely able to impart any of it to their peers, let alone to house staff or medical students. On the other hand, information seems to flow readily from house officers to medical students and from senior students to their juniors. A common characteristic among great teachers in medicine is an ability to uncover the learning receptors of students so as not to impede the flow of information down the gradient."

Olga Jonasson noted a change in the role of medical teachers: "They are encouraged not to teach, but to inspire students to seek out information they want and need. The hope is that this pattern of self-teaching will become a habit that will produce lifelong learning."

"A common mistake made by those in medical education," said Thorpe Ray, "is assuming that events such as graduation from medical school and completion of residency or fellowship mark the end of something. In reality, they mark the beginning of a career of perpetual study. The recent graduate should be prepared for his clinical training program, and the finishing resident should be prepared for his lifelong study. By this time, the habit of critical reading should have been established, as well as the self-evaluation and honest self-criticism that are essential for continued intellectual growth and maintenance of clinical skills. The source of useful knowledge and information for the physician is often self-instruction. Teachers help most by establishing sound reasoning and a disciplined approach to clinical problems. A good teacher should clearly demonstrate an approach that identifies the patient as an important and interesting person. The best teachers demonstrate that medicine is fun and learning is fun. They stimulate and attract students of medicine at all stages. Sometimes the manner of doing or saying something determines whether it will be remembered by students."

"Not all teaching experiences are pleasant or funny," according to Linda Clever. "I remember two nameless professors. They 'led' by bad example—and no one emulated them. The first asked the patient in a rheumatology clinic if she 'had any trouble with your tempero-mandibular joint.' Her puzzled look spoke volumes and reminded us to use lay language. The other professor asked an endocrine patient at grand rounds, 'How long have you looked like a frog?' Humiliation is never humorous, nor does it put anyone at ease."

John Askey recalled the words of a mentor at the University of Pennsylvania, O. H. Perry Pepper, who advised him one day as they rode to Pepper's home for an afternoon of tennis, "John, always have an 'arbeit.' " Askey remembers Pepper as a great stimulator who considered the main qualities of an investigator to be "the simplicity to wonder, the ability to question, the power to generalize, and the capacity to apply." At 86, Askey said that the virus for keeping him in contact with medicine continued.

Full-time Faculty

The teaching principles described by physicians in academia are equally applicable to the practicing physician.

"To me, teaching is essential for learning," said Saul Farber. "Throughout my adult life I have learned mainly through teaching. You learn a great deal from your students while trying to impart knowledge to them. I never go into a teaching session without being prepared. No matter how many times I present lobar pneumonia to medical students, I always read something about that subject the night before, and I never fail to learn something that I had not known before or to gain a new insight that had not occurred to me before, as, for example, about pathophysiology. When I return from a teaching session or rounds, I look up things that I think I should have known or try to find the answer to a question that has arisen. Preparation before and catch-up after the sessions have been very useful and extremely enjoyable."

The importance of preparation was impressed on Ralph Wallerstein during his training under William Castle, whose work on intrinsic and extrinsic factors in pernicious anemia led to the fundamental understanding of that disease. Late one night, Wallerstein noticed a light in Castle's office and, entering to say hello, found him busy studying and writing a presentation on pernicious anemia to be given to medical students. The fact that Castle, an international expert on pernicious anemia, felt it necessary to prepare for a lecture to students left a strong impression on Wallerstein.

As Lloyd Smith noted, "The subject matter of medicine is so vast that no one can master more than a part of it. Moreover, what we learn is eroded by new insights from basic and clinical research. One's most cherished aphorisms are continually being disproved by indisputable facts. Teaching requires a reappraisal of one's beliefs, a 'loosening of certainties,' as Will Durant said. You must defend your ideas once more both to yourself and, more important, to those being taught. Most of my teaching is done on ward rounds rather than as formal lectures. Fortunately, young people are remarkably forgiving of one's knowledge lacunae and are willing to play to one's strengths, if they can be found. This assumes that the teacher has a genuine interest in medicine (it cannot be feigned), is humble before the facts, and is a reasonable and secure master of ceremonies who brings out the best in all who participate in the complex sociology of ward rounds.

"When one is caught off base, which happens to all clinical teachers, it is imperative (a) to admit it, (b) to praise those who are better informed, and (c) to return the next day better prepared on the subject. Even when the clinical teacher is not well informed about a specific problem, he must remember that education is what is left when he has forgotten the facts. His personal interaction with the patient or general approach to the problem may be of more permanent value to those being taught than his instant recall of statistics and references."

Physicians should never be reluctant to acknowledge their limitations of knowledge, as one student learned from Julius Bauer. According to Samuel Rapaport, the student was presenting a case on rounds. He was doing very well, even as the questions got harder and harder. Finally, Bauer asked a question to which the student replied: "I am sorry, Dr. Bauer; I knew the answer to that question but I have forgotten it." Bauer countered: "I am sorry too, for you were the only person in the world who knew the answer to that question."

"The best self-education for clinical teachers is to remain conversant within a broad sweep of medical problems by being on the firing line frequently," said Lloyd Smith. "Preferably, they should teach in a way that encourages questions and alternative approaches. Unless their intellectual epiphyses have already closed, this approach will inevitably lead to their growth as teachers, physicians, and human beings."

"Multiple heads are far more important and productive than one head," in Saul Farber's experience. "No matter how uninformed a medical student or house officer is about a particular subject, his insight and curiosity often disclose an aspect of the situation that the teacher was unaware of." Arthur Fox pointed to yet another advantage of teaching: "Teaching demands knowledge of facts and communication skills. If one does not communicate ideas clearly, the loss of interest or the confusion of students and house staff is quickly apparent. If they are bright and aggressive, they will tell you when they do not understand or when they disagree. I learn from the bright young people who show me when I have not martialed my facts. Then I go back and read further to prove points."

The most important point, for William Waters, is never to give the same lecture twice. "Throw away your notes and start from scratch: reread, rethink, reorganize. The result is relearning, new learning, better information, new insights, and, of course, a much more spontaneous, enthusiastic lecture, seminar, or rounds." The technique that works for Marvin Turck is to "think of the two particular points that are clinically most relevant after I have read something, listened to a seminar, or interacted in a consultation. I then try to use those two points in teaching."

Ralph Haymond advised physicians "to associate with students with inquisitive minds, for they will stimulate you to keep current, even if only to avoid embarrassment. And if you never teach, you can assemble all the information you would need for a lecture, as a method of reviewing your own knowledge of a topic." Robert Manning's words summarized the consensus: "The old rule that you don't know something until you can teach it has a lot of validity."

Full-time Practitioners

For those near medical schools, a teaching appointment is invaluable in keeping up with new knowledge. Serving on the voluntary clinical faculty of a medical school may be an economic hardship, but it prevents obsolescence. "After World War II," related Rodney Rodgers, "I returned to three years of residency in medicine at Philadelphia General Hospital. I found myself shockingly ignorant, but was obliged to teach interns and medical students. The training was largely clinical and highly integrated with patient care. I spent all my spare time answering specific questions that arose while teaching house staff. It took six months of hard work before I caught up from my two years away from education. I resolved then to practice in a town with a medical school, to which I would volunteer my teaching services so as never to allow myself to decay again."

Physicians who practice at some distance from medical schools can still teach in local hospitals, as Alan Gordon does by conducting morbidity and mortality conferences. Although Richard Field has literally had to go to great lengths to maintain his ties with medical schools, it has allowed him to bring up-to-date general surgery to his community. As an Associate Professor at Tulane University and at the University of Mississippi School of Medicine, both of which are 100 miles away, he attends grand rounds and teaches students one day a month.

"The most important aspect of teaching," according to Saul Farber, "is the security of knowledge of the teacher. People in practice can feel secure by preparing in advance, and they can become as outstanding teachers as full-time academicians."

"Questions from students often point to inadequacy in your own knowledge," noted Sidney Howard. "Then pride forces you to update your information."

"The practitioner, perhaps without giving himself full credit, does a great deal of teaching and learning every day," said James Wyngaarden. "The kind of learning that appeals to me is that in which the roles of student and teacher are mixed, each learning from the other while working toward a shared objective. This is the kind that takes place on the wards with patients and in the laboratory with fellows. The mere transfer of information is certainly necessary to establish a joint knowledge base, but the kind of learning that is the most fun and the kind of teaching that is the most fun involve participatory collaboration." Major Bradshaw would like to capture the knowledge, experience, and skills of physicians who have retired, some at an early age, because of their disenchantment with managed care, but are unhappy about abandoning a profession that they clearly enjoy and find fulfilling. Bradshaw would like to find some mechanism to reimburse outstanding retired physicians for malpractice insurance, licensure fees, society membership dues, modest travel expenses, and the like. In return, the physicians would teach at a designated clinic or hospital for one-half day five days a week six months each year. These Senior Clinical Educators could teach, by word and example, the basics of professionalism, the importance of establishing rapport with the patient, and the skills of history-taking and physical examinations.

For James Young, working on projects and writing manuscripts are the best form of education. "I concentrate my continuing medical education activities on writing a variety of manuscripts, books, and book chapters and on creating other educational packages, such as video conferences, education slide lecture sets, and cyber sessions. My lectures, however, have been most valuable to me; while creating presentations that are educational and entertaining for others, I paradoxically learn the most. If I enjoy my own lecture and learn something new from it, I consider it a successful venture and don't give undue attention to criticism received from the audience. Nor do I take seriously compliments about presentations that I think miss the mark. Although this kind of continuing medical education is often considered to be solely the realm of academicians, I consider myself first a clinician. I believe that any clinician can pursue education in this way, and some of the most thoughtful and intriguing presentations I have heard have been by clinicians rather than academicians."

Writing and Speaking Richard Field liked to prepare at least one paper each year. "I usually invite a colleague to be a co-author. We try to stimulate our thinking and share anything we consider useful by publishing it. The writing is a wonderful learning experience, as is the presentation of exhibits at state medical meetings and at the American College of Surgeons' clinical congresses." Meeting interesting people and the pleasure of traveling are added benefits.

Teaching the Office Staff As James Wyngaarden noted, "The practitioner must do a great deal of teaching when interacting with patients, nurses, physical therapists, or other hospital staff. The physician must not be unduly impressed by rank; the concept of rank is one of the greatest deterrents to learning."

Brian Goodell, who has participated in in-service training sessions in community hospitals in his area, pointed to the reduction in turnover rate and the improved communication such sessions provide. "We make sure that the nurses have access to nursing journals in the library. I encourage them to give me articles from these publications because they are often very practical."

One of the provisions of employment for nurses in Richard Parkinson's office is participation in a continuing education program. "I devote about one-half hour three days a week to continuing education. The program, which consists of a review of basic science and clinical medicine, forced me to review all the subject material. The first nurse who came to work for me was an LVN whom I assisted in obtaining her RN license, and who, after further training, was able to pass the physician's assistant examination with a high mark. Another medical assistant who handled the business end of my practice was so fascinated by that nurse's progress that she entered the field of nursing. She is currently working on her nursing degree, and I try to keep ahead of her and to discuss with her the clinical significance of our cases."

* * * * *

The very nature of medicine requires that physicians be teachers. Teaching is an impetus for study; it requires the teacher to acquire, review, and organize the knowledge to be taught. In good teaching, teachers are also learners, and exchanges of ideas, challenges, and feedback make learning a lively affair.

The distinguished teachers we interviewed all stressed the importance of preparation. None was willing to rely totally on memory. The practicing physician who has the opportunity to teach will profit immeasurably from the experience. Those without access to medical school teaching services will benefit from participating in hospital staff meetings and from teaching nurses and office staff. Informal discussions are also an excellent way to gain knowledge. Physicians who devote time to teaching their patients will be amply rewarded by improved cooperation.

REFERENCES

1. Sénèque. *Lettres à Lucilius,* Tome I, text established by François Préchac and translated by Henri Noblot. Paris: Société d'Édition "Les Belles Lettres," 1945:21.
2. Mayo, CH. Quoted in: *Proc Staff Meetings Mayo Clinic.* 1927;2:233.

10

Analysis of Practice

• • •

> We physicians had need be a self-confronting and a self-reproving race; for we must be ready, without fear or favour, to call in question our own Experience and to judge it justly; to confirm it, to repeal it, to reverse it. . . .
>
> PETER MERE LATHAM[1]

We have long believed that the best needs-assessment for continuing education for physicians derives from practice analysis. Our lengthy interviews with practicing physicians have yielded a number of effective methods used to study individual practices and profit maximally from experience. Many used index cards and ledgers to note patient problems seen, treatments prescribed, and outcomes obtained; some recorded lessons learned from puzzling patients; and others studied their mistakes. All were dedicated physicians who developed methods to advance their learning from their clinical experience. The concepts they related continue to be valid and important today, although the computer has now replaced pen and paper for the recording and manipulation of data. Whether physicians view data electronically tallied and presented on a computer screen or manually recorded, sorted, and stacked on index cards, the information allows physicians to use their clinical experience to improve patient care. In fact, physicians developing such analytic methods should probably lay out their approach with pen and paper before selecting appropriate software.

It is the *concept* of practice analysis that we wish to encourage. We have noted that managed-care organizations, which include many practicing physicians today, produce data for billing and cost-containment that can also be used for practice analysis. Physicians should begin to look at those same data to identify knowledge deficits and to plan their educational activities as a means of improving patient outcomes.

William Budd's duties as a country doctor permitted him to make observations and collect evidence that typhoid fever was a communicable disease.[2] William Pickles tried to stimulate other country doctors to keep records of epidemic diseases: "We country practitioners are in a position to supply facts from our observation of nature, and it is, I feel most strongly, our plain duty to make use of this unique opportunity."[3] Sir James Mackenzie believed that research in the physician's office was a necessity, for the general practitioner "has opportunities which no other worker possesses—opportunities which are necessary to the solution of problems essential to the advance of medicine."[4]

In 1879, following an undistinguished career as a medical student, Mackenzie entered general practice in a small English town. "About 1883 or 1884," he wrote, "I resolved to begin a series of careful observations entirely for my own improvement, never dreaming of research, for I was under the prevalent belief that medical research could only be undertaken in a laboratory or, at least, in an [sic] hospital with all the appurtenances. I merely sought to find out something about the nature of my patients' complaints . . . . I had thus placed before me two definite objects, at which to aim: (1) understanding of the mechanism of symptoms, and (2) understanding of their prognostic significance. When . . . I look back upon my work, I can recognize that it was this simple resolution and these definite aims which guided me to such success as I have achieved. . . ." Mackenzie's detailed records of patients with heart disease enabled him to become one of the leading heart specialists of his time, and a pioneer in symptomatology.

The study and analysis of practice give physicians a reliable perspective and a formal record of their own work, thus permitting them to profit maximally from lessons learned. This, we think, is the most rewarding kind of continuing education.

The practice of medicine can and should be a scholarly and intellectual process. "The only way I have found to do that," said Warren Williams, "is through the study of the practice itself. I tried to develop my practice by emulating my medical school professors, who seemed to know exactly what they were doing. When I first started my practice, it seemed to be one sore throat after another, getting people in and getting people out. It was not intellectually stimulating until I started my practice study and analysis." John Fry found that simple, inexpensive methods of recording, reviewing, and analyzing everyday work not only yield better services, but add immeasurably to his enjoyment of medicine. Thus, practice analysis not only delivers the most benefit to physicians from their experience, but also heightens their zest for their work through greater immersion and more focused direction for future study. These advantages increase the likelihood of improving patient services and enriching professional life.

Physicians may organize their practice for study by:

- indexing patient charts by clinical problem, to permit a critique of aggregate experience in specific conditions;
- keeping statistics on the problems seen, drugs prescribed, and laboratory studies ordered;
- compiling and classifying salient clinical features observed in specific problems, diseases, and procedures, and recording mistakes and lessons learned;

- performing an audit of patient records;
- tracking, and reacting to, patient outcome;

All of these are facilitated by electronic technology.

INDEXING PATIENT CHARTS BY PROBLEM

John Fry kept a card index of all patients diagnosed with certain diseases, which permitted him to calculate incidence/prevalence rates and facilitated follow-up reviews on patients with particular diseases. He also collected the following sets of data: (1) day sheets that recorded all physician–patient contacts by patient's name, age, sex, diagnostic group, and referrals for studies or consultation, and (2) an age–sex register that provided the current population at risk. His studies enabled him to reduce his volume of work per patient and therefore to treat more patients, to lower his prescribing costs, and to minimize his referrals to consultants. It took him a few seconds per consultation to record the data, and a secretary entered the data weekly into a ledger. Fry's analyses of these data led him to be more conservative in the use of antibiotics,[6] and his studies of emotional disorders, acute back pain, hay fever, and hypertension in his practice prompted changes in treatment of these patients.[7] This recording system allowed him to set down his long-term experience in following patients in family practice, and the disease index provided information that led to his book *Common Diseases.*[8]

William Cooper has kept an index of all his patients categorized by disease. "If I read an article that does not quite agree with my recollection of my clinical experience, I can use the index to review my patients and compare my experience with the author's view."

Warren Williams once listed patients' names on cards by diagnosis so he could pull specific conditions for study. Each 5-by-8-inch file card was labeled with the name and code number of a disease, according to the *International Classification of Diseases, 9th Revision, Clinical Modification* (ICD 9CM). "Simply recording this information made me pay attention to details and ask certain questions that I had never before considered, such as: What is a 'problem'? What is worthy of being indexed? It was an intellectual process that had not been alive in me before." He also found his cards useful in constructing a practice profile. "Some years ago, I asked my receptionists to tabulate patients by their particular clinical problems while I was away at a cardiology meeting. On my return, I found a completed practice profile on my desk. Aside from smoking and obesity, the most frequent diagnosis was depression. I then searched for cardiology, and found it to represent less than one percent of my patients. It dawned on me that this was a beautiful tool to define the postgraduate education I required. I had not attended a single psychiatric meeting or read a psychiatric journal, and yet depression was one of the most common problems I encountered. I realized that if I wanted to do the most for my patients, I had better enroll in some psychiatric programs. Until then, I had been concentrating on subjects I liked, and now I had a tool for a more practical approach."

His original 5-by-8-inch cards have been replaced by more versatile and powerful computer systems, but he continues to benefit from maintaining his practice database. "I am now on the medical staff at St. Joseph's Community Health Center in Hillsboro, Wisconsin, a 10-bed hospital with an attached 65-bed nursing home, where I am the Medical Director. My office practice is about ten miles away in Elroy, a slightly larger town of 1300. I have been using Excel™ for cross-indexing during the past few years because it is fairly intuitive and easy to use. I can enter information myself, but retrieving data from Excel is laborious, at least at my level of expertise. Microsoft Access™ is much more sophisticated and has wonderful retrieval possibilities, but I have not had time to learn the fine points of programming it. I have hired a programmer to set up a customized version of Access, specifically to cross-index my patients, including the usual demographic data, diagnoses, medications, referrals, and procedures. I hope to be able to download into Access the data in the various Excel files so that they will not be lost or need to be reentered.

"I now cross-index not only the problem list or diagnoses, but also medications, including short-term medications, such as antibiotics. This addition has proved useful. The Food and Drug Administration (FDA) has removed previously approved medications from the formulary on several occasions, and I have been able to retrieve the names of all my patients who were taking those drugs, either by my direction or a consultant's, and advise them to discontinue the medication.

"It has also been helpful for me to have the medication cross-indexed because of the close relationship I have with Scott Larson, a young academic-minded pharmacist at our hospital. We discuss and review medications for the hospital and nursing home patients daily, and I use that information and his expertise in my office practice. The Palm Pilot™, with the drug information database ePocrates™ and the infectious disease database qID, also from ePocrates, along with the indexing, keeps me out of trouble. I maintain a list of all my hospital and nursing home patients on the Palm Pilot™, along with the clinical problem list and medication list. The drug interaction program from ePocrates is run monthly on each patient's medication list. The cross-index list of clinical problems continues to be helpful in the evaluation of my practice profile and answers the important question: What am I seeing, and where do I need to concentrate my continuing medical education to improve the quality of care for my patients?

"At the Swedish Hospital in Colorado, we would close the office and call in a consultant for our own Grand Rounds once a month. Using the diagnosis index, we assembled the records of patients with a specific problem and went through them with the consultant. We asked certain patients to be present for these sessions, and they loved it. The whole staff participated, and as a result we changed our ways of doing things, including more effective use of certain drugs and better patient education. We always asked the consultant for a composite, constructively critical written report on the Grand Rounds. Since we closed the office for a half day and paid the consultant, we lost income on that day, but this intellectual part of the practice was both enjoyable and instructive. The information gained in our Grand Rounds was 100 percent applicable to our practice, and the patients ultimately benefited.

"In my current practice, I plan to ask consultants at my primary referral centers, the University of Wisconsin and the Mayo Clinic, to participate in our Grand Rounds. I am getting to know a few of the consultants, some of whom are energetic and willing to teach an old dog new tricks. Physicians at both institutions have been helpful in giving their time for telephone consultations.

"The most difficult issue for me, here in rural practice, is the loss of immediate consultative help. A consultation at Swedish Hospital simply required someone to come up one floor or down two to see a patient, but here it means a helicopter ride or an hour-and-a-half ambulance ride. A consultation for an ambulatory patient requires a two-and-a-half-hour drive by car to the Mayo Clinic or an hour-and-a-half drive to Madison, and many of my patients are just not willing or able to do this. So the telephone consultation, which is not only documented in the record but is also cross-indexed in the computer, has been a boon. I am impressed with the willingness of the various distinguished physicians at these great institutions to help me on a moment's notice and without compensation. This is a view of medicine that the general public does not always see."

KEEPING STATISTICS ON CLINICAL PROBLEMS, MEDICATIONS, AND LABORATORY STUDIES

The Need

Through extensive work in identifying educational needs in physicians' offices, S. E. Sivertson and Thomas Meyer found that the average physician really did not know what his practice constituted. Said Sivertson, "Early in our work, we asked some physicians to predict their practice profile. They were unable to do it accurately. They were so far off, in fact, that we could not use their predictions to help plan their continuing education. The physician frequently told the consultant: 'This is the first time I have understood my practice and how my continuing education should be related to it.' In addition, older physicians would say, 'My practice and I are growing old together. I need to focus more on geriatrics.' "

In an experiment to see if feedback about ambulatory practice would influence the behavior of an internal medicine house staff, Reid and Lantz found that only 50 percent of resident physicians could correctly guess the relative frequency of types of patients they saw.[9]

Jeremiah Barondess kept a detailed record of patient visits in his practice. "For three months I kept track of the reason for each patient's visit along with the diagnosis. In nearly a thousand office visits over three months there were only two instances of nephrologic disease and five of hematologic disease, whereas nearly 350 patients had cardiovascular disease. There were relatively few gastrointestinal or infectious problems of major consequence." Every physician can profit from this type of study.

Aggregate data that permit analysis of the problems seen, drugs prescribed, and laboratory studies ordered facilitate the study of practice. If physicians also know the costs they generate, the time they spend with patients, and the reasons for their consultation requests and hospital admissions, they can improve their practice management. Managed-care organizations capture clinical data on individual practices when they compile claims data. If these are distributed for education and not for cost-saving alone, they will simplify data collection for physicians. "The effect of managed care on a physician's continuing education and lifelong learning," said Garrett Lynch, "has been a two-edged sword, albeit chiefly a negative one. The increased paperwork and telephone approvals for testing can drastically cut into the time physicians have to read, study, or attend conferences. The demands to see more and more patients for briefer and briefer periods has curtailed the time available to seek specific information during a patient encounter. One positive effect of managed care, however, has been the creation and implementation of patient guidelines, which permit physicians to keep abreast of current diagnosis and therapeutics for a specific disease."

Recording the Data

Cumulative data permit a description of practice activities, identification of patients with particular conditions for further study, description of patterns of laboratory test-ordering, and listing of medications prescribed. From such cumulative data, you can analyze your practice and compare it to similar practices in published reports as well as to local and national standards. You may find, perhaps with the help of consultants, that you are diagnosing certain conditions more often, or less often, than other physicians are. Such a finding would not necessarily mean that you are at fault, but might signal a need to reevaluate the implicit or explicit diagnostic criteria being used. If you are prescribing certain medications more, or less, than your peers are, it may be wise to learn more about these drugs, their efficacy, side effects, and contraindications.

You must, of course, be careful not to overestimate the significance of a small series of observations, which may help physicians focus on their practice, but should not give a false sense of security when the incidence of harmful effects may become apparent only in a large series. The compilation of outcome figures, however, is still useful because it allows physicians to compare their results with those of a larger series.

NOTATION OF SALIENT CLINICAL PROBLEMS

To facilitate learning from experience, some physicians keep notes on patients with certain problems, recording unusual manifestations, the value of certain laboratory studies, the effect of treatments, and lessons learned, so their cumulative experience can be coordinated and reviewed. From an analysis of the patient data Paul Dudley White recorded on 4-by-6-inch cards, he was able to determine the frequency of rheumatic heart disease and hypertension, among other conditions, and this information formed the basis of his first book. (See Reflections by Willis Hurst, pp. 43–56.)

For many years, Norton Greenberger used cards to keep notes on patients and to remind himself to read published reports about certain interesting diagnoses. He now uses the computer to record patient data, including the patient's name, hospital number, and major diagnosis or problems. When he reads pertinent articles, he abstracts them in a format that is suitable for slides and then downloads the abstracted material onto a floppy disk can use on PowerPoint™ software.

Telfer Reynolds categorizes his cards by disease. "We have thousands of cards in the file, divided into two sets: one comprising the consultations made by residents on my service and the other the cases I have seen personally. Any time a question arises about a particular disease, we can pull out 40 or 50 cards and spend a half hour sorting them. It is not real research—you would have to go to the charts to get the full data—but they often answer a question quickly on the basis of our past few years' experience. If I were starting today, I would use the computer to store more legible notes on instructive cases."

A valuable asset in clinical practice, in the opinion of Walter Somerville, is a memory aid to assemble the physician's personal experience in specific diseases or procedures. "The data cards originated by Paul Wood (Figure 1) are designed to tabulate the main features of selected conditions or procedures. A comparison of this information in the aggregate with the reported experience of others leads to logical decision-making. For example, salient features of each candidate of percutaneous transluminal coronary angioplasty (PTCA) are annotated by hand. Time-consuming minutiae are left to the detailed case record. Within weeks, impressions emerge, eventually to be confirmed or discarded. Keeping records like this helps the physician draw on his entire experience rather than only the past few cases."

Notes on Experience

Since her medical student days, Celia Oakley has kept notes on what she learned during the day. "As a student, this was a considerable amount, but I had the time and the inclination to review what I had written. Now I am busier, but I still jot down the things that I learn each day."

Bruce Zawacki noted in his diary any problem that arose in the course of practice or during presentations, after which he looked up material on the subject. Robert Smith records in a little book notes on his surgical patients, especially any unusual aspects of the operation. "I also record my contacts with the referring physicians, to make sure that we keep a good exchange and that I dictate letters. I can get about six months' use out of one book. I carry the book with me everywhere except the shower. With the pressure of all the administrative and patient-care duties I have, if I don't make notes and outline each day's schedule the evening before, I am apt to forget something. The diary has become my auxiliary brain. I really couldn't function

Form No. M598 PTCA SPECIMEN

NO.	NAME	S. AGE	PLACE	AP	MI	EX Test	L Main	AD	CX	RC				E.C.G.	X RAY	PTCA RESULT
1	SAKI	M/60	P	2	+	+	–	+	+	+				Ant MI	+	+
2	MANT	M/50	H	3	O	+	–	O	+	+				Inf MI	O	+
3	GOODS-BECK	F/65	H	3	+	+	+	O	O	+				N	O	–
4																
5																
6																
7																
8																
9																
10																

FIGURE 1. Card originated by Paul Wood and used by Walter Somerville to tabulate clinical data on patients having percutaneous transluminal coronary angioplasty. Clinical data can be similarly tabulated for patients with clinical conditions of particular interest. AP, angina pectoris; MI, myocardial infarction; EX Test, exercise test; L Main, left main coronary artery; AD, left anterior descending coronary artery; CX, left circumflex coronary artery; RC, right coronary artery.

without it. For our Grand Rounds or our weekly vascular conferences at Emory, it is also useful to look back through the book and quickly select a half-dozen interesting and unusual cases." Some physicians prefer a PDA device over the notebook.

Learning from Mistakes

Osler advised physicians to record their mistakes: "Begin early to make a threefold category—clear cases, doubtful cases, mistakes. And learn to play the game fair, no self-deception, no shrinking from the truth; mercy and consideration for the other man, but none for yourself, upon whom you have to keep an incessant watch. . . . It is only by getting your cases grouped in this way that you can make any real progress in your post-collegiate education; only in this way can you gain wisdom with experience. It is a common error to think that the more a doctor sees the greater his experience and the more he knows."[10]

Jane Somerville considers her study of mistakes to be the single most useful exercise she has undertaken. In the current climate of medical litigiousness, records of mistakes may be subpoenaed and used punitively. As a result, most physicians are now reluctant to record mistakes as such, just as, in the U.S. government, Presidents and their staffs do not like to preserve notes for fear that they will be subpoenaed.

TRACING AND REACTING TO OUTCOMES

Without a specific mechanism for follow-up, physicians are often unaware of the therapeutic results in their patients. In this sense, they know less about their practice and their performance than a football coach knows about the performance of players and their opponents. "Without statistics, we would be unable to maintain a high level of performance," said Tom Landry, former head coach of the Dallas Cowboys. "We use a quality control system to monitor our football team, that is, we set guidelines for our individual player's performance as well as for our team performance. Our quality-control coach accumulates all the data and alerts the staff when performance levels are below guidelines. We are then able to make adjustments to prevent possible losses in future games. Our most vivid results come when we fall into a slump late in the season. We then concentrate on weaknesses and apply proper adjustments. This usually corrects the weaknesses and returns us to the winning path. Without statistics, however, we would not be able to identify the problems."

Coach Joseph Paterno of Pennsylvania State University also found that recording and analyzing data are invaluable. "We do not practice without a doctor on the field. He records in a diary everything that happens at each practice. We keep a record of the temperature, the type of drills, the number of injuries, and so on. We can tell if more injuries occur when we scrimmage two days in a row or when we have a one- or two-day break between scrimmages. If we are having more sprained ankles than usual, we can review our records and compare the current year with past seasons. Statistics help us keep our team healthy. I use medical statistics to make determinations about equipment, style of practice, type of drills, and when not to practice.

"We also use statistics on the performance of other teams to determine their tendencies and therefore our best strategy in certain field positions and at certain downs. We are constantly reviewing our computer kickout for a better evaluation of the other team."

Medicine is admittedly more complicated than athletic enterprises, but the analogy illustrates the value of analyzing one's performance. Once problems are identified, solutions can be sought. A study of results requires a routine method of tracing patient outcomes.

E. A. Codman was a strong advocate of the "End Result System." "In brief," he wrote in 1918, "it is this: That the Trustees of Hospitals should see to it that an effort is made to follow up each patient [the staff treats], long enough to determine whether the treatment given has permanently relieved the condition or symptoms complained of.

That they should give the members of the Staff credit for taking the responsibility of successful treatment and promote them accordingly. Likewise they should see that all cases in which the treatment is found to have been unsuccessful or unsatisfactory are carefully analyzed, in order to fix the responsibility for failure on:

1. The physician or surgeon responsible for the treatment.
2. The organization carrying out the detail of the treatment.
3. The disease or condition of the patient.
4. The personal or social conditions preventing the cooperation of the patient.

This will give a definite basis on which to make effort at improvement. . . .

"The Idea is so simple as to seem childlike. . . . It is simply to follow the natural series of questions which any one asks in an individual case:

What was the matter?

Did they find it out beforehand?

Did the patient get entirely well?

If not—why not?

Was it the fault of the surgeon, the disease, or the patient?

What can we do to prevent similar failures in the future?

"We believe that the general acceptance of a system of hospital organization based on the truthful record of the answers to these questions means the beginning of True Clinical Science."[11]

Some surgeons send questionnaires to their patients at intervals of three, six, or 12 months to determine the success or limitations of their procedures. Michael DeBakey writes to his patients or the referring physicians at regular intervals to inquire about their progress.

From his analysis of results so obtained, he has been able not only to monitor and report on his clinical experience continually, but to recognize certain patterns of disease that have led him to devise new surgical treatments, such as excision of aneurysms, coronary artery bypass, and others.

Bruce Zawacki maintained an alphabetized file of operative notes, supplemented with review articles on new techniques. "Before performing a procedure not done regularly, I use this file to review my experience and the articles I have collected. I also often present a particularly difficult preoperative case at a regular medical school conference. At our monthly mortality and morbidity conference, invited guests critique our approach, and we review any untoward events. We identify problems, plan solutions, and assign certain physicians to implement those solutions. Yearly, we have an outcome review, in which our current mortality and morbidity data are compared to those of all previous years for possible trends."

Gustavo Kuster sends every surgical patient a follow-up letter or questionnaire six months after the operation and every year thereafter. "I have about 20 different kinds of questionnaires, coded according to the operative procedure. These questionnaires allow me to be precise in answering questions about our operations and to improve my patient care. Through the questionnaires, for example, I found that in repair of hiatal hernia, it was postoperative bloating that made the patients most unhappy. I reviewed this technique more carefully, visited other medical institutions, and then modified my techniques slightly by making the fundal plication extremely loose around the esophagus. That practically eliminated the unpleasant side effects of the procedure."

We have given examples of recording elements of practice experience on index cards, as ledger book entries, and as tabulations on a chart to crystallize the concepts. Current computer software simplifies data entry and access, and new products are continually being introduced. When searching for software, you should ensure that the functions described in this section are available.

ENLISTING HELP IN THE ANALYSIS OF PRACTICE

> Nothing is so difficult to deal with as a man's own Experience, how to value it according to its amount, what to conclude from it, and how to use it and do good with it.
>
> PETER MERE LATHAM[12]

Most people find it threatening to have their work reviewed. For professionals, the threat may be real, since society often judges their shortcomings harshly, resulting in regulatory, even punitive, solutions. A few physicians may, indeed, require regulatory sanctions, and all can benefit from reminders of their errors of omission and commission. Careful, constructive analysis of events in practice can motivate physicians to continue their education, whereas draconian penalties may drive some underground. The data on their practices then become unreliable, and the opportunity to profit from experience is lost. We distinguish clearly between formal external quality-assurance mechanisms and the improvement in medical practice that ensues from a well-motivated physician's voluntary analysis of personal practice.

One byproduct of managed care is the collection of information on individual practice from claims data. Most managed-care organizations can supply physicians with information on the sex ratio and predominant age group of patients seen, the most prevalent ICD9 diagnoses made and procedures performed, and, in some cases, the medications most frequently prescribed. Unfortunately, these statistics are not always presented to the physician, but they do provide an outstanding opportunity to study, and gain from, one's clinical experience, especially when physicians discuss the statistics with peers.

The National Committee for Quality Assurance (NCQA), an independent nonprofit organization, evaluates and reports on the quality of managed-care organizations in the United States through the Health Plan Employer Data and Information Set (HEDIS).[13] HEDIS collects information for the Health Care Financing Administration (HCFA) and audits five domains to assess the quality of a health plan, including effectiveness of care, as measured by such HEDIS standards as breast-cancer screening, beta-blocker treatment after a heart attack, and eye examinations for diabetes. Other markers assess access/availability of care, health-plan stability, use of services, and information on the Board certification of participating physicians. The study of practice has been enhanced by HEDIS.

John Walther practices in an HMO in Ohio, a professional corporation of some 50 physicians, which decided to have its medical records scrutinized for compliance with various quality indicators of HEDIS. As an incentive, the group agreed that 20 percent of their salary would depend on compliance with the various quality indicators and the other 80 percent on production (the number of patients seen). Of the portion related to quality, 35 percent concerns accurate and complete coding, defined by the 1999 HCFA Coding Guidelines, and 20 percent concerns quality of outcomes. For simplification of the audit, one disease is selected each month. For example, the Internal Medicine/Family Practice audit in January might be: "Is the patient with diabetes assessed yearly for microalbuminuria?" and in February: "Is the patient with a diagnosis of congestive heart failure prescribed an angiotensin converting enzyme (ACE) inhibitor?"

Another 15 percent of the quality evaluation is concerned with preventive medicine, including the following items:

- mammograms every two years for women age 50–70 years,
- Pap smears every three years for women age 20–65 years,
- colorectal screening yearly after age 50 years,
- flu vaccine yearly after age 65 years,
- tetanus every 10 years after age 18 years.

Other quality criteria relate to proper recording: 10 percent for diagnosis sheets; 10 percent for medication sheets; 5 percent for vital signs and for minutes patients waited to see physicians (threshold 30 minutes or less), and 5 percent for attendance at site quality meetings. The audit is conducted by a full-time registered nurse with a rank just under the vice-presidency.

The system encourages Walther to check more carefully on the patient's diagnostic criteria and therapy. For example, if he is seeing a patient with congestive heart failure, he will review the chart carefully to be sure that the patient is taking an ACE inhibitor, if indicated. The most difficult aspect is the coding. In the beginning, Walther resented the system, but now believes that he is practicing better medicine because of it. This system provides an incentive for the physician to avoid overlooking certain details of care. Other groups may prefer computerized reminder systems.

Arnold Goldschlager described meetings that one Independent Physicians Association (IPA) conducts monthly. The IPA medical director attends each meeting with an agenda; a practicing physician is selected as leader. Physicians who miss a meeting are fined $190. Meetings focus on a particular subject, such as common eye problems that do not need a specialist referral, common skin conditions for which liquid nitrogen is used to remove the lesion, and a review of patients who visited an emergency room instead of making an office visit.

Physicians are given report cards that analyze cost data. Those whose costs are more than the group's average are not considered to have cost-effective practices. Referrals are encouraged to those surgical consultants who generate the least costs. Physicians are taught how to instruct patients on therapeutic exercises and thus avoid referrals to physical therapy. These policies encourage or enforce cost-saving measures, with less emphasis on the quality of care, although the administrators would argue, sometimes correctly, that this approach can provide equal or superior service. In any case, data collected on individual practices can be used to discuss real events in practice at these meetings and can generate ever-improving patient care with cost containment receiving just attention. We stress the discussion of practice data as a major educational tool.

The Norwegian Medical Association has developed a method (SATS) using the PDSA (Plan–Do–Study–Act) cycle, which is applicable to both quality improvement and self-directed learning. Tor Carlsen described the approach: "This method combines three elements: (1) defining quality indicators, (2) selecting computer software that enables simple input and retrieval of data from the electronic patient record, and (3) organizing study groups to discuss practice data. Four topics were chosen for testing the method (clinical use of the laboratory, and diagnosis and management of sore throat, migraine, and diabetes).

"The groups, whose members were general practitioners with 10 to 20 years of practice, started discussing the need for improvement in their own practice, and agreed on quality goals (how often quality criteria should be met). Next, clinical performance was recorded in the computer system. Reports were presented to the group, differences were analyzed, and needs for improvement were identified. The group members provided ideas on how to effect change in practice. A second period completed a cycle of six to 12 months.

"The first trial, carried out in 1995–1997, included about 200 family physicians in 30 peer groups. Nearly all participants showed improvement, those with the lowest initial scores showing the most. Participants reported that SATS provides an attractive learning environment and expressed high motivation for peer group work. The fact that actual observations of practice were the focus of discussion, not subjective opinions, enhanced awareness of the need for change. The confrontation with facts, although unpleasant for many, was a major driving force."

Some academic institutions are using the computer to analyze various aspects of practice. Lawrence Cohn described a system in place at Brigham and Women's Hospital: "At our institution we have a highly developed computer database system that can analyze all elements of patient practice. In this cost-conscious era, I believe that this is instrumental in reducing not only cost but waste, improving practice techniques, and discovering where problems exist in the institution or individual practitioner. We are able to analyze our Intensive Care Unit (ICU) experience in terms of laboratory studies, expensive and inexpensive medications prescribed, procedures performed, length of stay, operating times, blood use, and patient outcomes. We consider this to be extremely important, and we should look upon it as an impetus to improve practice techniques rather than as an onerous "big brother" oversight of activities. In addition, we compare our own practice with that of our sister hospitals in the same health system. These techniques may improve the outcomes for the same disease or procedure in a hospital that has less positive outcomes than others. A simple adjustment and consultation with the other team may lead to a safer and more cost-effective technique, with better patient outcomes."

The American Board of Family Practice conducts an office record review that may be part of the certification process. Information that should be available in the office chart includes the patient profile, possible risk factors, presence or absence of allergies and drug intolerance, past history, current immunization status, clearly stated primary and associated health problems, current medications, laboratory results, conclusions, treatment, and patient education plan for each problem. Four patient charts representing conditions frequently seen in the family physician's office are required. Physicians complete data scan forms based on their review of patient charts. The Board may require physicians to submit photocopies of portions of patient charts from which the data scan forms are completed. An individual computerized report containing tutorial statements about recommendations for management and record-keeping for specific problem categories is generated and mailed to each candidate. The reports identify any discrepancy between the records provided and the recommendations of the appropriate advisory committee.

* * * * *

To profit most from experience, physicians must know what their practice consists of and what results they obtain. The methods of study outlined in this chapter are, unfortunately, used by relatively few physicians. The potential dividends in improved patient care and physician satisfaction, however, are great and well worth the invest-

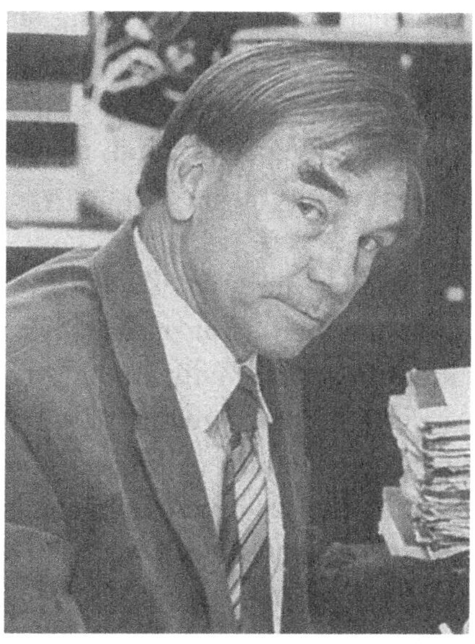

Evidence-based medicine has certainly added a new dimension to empirical medical practice, but it should complement, not replace, the conventional skills of the practitioner.

IAN R. MACKAY, M.D.
Professional Fellow
Biochemistry and Molecular Biology
Monash University
Clayton, Victoria, Australia

ment of time in practice analysis. To be most useful, the physician's experience should be compared with that of others reported in publications, at meetings, and in discussions with colleagues.

We suggest that physicians not now engaged in analysis of their practices consider establishing a simple method of indexing patient charts by problem or diagnosis and periodically reviewing the charts with a respected colleague to discuss diagnostic approaches and therapeutic plans for specific common conditions, such as hypertension.

In addition, physicians can profit from keeping simple notations on cards, like those designed by Paul Wood, on one or two conditions or procedures that interest them. Once the concepts recorded on index cards and ledger entries are clearly in mind, most physicians will do better to seek computer software to record, analyze, and access their practice data.

Data collected by HMOs and HEDIS can be useful in helping physicians review their practices. For maximum and sustained educational value, the identification of educational needs from events in practice should avoid intimidating programs that may lead to defensiveness and inhibit the physician's willingness to participate in assessment of performance. Preserving the buoyant spirit in physicians is important, so that they will continually strive to offer their patients better care. External sources must therefore be careful not to stifle enthusiasm for practice.

REFERENCES

1. Latham PM. General remarks on the practice of medicine. In: Martin R, ed. *The Collected Works of Dr. P. M. Latham.* London: New Sydenham Society; 1878:466.

2. Budd W. *Typhoid Fever. Its Nature, Mode of Spreading, and Prevention.* New York: George Grady; 1931. Reprint of 1874 original.

3. Pickles WN. *Epidemiology in Country Practice.* Baltimore: Williams & Wilkins; 1939:9.

4. Mackenzie J. *Principles of Diagnosis and Treatment in Heart Affections.* Joint Committee of Henry Frowde and Hodder and Stoughton. London: Oxford Univ Press; 1916:1–2.

5. Wilson RM. *The Beloved Physician: Sir James Mackenzie.* New York: Macmillan Co; 1926:51–52.

6. Fry J. Information for patient care in office-based practice. *Med Care.* 1973;11(Suppl 2):35–40.

7. Fry J. On the natural history of some common diseases. *J Fam Pract.* 1975;2:327–331.

8. Fry J. *Common Diseases: Their Nature, Incidence and Care.* Ridgewood, NJ: George A. Bogden & Son; 1983.

9. Reid RA, Lantz KH. Physician profiles in training the graduate internist. *J Med Educ.* 1977;52:301–307.

10. Osler W. The student life. A farewell address to Canadian and American medical students. *Med News.* 1905;87:629–630.

11. Codman EA. *A Study in Hospital Efficiency: As Demonstrated by the Case Report of the First Five Years of a Private Hospital.* Boston: Thomas Todd Co; 1918:8–9.

12. Latham PM. General remarks on the practice of medicine. In: Martin R, ed. *The Collected Works of Dr. P. M. Latham.* London: The New Sydenham Society; 1878:465.

13. Health Care Financing Administration. Medicare HEDIS® 3.0/1998 Data Audit Report. Available at: /http://www.hcfa.gov/ quality/3i2htm. Accessed Sept 13, 2000.

REFLECTIONS

• • •

Dr. A. McGehee Harvey received his M.D. degree, as well as his intern and residency training, at Johns Hopkins University School of Medicine. He had served as President of the Association of American Physicians, and was a Fellow of the American Academy of Arts and Sciences, Royal College of Physicians, and Royal Society of Medicine. The American College of Physicians honored him with the Distinguished Teaching Award. He was also Editor of *The Principles and Practice of Medicine*[1]. According to Dr. Sherman Mellinkoff, Dr. Harvey, a respected scholar of medical history, brought to differential diagnosis "a blend of sagacious empiricism and the scientific method, a combination that reflects . . . his motivation: an abiding devotion to the dispassionate exercise of logic and reason."

REFERENCE

1. Harvey AM. *The Principles and Practice of Medicine.* Norwalk, CT: Appleton & Lange; 1998.

Personal Responsibility for Learning

A. McGehee Harvey, M.D. (1911–1998)
Former Distinguished Service Professor of Medicine
Johns Hopkins University School of Medicine
Baltimore, Maryland

To be a good physician, you have to make medicine your number one priority. You cannot enter medicine with the soul of a money-changer. You must love it and must develop your own expertise through creative scholarship. That ideal alone will make you an outstanding physician. It is a matter of developing the habit of learning so that it becomes second nature and not something you turn on and off at certain times. If you can keep your curiosity about medicine alive, it will sustain you when you are in the middle of a difficult problem.

PERSONAL RESPONSIBILITY FOR LEARNING

Education must be pursued actively, not through the passive receipt of information distilled by someone else. I require all students, during their medical quarter, to choose a clinical problem that has no ready answer but for which an answer is possible by examination of patient records or by review of the literature. At the end of the quarter, they present the results of their studies to their classmates. This exercise establishes education as primarily the student's responsibility. You can motivate students to make the most of their experience by adding the experience of others, as recorded in publications or other medical records. That principle was enunciated by William Henry Welch and later became a precept of the Western Reserve experiment in the mid-1950s.

When physicians go into practice, they become members of the medical community. If each physician presented personal experiences on a particular subject to colleagues at a local medical meeting, all would have a continuing flow of useful information, which would not only improve their patient care but would constantly emphasize the importance of keeping abreast of new knowledge. Special courses are important, but what you get out of them is governed largely by your motivation and the time and effort you invest in them.

Making self-education a habit—a part of your routine activities—is important. The foremost principle is that no one else is going to provide your continuing education; you must do it yourself. One way to do this is to select certain key journals for regular review. Another is discussions with colleagues, whether at lunch or at other times. You can learn a great deal from your own cases if you share your experiences with others.

PUZZLING CASES

We used to keep a puzzling-case book and a mistake book at our weekly resident rounds. It was surprising how often another case would later come along about which you could learn something by referring to the previous one. By presenting your mistakes to your colleagues for discussion, you can often find out why you made the mistake, and you can avoid a repetition of it.

Medicine is an exercise in problem-solving, and the same basic techniques used in the scientific laboratory to approach an unknown are applicable to clinical problem-solving. In differential diagnosis, you have to gather information systematically from the moment the patient enters the room. You can get ideas each step of the way, and those, in turn, will create new questions to be answered.

Most important for students to understand is that they must remain curious, alert, and eager for new information. Learning to organize, assess, and transmit information clearly to consultants is a distinct advantage. A teacher can provide motivation and an environment for learning, but it is still up to the student to be an *active* learner.

11

Social, Ethical, and Economic Problems in Medicine

• • •

> The exceptional advances of modern medicine have restored to productive life many patients with previously fatal or disabling diseases, but these very successes have raised a host of troubling ethical and economic questions. Reconciling society's increasing demands on medicine with the realities of inflation, governmental regulations, changing social values, and an aging population poses knotty problems.
>
> MICHAEL E. DEBAKEY, M.D., AND LOIS DEBAKEY, PH.D.[1]

OPPORTUNITIES FOR INVOLVEMENT

The methods and approaches physicians use to learn from their clinical experiences not only perfect their skills, but heighten their personal satisfaction and passion for practice. Such activities can no longer be limited to the study of clinical findings, diagnosis, and therapy, for extraordinary medical innovations have raised a rash of problems—economic, social, legal, moral, and ethical. Can we afford the advances? How do we control the escalating costs? How do we provide the new services for the economically deprived? How do we reconcile society's ever-increasing demands and expectations of medicine with its increasing criticism of rising costs? What role should medical and professional judgment play in ethical quandaries? How do we define the difference between prolonging living and prolonging dying? All segments of society have become interested in these questions and problems.

"These issues have raised physicians' interest in the problems and have stimulated the desire to learn," said Philip Lee. "The changing responsibilities have begun to affect physician attitudes. I believe that the time has come to address these questions actively. Physicians must learn what the problems are and seek objective information, not base their judgments on the often biased discussions provided through give-away journals or special-interest journals. Physicians must seek out other sources of information, review and evaluate them, and then make their own decisions."

"Medical ethics is fascinating and important," in Albert Jonsen's view, "but the way it is now taught to physicians poses some problems. Because ethics is based on academic philosophy, it can be, and often is, presented purely theoretically. Moreover, when the ethicist has little clinical experience, his approach may be abstract and simplistic. Competent teaching of medical ethics requires concreteness and practicality. It should result in broadening of vision as well as have clinical relevance." Physicians can use some of the methods discussed in this book to address economic, social, and ethical issues. How can they proceed?

INDIVIDUAL INVOLVEMENT

Bruce Zawacki explained how the clinician can stay abreast of advances in the field: "Today, ethical problems, experienced most poignantly at the bedside, are found to have their root causes as often in healthcare organizations (HCOs) and systems as in the ethical values and skills of a few professionals, such as physicians, nurses, and the clergy. Moreover, administrators and other members of the healthcare team have greatly increased their social and economic power, as well as their ability to be heard. What used to be called 'medical ethics,' therefore, is now more functionally labeled 'healthcare ethics' and requires use of ever-broadening resources.

" 'Doing ethics' is in many ways like 'doing surgery' because it is at least as much a skill to be practiced as a body of knowledge to be learned. Ethicists are earnest, reflective, scholarly, and enthusiastic, regularly engaging in face-to-face ethical discourse and in reflection on how to improve. For physicians, this usually means joining the best healthcare ethics committee (HEC) available. The major, often funded, mission of HECs is self-education. In teaching ethics not only to one another but also to their patients and their HCOs, the physicians teach themselves. The National Reference Center for Bioethics Literature and the Bioethicsline databases option on the National Library of Medicine Internet Grateful Med Web site (www.igm.nlm.nih.gov) are additional sources of assistance in such learn-while-teaching efforts.

"Of the serials most widely and routinely read by physicians, *The New England Journal of Medicine, The Journal of the American Medical Association,* the *Archives of Internal Medicine,* and *The New York Times* provide the most authoritative, readable, and consistently relevant articles and editorials about healthcare ethics. Those wishing to satisfy a special interest or develop a special facility in dealing with ethical issues will find the *Journal of Clinical Ethics,* the *Hastings Center Report,* the *Healthcare Ethics Committee Forum,* and the *Cambridge Quarterly of Healthcare Ethics* to be most helpful. Finally, such enthusiasts will find the Web site http://www.asbh.org/ to be helpful, and at least biannual attendance at the American Society of Bioethics and Humanities multidisciplinary convention to be not only challenging but also collegial and encouraging. And we all need that kind of collaboration in our self-education."

"Consult other physicians or professionals regarding particular ethical problems you face in caring for individual patients," advised Philip Lee. "Some physicians in university medical centers may consult chaplains, philosophers, or others with particular expertise in ethics, for example, regarding a decision not to resuscitate a patient who has cardiac arrest. When should the decision not to resuscitate be discussed with the patient? When should the family be involved? In the case of a hospitalized patient, when should the nurses or other members of the staff become involved? In short, the very process of deciding who should be involved in the decision and what rights the patient, family, hospital staff, and attending physician have will help to educate the physician about the issue."

Thomas Hunter pointed out the need for physicians to educate other groups, both lay and law, to the realities of medicine and biological science and for physicians to listen to the concerns of these groups. "The trust in physicians and scientists has been badly eroded for many reasons beyond our control, partly because of the general mistrust of authority since the 1960s. But our resistance to participation by the laity in policy decisions has also played a part. We need to recognize that ultimately we are responsible to the public and that we must work actively with them in formulating ethical and social policy." Zawacki suggested that the attending staff should be encouraged to include such considerations in their daily bedside teaching.

ORGANIZED MEDICINE

Robert Glaser urged medical organizations and academicians to sponsor seminars, symposia, and conferences on ethical, social, and economic problems. "The professional media also have a role in publishing thoughtful, informative articles on these subjects."

County and state medical societies offer the opportunity for grassroots participation on committees studying and formulating policies in sociomedical and economic problems. Philip Lee thinks that physicians often deal with the broader issues through professional organizations such as county and state medical associations, the American Medical Association (AMA), and specialty societies. "These bodies often conduct policy studies and communicate the information to members for further consideration of the policy position with respect to the impact on an individual physician's practice. Mechanisms for representing the views of physicians, although imperfect, fit very well with our pluralistic approach to public policy and the kind of influence accorded special interests, including the medical profession."

Most medical societies have capable staffs that research pertinent issues and distribute bulletins and newsletters to their constituents. The AMA, for example, publishes the *American Medical News*, and the American College of Physicians publishes *The Observer.* These publications help the busy physician who cannot spend time reading all published material on these subjects.

* * * * *

Advances in medical science and practice, while improving patient care, have also raised countless social, ethical, and economic problems. Their significance demands that physicians devote some time to studying the issues and contributing to their solutions. When ethical problems arise in the care of individual patients, the physician should discuss the issues with colleagues, the clergy, the patient's family, and, in certain circumstances, an ethicist. Formal consultations may be in order. The leading medical journals now have regular features that discuss the issues authoritatively, and the public media also devote considerable space to these topics, so the physician can be aware of current thinking on important issues. Medical societies are becoming increasingly involved; some have formulated formal positions on specific issues, and most publish newsletters and bulletins to keep members informed. Despite time limitations, physicians must actively participate in the solution of social, ethical, and economic problems in medicine if they are to remain effective advocates for excellent patient care. In Saul Farber's words: "We are part of a great profession; we must work to preserve it."

REFERENCE

1. DeBakey ME, DeBakey L. The ethics and economics of high-technology medicine. *Compr Ther.* 1983;9:15–16.

REFLECTIONS

• • •

Dr. C. Rollins Hanlon received his M.D. degree from Johns Hopkins University and attained the rank of Associate Professor of Surgery there after U.S. Navy service in World War II. Thereafter, he was Chairman of the Department of Surgery at Saint Louis University for 19 years before his 17-year tenure as Director of the American College of Surgeons. During 49 years of Fellowship in the College, he also served as Governor, Regent, and now Executive Consultant.

An extraordinarily literate physician, he holds honorary degrees from four universities, honorary membership in 10 national medical specialty societies, and honorary fellowship in five English-speaking Surgical Colleges. His honors include the DeBakey International Surgical Society Award and the Fleur-de-Lis Award of Saint Louis University. He has served as President of six national and international surgical societies, of the Council of Medical Specialty Societies and, currently, of the Warren and Clara Cole Foundation, which he established in 1987. Widely known as a distinguished scholar and aficionado of *belles-lettres,* he has had a long-standing and active teaching career in the liberal arts related to medicine, and is Editor of the Ethics Section of the *Journal of the American College of Surgeons.*

Early Influential Habits

C. Rollins Hanlon, M.D.
Executive Consultant and Former Director
American College of Surgeons
Chicago, Illinois

The challenge to write about surgery as a lifelong, passionate encounter recalls a comment of William F. Buckley, Jr. in his book, *Nearer My God*,[1] that for him to write about his faith would put his faith at a fearful disadvantage. In the same way, describing my fascination with continuing education in surgery as a pattern for possible emulation risks being inadequate or self-serving.

But my own inspiration from the biographies and anecdotal recollections of other surgeons emboldens me to set down certain experiences and personal lessons that might be useful to some now early in their careers. As a start, I stress the essentiality of the habit of reading, not merely in all aspects of medicine and science, but in the humanities—biography, history, and philosophy. These liberal arts enhance and deepen the physician–patient relationship.

Many physicians have exemplified how a medical education, with its unique window on the human condition, can lead to a distinguished literary career. Somerset Maugham and Walker Percy come readily to mind, as well as other classic authors such as Chekhov and a host of present-day physicians who have published novels and essay collections about the medical career and life in general.

Kathryn Montgomery Hunter, in *Doctors' Stories,*[2] has cogently portrayed how physicians rearrange the patient's narration into a "doctor's story" that describes a recognizable clinical entity. Such reformulations may, however, risk the loss of those idiosyncratic particulars that individualize each patient's illness. Similarly, a physician's personal story is calculated to provide not an exact template for other physicians' careers, but rather some biographic snippets that may stimulate emulation.

The revolution in electronic packaging and transmission of data has led some to predict obsolescence of the book. I do not concur. Nor do I believe that early mastery and continuing cultivation of reading skills may be abandoned. It seems scarcely necessary to defend the book as a simple, durable, easily portable instrument to put us personally into happy communion with the sages, free of encumbering technology. Moreover, an early mastery of reading the printed word can facilitate comprehension of the electronic monitor display. And recent studies of cerebral function challenge the classic dictum that we are born with all the brain cells we will ever have; there is even a hint that such cellular recruitment may occur not merely in infants but in those of us at the age when Alzheimer's disease threatens.

Every medical student faces the daunting body of anatomic, physiologic, and other data to be absorbed in a limited time and kept at the ready for application to the diagnosis and treatment of patients in the consulting room or hospital bed. Praise of the book in no sense diminishes the marvel of ready electronic retrieval of the vast holdings of the National Library of Medicine and Internet resources for reliable guidance in medical dilemmas. This requires a mastery of computer and reading skills to supplement, rather than replace, the basic diagnostic process by which facts are marshaled to support or reject a clinical hypothesis.

We must recognize, as well, the challenge of sophisticated patients who arrive in the office not with newspaper or magazine clippings, but with downloaded pages of sometimes questionable data that prompt them to ask searching questions. For today's urgent need to keep abreast, the Internet search engines make it easier for physician and patient, but both should view such information with a critical eye.

My Father never attended college, but as an inveterate reader he accumulated a large number of wisely selected books, housed in glass-fronted sectional bookcases lining three walls of the room we called "the library." When the family built a smaller house, my brothers and I split up the literary holdings; my part included the incomparable 11th edition of the *Encyclopaedia Britannica,* still frequently consulted. The parochial school nuns gave us heavy reading assignments, and Baltimore's Enoch Pratt Free Library was only a 30-minute walk from home. On Saturday mornings, we would often pause in a nearby park after our library visit to read one or more of the generous five-book allowance, so we could sign out others before finally heading home with full cargo.

As one of the various educational "clubs" my father formed for us at home, the poetry branch had us commit to memory extended works, such as "Hiawatha" or "Gunga Din," to be recited on demand for a small reward. The Jesuit high school introduced me to extended Latin and Greek studies, continued in college, along with membership in the debating society and editorship of the school newspaper. The painful obligation of two editorials for each weekly issue instilled an early appreciation for deadlines.

In the laboratory of a distinguished Jesuit biologist, I had the good fortune of completing a summer college research project on the behavior of paramecia. An equally fortunate association with a medical school classmate, William P. Longmire, Jr., brought us together as volunteers in pathology during the summer after our first year. W. G. MacCallum and Arnold R. Rich taught us the rudiments of gross and microscopic pathology, and multiple, carefully studied autopsies helped us correlate the clinical story and the final anatomic report. I shared with Longmire the surgical internship and a subsequent research fellowship to study surgical shock under the incomparably meticulous Philip B. Price, whose 12 years as a missionary surgeon in China included an investigation of de-germing the surgeon's hands that will never be matched for sheer tenacity.

Longmire's distinguished career in launching the Department of Surgery at the University of California at Los Angeles and his fraternal help in getting me a position with Alfred Blalock led to my own Chairmanship of the Department of Surgery at Saint Louis University School of Medicine. Much later, I worked with Longmire in various capacities at the American College of Surgeons. This personal and professional association over more than 65 years illustrates the benefits of a collegial relationship that began early in medical school and grew steadily more vital in ensuing decades.

An early interest in medical history began when the great Swiss medical historian Henry Sigerist came to Johns Hopkins as Chairman of the W. H. Welch Institute for the History of Medicine. Six first-year medical students had the unparalleled opportunity to join Sigerist in close colloquy every week. These remarkable seminars generated a keen appreciation of historiography, without necessarily inculcating the master's socialist philosophy. Sixty years later, I was privileged to oversee seminars at Northwestern University with bright freshman and sophomore medical students, sharing an analysis of the complex issues posed by today's technical and sociologic issues in medicine. A continued mentoring relationship with some of these students is another treasured reward.

A long administrative experience with the American College of Surgeons has provided a front seat at the unfolding drama of the Surgical Education and Self-Assessment Program (SESAP). Started 29 years ago with the benefit of generous advice from the American College of Physicians and their Medical Knowledge Self-Assessment Program, SESAP has been a resounding success in stimulating myriads of surgeons to keep abreast of advances in surgery by a process that stresses individually directed learning and comparison with the performance of one's peers.

In addition, the American College of Surgeons has sponsored extended seminars on "teaching surgeons to teach" and on the mastery of new technical procedures by simulation and by hands-on instruction. The worldwide dissemination of skillfully designed and administered courses in Advanced Trauma Life Support is a gratifying demonstration of personal learning modes that have improved public health internationally.

Medical ethics is an increasingly relevant aspect of modern healthcare that is moving from its philosophical roots to a more pragmatic, case-based focus necessitated by technical and economic developments. Surgical journals now publish special articles on ethics, and a splendid book, *Surgical Ethics*,[3] includes chapters written jointly by clinicians and ethicists or philosophers. The growing stress on patient autonomy and the bitter criticism of paternalism may have gone too far. A more judicious approach would permit patients to participate actively in decisions about their care, but would not discourage clinicians, with their special education and training, from advising patients what is in their best interest. Taking time to know the patient gives at least a secular humanistic approach to the communication between physician and patient, and there is room beyond that for a spiritual, or even overtly religious, dimension to this therapeutic relationship.

REFERENCES:

1. Buckley WF Jr. *Nearer, My God: An Autobiography of Faith.* New York: Doubleday; 1997.

2. Hunter KM. *Doctors' Stories: The Narrative Structure of Medical Knowledge.* Princeton, NJ: Princeton Univ Press, 1991.

3. McCullough LB, Jones JW, Brody BA, eds. *Surgical Ethics.* New York: Oxford Univ Press; 1998.

12

The Physician–Patient Relationship, Physical Examination, and New Procedures

• • •

> The relationship between doctor and patient partakes of a peculiar intimacy. It presupposes on the part of the physician not only knowledge of his fellow men but sympathy. . . . This aspect of the practice of medicine has been designated as the art: yet; I wonder whether it should not, most properly, be called the essence.
>
> WARFIELD T. LONGCOPE[1]

Gene Stollerman would like to see continuing medical education emphasize clinical skills.[2] He deplores the growing gap between medical technology and clinical skills, in which advice based on the interview and examination is replaced by that based on results of laboratory studies and technical procedures. The development of clinical skills, he points out, enables physicians to obtain a better understanding of the patient's problems and gain confidence in their own ability to determine what technologic tool is required to substantiate the clinical findings and what consultations would be to the patient's advantage. Learning about new tests and procedures, unfortunately, is much easier than discovering how better to examine a patient. Richard Lewis emphasized the value of the clinical history: "The importance of the clinical history cannot be overestimated. The physical examination cannot be done in a vacuum; the history is critical to alert the examiner to possible abnormal physical findings. Subtle abnormalities are discovered only when specifically searched for as a result of the history."[3]

PHYSICIAN–PATIENT RELATIONSHIP

Stuart Yudofsky recalled: "During a required rotation in psychiatry in my third year of medical school, I came under the supervision of Hilde Bruch, a psychoanalyst and international expert in understanding and treating patients with anorexia nervosa. Her demanding and perspicacious tutelage[4] introduced me to a whole new universe of understanding and providing meaningful help to those who suffer from disorders of mood, behavior, and thinking. She considered every patient, regardless of any primary psychiatric illness, as a whole person whose medical complaints and dysfunctions must be understood through a matrix of biological, psychological, social, and spiritual domains."

Many patients feel intimidated by the very presence of a physician and are reluctant to ask questions or even discuss fully the nature and extent of their complaints. They may hesitate to impose on the physician's time; they may be embarrassed to expose their inner selves; or they may be fearful of the consequences of their illness. Eliminating these patient inhibitions requires special skills in interviewing and communication.

Physician–Patient Relationship as a Therapeutic Tool

The physician–patient relationship is, of course, a powerful therapeutic tool that the physician should learn to use skillfully. Richard Reitemeier gave this example of its importance: "J. Arnold Bargen was one of America's pioneers in the study and management of inflammatory bowel disease. When he began this interest in the mid-1930s, he recognized the terrible plight of such patients and did all he could to help them. Because of that interest, many patients were referred to his care. I suspect they were referred with some gratitude on the part of their own physicians, since the management of the disease was a great challenge and usually extremely frustrating. Bargen welcomed the opportunity to care for such patients, and, as one of his assistants in the hospital in the early 1950s, I recall seeing a remarkable demonstration of the effect of that kind of welcome on an ill person.

"A young woman with severe ulcerative colitis of several years' duration was admitted to St. Mary's Hospital several days before Bargen was to begin his term as the consultant in charge of such cases. She arrived emaciated, with a high fever, considerable abdominal pain, and the usual raging diarrhea. We did all that we could to make her comfortable, but her symptoms continued without change until the morning Bargen met her. He walked across the room and stood at the bedside of this patient, reaching out to grasp her right hand with his and placing his left hand on her forearm. Looking her straight in the eye, he said, 'I am so glad you have come! We are going to make you better!' He then went on with the usual interrogation of her history and a physical examination. However, we all noted that the very moment that he greeted her with that welcome assertion, she seemed to relax. As the day wore on, I was gratified and intrigued to watch all of her clinical signs improve. The fever abated, her diarrhea and abdominal pain quieted down, and indeed she did get better. I have always thought that the magic of his greeting was transferred to that woman through the warmth of his handshake and his evident honesty. He really did care about her."

Understanding the Patient's Point of View

The patient's perception of the hospital may be quite different from the physician's, as Francis Moore learned. "As a senior resident in a Boston hospital in a largely Italian-speaking neighborhood, I encountered a woman admitted for headache. Because all the simple tests were negative, she was scheduled for the more rigorous tests that we had in those days, including an encephalogram and a ventriculogram.

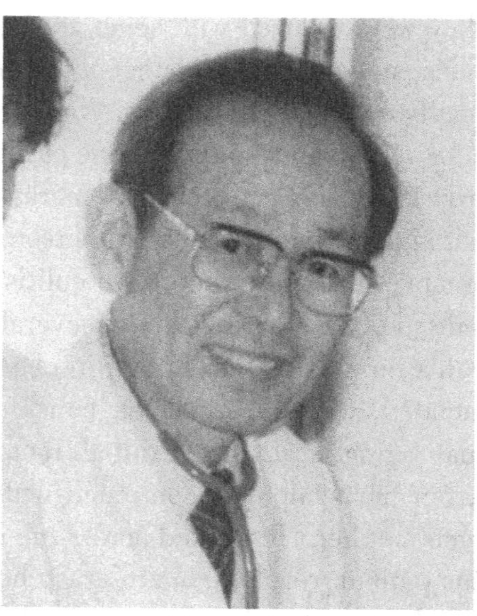

Things that seem trivial to the physician may have great significance for the patient.

KUNIO OKUDA, M.D., PH.D.
Director, Department of Medicine
Chiba University
Chiba City, Japan

One morning, as I was coming around with my white-suited junior resident troupe behind me, she said, 'Doctor, you know, I think I am just too sick to be in the hospital.' There was no response from the dumbfounded residents. She continued: 'I would like to go home for a few days until I feel a little better. Then I will be happy to come back to the hospital for the tests. But right now, I am just not feeling well enough.' How many patients she unwittingly spoke for!"

"One incident served to teach me," recalled Kunio Okuda of Japan, "that things that seem trivial to the physician may have great significance for the patient. As a young resident at the Chiba National Hospital, I was in charge of a ward room with five middle-aged women with chronic diseases. I made it a rule to see them in the morning, starting from the right side of the door. One day, for no reason and without thinking, I started seeing them from the left. I later learned from the nurses that the woman on the right whom I used to see first and the one on the left whom I saw first that particular day had a big fight in the afternoon. I realized that I had been concentrating on the patients' diseases and had been negligent of their feelings and personalities. I learned an important lesson."

Most physicians are relatively content with their clinical skills, not realizing that even basic skills need to be analyzed to avoid bad habits and omissions. There is even need to improve continually one's ability to listen intently and actively to patients. A common mistake made by medical students is to refer to the patient as "a poor historian." "Walter Cherny has always been a stickler for precise language," said Arthur Christakos. "Whenever students or residents make the mistake of referring to the patient as a historian, Walt is always quick to remind them that the one who records the history is the historian, and most of the time, he agreed, the historian was poor."

The physician–patient relationship, moreover, is constantly changing in response to societal changes as patients become more aware of medical matters. Currently, the trend is to make the patient more of a partner in health decisions. To adapt to these changes, the physician must be ever alert to the human side of medicine, and daily learning must therefore include improvement in the physician–patient relationship, as well as in clinical skills.

Rebecca Kirkland noted how the Internet is affecting the physician–patient relation: "When a patient calls or enters the office with documents printed from the Web, what is the appropriate protocol? If the article is correct, the physician can volunteer to interpret the information; if it is not accurate, he can refer the patient to reliable Web sites. The primary focus should always remain the patient, and winning the confidence is worth the time expended."

Charles Parker lamented the diminishing opportunities to gain the personal satisfaction that the physician–patient relation brings: "Indeed, many traditional customs have succumbed to cost-effectiveness. The pleasure, for instance, of follow-up visits or suture removal, which permitted precious moments to chat with the well patient, have become the domain of the nurse-practitioner or the physician-assistant. The days when a physician had the discretion to take an extra 20 minutes to explore the family life or a school problem have vanished with managed care. Now a curt, anonymous telephone voice reminds us that only a 10-minute visit is allowed. As the physician arrives at the clinic for his morning rOutine, he is greeted not by a pleasant smile from the receptionist, but by an indifferent printer spitting out the daily schedule: name, time, and chief complaint.

"It seems to me that the physician–patient relationship no longer allows enjoying the fruits of your labors because someone else sees the happy, healing patients. The passion is now dependent on the moment at hand and satisfaction from learning and understanding the patient's problem."

Maurice Bernstein believes that most changes in the physician–patient relation involve time, access to resources, and multiple health-care personnel: "Time seems to be limited in the physician–patient relationship in this era of managed care. I say 'seems' because I think it doesn't have to be in all cases. Time to allow the patient to talk is something we try to teach first to our students. It also involves time for the physician to listen. Students new to interviewing sometimes give the patient only a few seconds between the initial open-ended question and the student's follow-up direct questioning. This behavior is not, however, limited to new students but includes physicians in practice. The solution is for the physician to learn how to use the time available more efficiently, allow more time through novel scheduling techniques, and simply take the time to help the patient and let the chips fall where they may.

"Access to resources is clearly more difficult in managed care. Although there are examples of the non-beneficial effect of resource limitations, there are also examples of the wisdom of not doing a procedure. In practice, even if the patient is seemingly 'informed,' time limitations imposed on the physician cause inadequate discussion of the benefits and burdens and may cause the patients to demand approaches that are unnecessary or, worse, harmful. Screening for approval by a utilization committee of physicians can be beneficial.

"Time limitations may also cause poor communication among members of the healthcare team, leading to confusion about the medical goals expressed to the patient or family by each team member. One physician must remain the attending physician.

"The hospitalist, an old profession overseas, is new and developing in the United States because of the need for more specialized hospital care and the need, in this managed care age, to reduce the number of hospital days to a minimum. The relationship between the patient and the office-based physician can be disrupted, although my experience is that many patients are satisfied with the hospitalist but are eager to return to their own primary care physician. The disruption often occurs because of limitation of time, the inability of the office-based physician to communicate the history to the hospitalist, and the inability of the hospitalist to provide the primary care physician with timely feedback about the patient's hospital course. This is generally recognized as a systemic problem with the hospitalist system and has yet to be solved.

"I look at the problem of time in medical practice as the major factor to establish, but also to destroy, the physician–patient relationship. I worry that those in managed care find that the 'bottom line' has more to offer than time."

"Has the passion been drained from medicine?" asked Robert Moser. "I think not. But there has been seepage. Medicine will always be conducted on a human-to-human basis, but the interposition of technology has been a mixed blessing. 'Laying on of hands,' the paradigm for personal communication, alas, has become a time-consuming anachronism. In this wondrous era of molecular biology and instantaneous transmission of electronic data, our capability to help our patients has soared to unprecedented heights. Yet never has our reputation, respect, and esteem been lower in the public mind. Why this unseemly paradox? Simply put, they expect even more than we can deliver; they want the vaunted science of medicine to be repackaged into thoughtful care. It is an impossible immediate transmutation. It will take some pain and more time."

Methods That Hone Clinical Skills

Seminars Michael Balint pioneered research seminars to study the psychological implications in general medicine. His discussion groups, first organized at the Tavistock Clinic in England, consisted of eight to ten general practitioners and two psychiatrists. Balint noted that, at first, the general practitioners tried hard to entice the psychiatrists into a teacher–pupil relationship, but for many reasons it was thought advisable to resist this. Instead, he strove for a free give-and-take atmosphere, in which everyone could discuss clinical problems and receive assistance based on the experience of the others. The chief purpose was an examination of the ever-changing physician–patient relationship. Physicians' recent experiences with patients, reported by the physician in charge, provided the material for Balint's discussion groups. The physicians reported freely on their experiences, using clinical notes and including an account of their emotional responses to patients.[5]

File of Clinical Biographies and Writing In addition to participating in seminars that focus on physician–patient conversations and interactions, Gayle Stephens also maintains a file of "clinical biographies" of patients in his practice—narrative descriptions of patients' longitudinal experiences with illness. He also teaches and writes about interviewing and the physician–patient interaction.

Keeping Abreast of Changing Attitudes Physicians need ways of ensuring that they are reacting constructively to the changing attitudes of their patients toward medicine. Stephens recommends that physicians develop a circle of friends who are *not* physicians and listen to their stories about physicians and hospitals. Reading lay articles about health in newspapers, magazines, and books and watching television programs and advertisements about health and related issues can be helpful. Stephens advocates a nonjudgmental listening style so that patients will be uninhibited in their conversations with physicians. Never should a physician deride or humiliate a patient for doing something unorthodox.

"Listening is the most important way to learn what the changing attitudes are," said Jonathan Rodnick. "I serve on the Board of Directors of a community-based health organization that has predominately laymen on its Board, and listening to their views makes me aware of the public's attitudes. If I were unaware of my patients' changing attitudes, however, I would hope that they or my staff would constructively point out my inappropriate assumptions and actions."

John Geyman advocates self-study to improve knowledge about patients' attitudes. "Increase your knowledge of the community, the occupational settings, and the home environments. If, for example, you practice in a logging town, visit the local lumber mill and make occasional home visits. Encourage your patients to take an active role in the decision-making concerning their health care."

Videotaping or Audiotaping Physician–Patient Encounters Each physician should have the benefit of being videotaped periodically, or at least audiotaped, while interviewing a patient and having the tape reviewed later with an expert. Both profit from the exercise. The human interaction that takes place in medicine is too important to be neglected in lifelong learning. Some medical schools offer courses in this subject, but hospitals and specialty societies could do more in this regard.

I. R. McWhinney considers videotapes of the physician–patient encounter to be one of the most powerful tools we have. "The ideal is for a learner, whether student, resident, or practicing physician, to review the tape with a colleague skilled in the art of interviewing."

Self-observation For those physicians without access to videotaping facilities, self-observation can be useful. Geyman periodically audits himself during a patient encounter. "I remind myself of the need for a relaxed, approachable manner; open-ended questions and active listening; and avoidance of distractions. I try to learn something new about the patient as a person in each encounter, that is, beyond information related to his medical problems. I also ask myself whether the patient has had sufficient opportunity to participate in decisions about further diagnostic steps, management, and follow-up. In addition to self-audit techniques, it is useful to observe the patient's reactions to me as a physician, as well as the reactions of residents and students to me as a teacher."

Teaching Observing and teaching medical students at the bedside increases the physician's understanding of the basic techniques of the physician–patient relationship. As part of the family practice residency program in which Rodnick participates, residents are observed and videotaped while interacting with patients. Rodnick explained: "By observing young physicians with patients, analyzing their styles, and trying to give constructive feedback, I subsequently analyze my own office behavior. This self-analysis gives me ideas to improve communication in my practice and helps me understand both verbal and nonverbal physician–patient communication. The adage that the teacher learns as much as the students is certainly apt in this situation."

THE PHYSICAL EXAMINATION

According to Richard Lewis, "[T]he physical examination provides information that improves clinical decision-making and reduces costs by eliminating redundant testing."[3]

A master clinician can gain astonishing information from a physical examination. "I often think of the best teaching that I ever had in medical school," said Marvyn Elgart. "It was the introductory demonstration by David Barr, Professor of Medicine at Cornell University. An eminent clinician, Barr told us that he was going to show us all the things that we could learn from a patient without having the patient disrobe. He then had a patient come into his office, stood up to greet him, and then stopped and turned to us. For the next 40 minutes, as he and the patient remained standing, he pointed out from an unending fountain of knowledge all the things he had discerned about the patient's eyes, skin, touch, and gait, as well as all the disease possibilities that had entered his mind during those few minutes. It was remarkable. In novels, only Sherlock Holmes came close."

Bill Bennett recalled the considerable influence of Howard P. Lewis, father of Richard P. Lewis, and an outstanding physical diagnostician, on the medical career of every student he touched. "Twice weekly at a two-hour conference with interns and residents, Lewis would elicit a history and do a physical examination. He would construct a differential diagnosis brilliantly and would predict findings that would be verified at operation or on chest x-ray. One need only recall the dullness over Kernig's isthmus, signifying scarring from tuberculosis, or percussion of dullness over Traube's space, signifying enlarging of the spleen, to realize his lasting impact on a young intern. It would be interesting to pit this consummate clinician's physical diagnostic skills, painstakingly developed over a career, against modern imaging devices. In cost-effectiveness, I suspect that Lewis would win hands down. After retirement, he remained very active for some time in the teaching of physical diagnosis to medical students and house officers. It is clinicians like Lewis who signify excellence in the art of medicine."

Once physicians have completed formal training, they have few opportunities to improve their techniques of physical examination. Most formal courses do not address this problem. Many physicians slip into faulty habits that could easily be corrected. Being observed by a colleague while performing a physical examination helps the physician avoid careless and sloppy approaches to physical diagnosis.

Experts' Need for Advice on Fundamentals

One might wonder if being videotaped during a patient interview and being observed in performing a physical examination is not too basic for experienced physicians. Everyone, however, can profit from expert advice and exhortation. In athletics, coaches help team members perform their best. In sports such as tennis, even the champions continue to receive instruction from coaches. In 1964, Charles MacKinley and Dennis Ralston were preparing for a Davis Cup match at the Los Angeles Tennis Club with the help of Pancho Gonzalez. MacKinley, Wimbledon winner the previous year, was considered the number one tennis player of the day. Watching the great Pancho Gonzalez, one of the masters of the game, give a lesson to two champions offered spectators the promise of learning some of the fine points of the game. But Gonzalez's first remark to MacKinley during a rally was the basic "Watch the ball," followed a little later by the admonition, "You're not bending your knees!" So even champions need reminders about the fundamentals.[6]

Louis Kettel received a valuable reminder from a patient. "I once volunteered for an evaluation of my history, physical examination, and diagnostic skills using the patient–instructor program put in place for competency evaluation of our medical students and house officers. This program uses patients with well-established illnesses and physical findings and with considerable knowledge of their diseases, along with a validated, structured, gradable analysis form. In the process, I fully expected to find that I lacked some skills, since I have been an administrator for a number of years. I was taken aback, however, by the major critique. In analyzing my overall skills, the patient informed me that I had neglected throughout the examination to recognize that he was, in fact, a human being and that on no occasion had I called him by name. What a depersonalizing experience for the patient! Were I to function in the role of Dean in the absence of so simple a social grace, I would surely deem myself a failure. I assure you I corrected that behavior."

Peter Lee cited an example of the value of being observed: "To prepare for his discussion of the physician–patient relationship with medical students, Seymour Pollack, then a young psychiatry faculty member, asked to accompany me on ward rounds. Having recently returned to clinical medicine after several years of almost full-time administration, and therefore needing some positive reinforcement, I agreed, assuming that he would compliment me on my sensitivity and skill. On the designated morning, Pollack accompanied me, my resident, and two interns. We reviewed the problems of the patients, discussing the appropriate publications and recommending plans for diagnosis or management. At the end of the rounds, Pollack and I stepped into a conference room, and I asked him for his observations. I vividly remember his first sentence: 'Pete, I'm shocked.' He then described the several ways in which my behavior on rounds had not only been rather oblivious to the feelings of patients but, in some cases, actually offensive. In one instance, I had examined a woman in a ward with four or five other patients without pulling the curtains around her bed, and, in another, I made what I felt was an appropriate witticism across the bed of a patient who had no way of knowing that the joke was not about him. In still another case, directly across the supine body of an anemic patient in whom the question of tapeworm disease had arisen, a resident and I thoughtlessly discussed acquiring tapeworms from working in unsanitary mines. The impact of Pollock's honest description of my behavior at the bedside of patients was profound. Over the succeeding years, I have been followed by the ghost of Seymour Pollock as I have made rounds. The sensitivity I gained from having my ward rounds observed by a friendly critic forever changed my way of making rounds and greatly improved my bedside behavior."

NEW PROCEDURES

Physicians have too few opportunities to learn procedures that were developed or perfected after their formal training. A surgeon usually "scrubs in" with a colleague trained in the procedure. A few specialty societies offer programs for this purpose. Since 1977, for example, the American Academy of Orthopaedic Surgeons has included laboratory components in courses on surgical skills, with hands-on experience (see p. 356). Programs include Rotary Instability of the Knee, In-

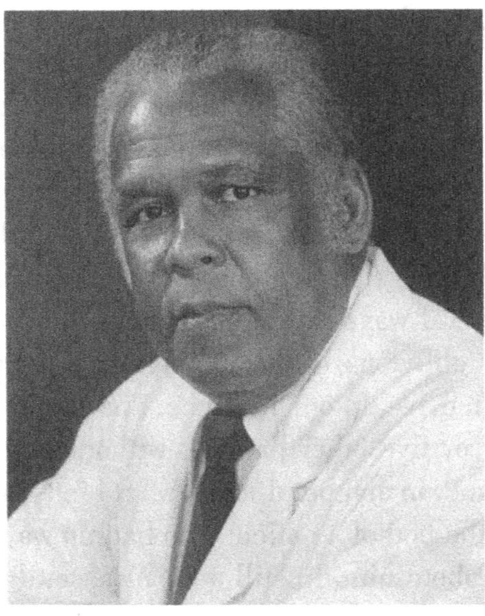

Students and residents are becoming the high priests of radiographic and laboratory triage. In the presence of negative imaging and laboratory reports, they may ask: "How could the patient be sick?" Technology has its value, but also its limitations; it is more important to cerebrate than to viscerate. Learning, thinking, and analyzing must be a budgeted part of our daily lives if we are to be true professionals.

CLAUDE H. ORGAN, JR., M.D.
Professor of Surgery
Chairman, East-Bay Surgery Program
University of California, San Francisco

tramedullary Nailing, Shoulder Disorders with Arthroscopy, and Arthroscopy of the Knee.

* * * * *

In all professions, basic skills need to be refined. But, embarrassment and pressures of practice prevent most physicians from actively seeking to hone their skills in interviewing or doing a physical examination. Few formal courses address these issues. Physicians can, however, ask a skilled colleague to observe them during these activities and then solicit suggestions for improvement. Observing a videotape of oneself in action and noting the problems recorded can also be instructive. New procedures may be difficult for the average physician to learn, but colleagues are usually willing to help, and medical societies are becoming more active in providing such instruction.

REFERENCES

1. Longcope WT. Methods and medicine. *Bull Johns Hopkins Hosp.* 1932;50:20.
2. Stollerman GH. Care of your clinical skills [editorial]. *Clin Exp.* 1984;1:11–12.
3. Lewis RP. Cardiac examination pearls. *Cardiol Rev.* 1996;4:34–46.
4. Yudofsky SC. Tribute to Hilde Bruch, the teacher. *JAMA.* 1987;257:196.
5. Balint M. *The Doctor, His Patient and the Illness,* 2nd ed. New York: Pitman; 1964.
6. Manning PR. Continuing education, physician competence, physician performance. *Fed Bull.* 1978;65:227–235.

REFLECTIONS

• • •

Dr. Steven Clemenson is a "country doctor" in northern Minnesota who received his M.D. degree from Saint Louis University School of Medicine and his residency training in Internal Medicine at Hennepin County Medical Center, Minneapolis, Minnesota. The frustration of increasing paperwork, combined with the difficulties inducing physicians to use guidelines in their daily practice, directed him into the new discipline of Medical Informatics, defined as "the intelligent use of computers to improve medical care." After spending time in academia in Boston, he is now helping direct research to determine if Form-Based Clinical Guidelines within the Electronic Medical Record can improve healthcare delivery. He is also leading the implementation of the Electronic Medical Record and Physician Order Entry at the MeritCare Health System.

Using E-mail to Enrich the Physician–Patient Relationship

Steven G. Clemenson, M.D.
MeritCare Health System
Bemidji, Minnesota

When we embark on a career of medicine, we feel genuine excitement at the prospect of helping our patients through health and illness. Unfortunately, far too much of this idealism dissipates as we progress through our training and professional lives. As we enter the everyday world of practice, the realities of managed care, insurance hassles, regulators, and other burdensome paperwork conspire to distance us from the wonderful, strength-giving physician–patient relationship.

When you practice in a small town, you converse with your patients every day—at the store, on the street, and at the corner café. In these interchanges, you learn much about your patients that is not disclosed in the examination room, but is part of the joy of being "my doctor" for your patients. As our world has become more urban, specialized, and scientifically sophisticated, we have lost some of the respect, trust, and, yes, love of our patients. How can we regain and nurture that special bond between physician and patient?

Can we use today's technology to regain the warm feeling that comes from a true connection with our patients? I think we can. E-mail is a start—a way for physicians and patients to gather information, ask and answer simple questions, and determine whether, and how urgently, a face-to-face meeting is needed. Of course, our staff and nurses will need to help assess and direct these communications, just as they have always done with telephone calls. The primary principle is to remove the barriers that have formed between physicians and patients. If we do not, others, not always qualified, will step in and assume our role.

We can also use the power of the Internet, along with our medical knowledge about a specific patient, to regain the role of trusted advisor and source of reliable information for our patients. There are many faceless commercial enterprises that are trying to claim this hallowed ground. Some have merit, but many are contaminated by the conflicting interests of profits, drug sales, insurance companies, and advertisers. The question for them is: What is the higher goal—the health of the patient or the health of the corporation and its advertisers?

To regain the privileged position of trusted advisor, physicians must make pertinent and valid information on healthcare available to patients and then be prepared to answer resulting questions. Such availability may be unsettling because it can be abused, but no more so than when the small-town physician is stopped on the street to answer patients' questions. The advantage of the electronic interchange is that physicians can have accurate information before them when they record the answer, whereas on the street they must rely on memory and horse sense.

We need to establish health-system-based Web portals where patients can review their medications and problems in understandable terms and then can be referred to medically correct and reasonable educational materials for those problems. The "Wild Wild Web" is an unregulated frontier where there is much that is good, but also much that is biased, incomplete, dated, or unreliable. Telling the difference is not always easy for lay persons or even for physicians in subjects outside their expertise. We need to ensure that only current, valid information is supplied. Why? Because it is part of our medical duty to improve the health and quality of life for the patients and the communities we serve. And it can also help us recapture the joy and passion for helping patients, which is the core of a rewarding career in medicine.

REFLECTIONS

• • •

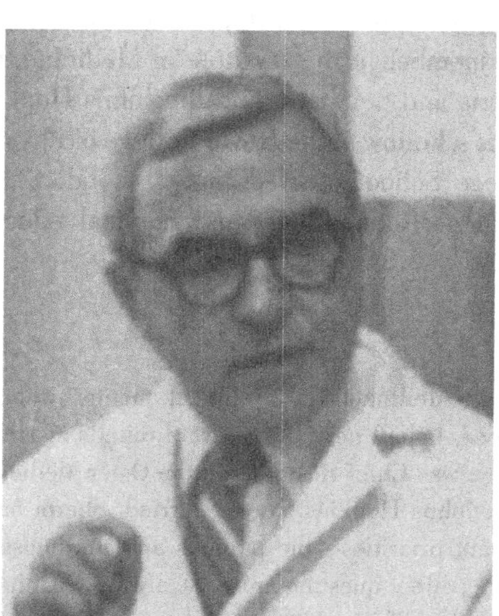

It is useful for physicians to have little groups that provide someone near at hand with whom to exchange ideas and discuss patients or published articles.

SHERMAN M. MELLINKOFF, M.D

The remarkable march toward excellence of the University of California at Los Angeles School (UCLA) of Medicine was in no small measure due to Dr. Sherman Mellinkoff's wise and persistent guidance during his deanship, 1961–1986. His outstanding contributions in the fields of medical education and gastroenterology have brought him recognition in the United States and in Europe. Among his awards are an Honorary Doctor of Humane Letters, Bowman Gray School of Medicine; the Ad Astra Award, University of Louisville; Physician of the Year Award, University of California; Abraham Flexner Award, Association of American Medical Colleges; and Honorary Alumnus Award, UCLA. Dr. Mellinkoff has received the J. E. Wallace Sterling Distinguished Alumnus Award, Stanford University School of Medicine and the Distinguished Medical Alumnus Award, Johns Hopkins University School of Medicine. He is a member of the Institute of Medicine, the American Academy of Arts and Sciences, and the Johns Hopkins Society of Scholars, and is a Fellow of the Royal College of Physicians and the Imperial College School of Medicine in London. His numerous publications in gastroenterology and medical education include several books.

* * * * *

> Sherman Mellinkoff is a clinical mentor who never preached. I shall never forget ward rounds as an intern while he was Chief Resident on the Osler Medical Service at Johns Hopkins. Never hurried, Sherm had two important priorities—the patients and the house staff. When a patient question arose, he always examined the patient himself and later shared new clinical insights with us in his gentle, wise way. His manner was invariably good-humored. We especially looked forward to his evening visits, when he became not only an able consultant but also a special friend who inspired us to prove worthy of our patients' trust. A caring physician, a wise academic leader, and a trusted friend for many faculty, students, and patients, he gave generously of himself to his family, his profession, and his colleagues. By example, he demonstrated the science and art of medicine as well as the best of personal human qualities.
>
> CAROL JOHNSON JOHNS, M.D.

Medicine: A Collegial Profession

Sherman M. Mellinkoff, M.D.
Emeritus Professor of Medicine and Former Dean
University of California, Los Angeles School of Medicine
Los Angeles, California

Continuing learning in medicine is an individual matter; the human mind is so complex that there are many different ways to approach this subject. Most important, I think, is to maintain curiosity about patients. To like patients and to be intrigued by their problems brings to medical practice both an emotional and intellectual attraction.

Looking at each patient independently before seeking opinions and comments from others fosters learning. Sometimes, medical students believe that they are not going to succeed unless they read the write-up in the chart and decide, on that basis, what they should record or say to the attending physician. On the contrary, to make the wrong guess independently and to find out why it is wrong through reading and discussion represent a good path to continued learning from experience.

This approach to patients was encouraged by George De Forest Barnett, who taught physical diagnosis at Stanford around 1940. He was a great bedside teacher. Although he did not publish a lot, he kept abreast of progress and was always an inspiration to his students. Another Stanford teacher to whom I am indebted was Arthur Bloomfield, a profound scholar who always began his discussion of a patient, after the diagnosis was firmly made, by reviewing trenchantly the history of that disease. Understanding what was known about a disease in the past and how the present state of our ignorance or enlightment was reached is helpful to continued learning.

A great teacher of mine who was a distinguished medical historian, as well as a master of differential diagnosis, was A. McGehee Harvey of Johns Hopkins. He inspired one's best effort to be rational and thorough in every clinical problem and to understand its historical and physiological implications. Another great bedside teacher at Hopkins was Philip Tumulty. I have never known anyone who more completely won a patient's confidence. Confidence is a tremendous asset, not only in caring for the patient, but also in obtaining an accurate history.

In gastroenterology for many years, I was lucky to be associated with Morton Grossman, a veritable gold mine of information and a sagacious interpreter of new developments. Mort started a program at the University of California, Los Angeles that was immensely helpful in continuing education. Major topics covered annually at the meetings of the American Gastroenterological Association were discussed at open-to-all gatherings, with most of the time spent on critical questions and answers.

Once when Mark Ravitch and I were seeing a patient with jaundice, he told me a story about William Thayer's collar button. Dean Lewis, who was described as the poor man's Halsted, had taken Halsted's place. Lewis was a good surgeon, but down-to-earth and not particularly eloquent. Thayer, who had taken Osler's place, was a Boston Brahman, and there was an imperious relation between him and Lewis. One Sunday, Thayer telephoned Lewis to say that he was sending his laundress into Johns Hopkins Hospital for an appendectomy and asked Lewis to attend to the matter. Lewis agreed to do so.

Some time later, Thayer was in the amphitheater and, to his consternation, he observed Lewis operating in the right upper abdominal quadrant. He asked, "What are you doing?" Lewis replied: "Well, I asked the patient what she was doing when her pains started. She said 'I was putting a collar button on one of Dr. Thayer's shirts.'" The point is that when a pain is really sudden, as it often is with a gallstone getting lodged somewhere, the patient remembers exactly what is going on at that time. But if the pain sneaks up, as it does with appendicitis, no such precise answer will be forthcoming.

A complementary point was often made by Phil Tumulty: "Don't be overly precise. There are times to ask specific questions (What were you doing when the pain started?), but there are other times when it is best simply to let the patient ramble, and although it may appear that it is a waste of time, it sometimes yields information that would not be elicited by direct questioning."

Physicians' biographies periodically re-ignite love of the art. The series that Mac Harvey wrote about the great pioneers at Johns Hopkins[1,2] stimulates the reader's appetite for continued learning.

I read articles in connection with the patients I have seen or heard about, and that makes what I read come to life for me. Similarly, when I am puzzled (and that is often), I like to discuss individual patients, articles I have read, or ideas with colleagues who are more familiar with the subjects than I am. I test new ideas in the same way.

In consultations, it is best to rely on what Dryden called the "plain style," that is, clear, precise, trenchant English. But we cannot all expect to be Drydens. It is sometimes more helpful, therefore, to obtain the consultation report through conversation. One of the worst wastes is, for example, to send a patient with lupus erythematosus to the radiology department with the request merely for a chest x-ray or an x-ray of some bone. The radiologist ought to know what the patient's problem is and what question is being asked about the patient.

I have a file at home of landmark articles to which I often refer. I review my reprint files periodically and am sometimes amused that an article I once considered important may no longer seem so. At other times, I am refreshed and amazed at how classical a particular paper has turned out to be. My file is extremely simple: I use a filing cabinet and manila folders and classify the material primarily by topic, but I file some articles by authors' names because I will remember them that way.

As biomedical discoveries multiply in the opening decade of the 21st century, information will be more readily accessible electronically. The worldwide library has been greatly expanded, and its resources are more immediately accessed. For the answers to some questions, this kind of electronic search is exceedingly helpful. Generally, however, questions do not come in a vacuum; they arise in a rational mind seeking explanations. For the clinician, most questions begin with the patient's story and appearance, which may lead to a search for information and to interpretation of the findings by consultation or informal discussion. We are still a collegial profession. We all need help; no one knows everything. And this obligatory interdependence helps preserve the passion for medicine and for continued learning.

REFERENCES

1. Harvey AM. *Science at the Bedside. Clinical Research in American Medicine, 1905–1945.* Baltimore: Johns Hopkins Univ Press; 1981.
2. Harvey AM. *Adventures in Medical Research. A Century of Discovery at Johns Hopkins.* Baltimore: Johns Hopkins Univ Press; 1974.

13

"Medical Errors" and Other Problems in Practice Unrelated to Medical Knowledge

• • •

If anything can go wrong, it will.

MURPHY'S LAW[1]

Murphy was an optimist.

O'TOOLE'S COMMENTARY ON MURPHY'S LAW[1]

Physicians who review their practice continually will serve their patients well, but good health care requires more than medical knowledge. At every step, extrinsic phenomena, errors, and omissions may adversely affect medical practice despite the physician's superb knowledge. "The best performance is built upon sound information," said George Miller, "but sound information is no assurance that it will occur." John Williamson found, for example, that highly informed physicians often did not respond to an unmistakably abnormal laboratory report.[2] About two-thirds of the abnormal results of three routine screening tests (urinalysis, fasting blood glucose, and hemoglobin) elicited no response from the physicians in his study, even after they attended a specially designed continuing education workshop and received reminders about the problem. The simple device of obscuring the abnormal findings on the laboratory report with a piece of removable fluorescent tape, however, significantly improved the response.

Starfield and Scheff illustrated that many of the problems interfering with patient care are unrelated to the physician's knowledge.[3] In only 14 of 53 children with low hemoglobin identified by a review of medical records and home interviews was the abnormality recognized, diagnosed, and treated, and the test subsequently repeated. The reasons for the oversights in the remaining 39 children varied. The low hemoglobin was unrecognized in 24 patients, was recognized but undiagnosed in six, was diagnosed but untreated in one, and was treated but not reexamined in four. Four patients were diagnosed correctly, but did not keep their subsequent appointments. Patient care can thus go wrong at any stage.

Morehead and Donaldson, after studying the care of patients with serious diseases in 40 neighborhood health centers, concluded that major problems resulted from failure to follow up on abnormal laboratory or roentgenographic reports, failure to implement the suggestions of consultants and others, and poor patient compliance.[4] In a study of emergency room care in an inner-city hospital, Brook and Stevenson reviewed the medical records of patients referred to the radiology department for upper gastrointestinal series, oral cholecystography, or barium-enema study.[5] Of 136 patients for whom adequate data were available, 30 (22 percent) did not receive appointments for treatment after completion of diagnostic procedures. Of the 106 patients who did receive appointments, only 54 (51 percent) kept them. Furthermore, only 37 (38 percent) of 98 patients interviewed who had had radiologic examinations could recall being told the results. The authors concluded that effective care had been provided to only one-fourth of the patients.

Gonnella and coauthors studied the detection of urinary tract infections at a university outpatient clinic.[6] An interview designed to elicit historical information about symptoms and signs of urinary tract infection was used on 133 patients, and urine samples were obtained from all of them. Thereafter, all patients were seen in the medical clinic by the regularly assigned student-attending team, which was unaware of the preliminary study. Eighteen patients with significant bacilluria (10^5 colonies/ml urine) were discovered by the preliminary history and screening, whereas only eight had correct diagnoses on the regular clinic routine. Yet when the knowledge of staff members was tested, their average score of 83 percent on the diagnosis and treatment of this condition showed that the problem was not primarily a lack of knowledge but failure to perform.

These and other studies show that medical practice is subject to oversights, lack of follow-up, and poor communication between physician and patient. Such quality-degrading incidents occur in any complex organized system, whether involving medical practice or a large engineering project. According to Chris Kraft, former Director of the National Aeronautic and Space Administration (NASA), a constant vigil is maintained in the space program to prevent errors of omission, misinterpretation, and lack of inspection: "After our initial years of experience, we recognized that redundancy checks were required to prevent termination of an otherwise perfect mission. Hundreds of examples of human error can be cited, including the problems of the Space Shuttle.

"We used color coding on liquid gas transport lines to warn of their contents and to ensure proper attachment. In the Space Shuttle, we even used different threads at junctions to prevent technicians from assembling the support equipment improperly. Unfortunately, they misassembled them anyway, forcing the lines together and causing damage to the system.

"In many instances parts were omitted from an assembly, despite required inspection points and a recording as each step was completed. When such an omission occurred in a pressure regulator of a space suit, we had to cancel a planned event on a 1982 Space Shuttle flight. We have had parts assembled backwards, an error that eventually caused a profuse leak in a system and required the complete redesign of a hydraulic actuator at great cost because the space team lost confidence in the equipment." In September 1999, the $87 million Mars Climate Orbiter (MCO) failed because navigators used English units of pound-seconds instead of metric newton-seconds in guiding the space-craft. For this error, *Science* designated the incident the "blunder of the year."[7]

After the tragedy of *Apollo 1,* in which astronauts Grissom, White, and Chaffee died in a fire while in a space capsule, Gene Kranz, a flight director in NASA's Mission Control, said, "From this day forward, Flight Control will be known by two words: 'Tough and Competent.' *Tough* means we are forever accountable for what we do or what we fail to do. We will never again compromise our responsibilities. Every time we walk into Mission Control we will know what we stand for.

"*Competent* means we will never take anything for granted. We will never be found short in our knowledge and in our skills. Mission control will be perfect."[8] The fate of the *Columbia* highlights the importance of this pledge.These principles, and the dire consequences of ignoring them, also apply to all healthcare professionals.

The Institute of Medicine highlighted medical mistakes in a report entitled *To Err is Human: Building a Safer Health System*[9]; in one study, medical errors were said to kill some 44,000 people in U.S. hospitals, but in another study, the number was 98,000, an inordinately broad range. Although McDonald and coauthors[10] make compelling arguments that the Institute of Medicine report exaggerated the frequency of the problem, everyone wants to reduce medical errors to a minimum, regardless of their source.

A powerful analogy to the diminished effectiveness in complex organized systems, whether medical practice or space missions, comes from the second law of thermodynamics: energy spontaneously becomes less concentrated, that is, more diffused, in closed systems, and inanimate matter tends to become random rather than remaining neatly ordered and organized. As Frank Lambert noted: "Complex human activities are inherently subject to becoming disorderly—just as orderly groups of molecules in a high energy system are unstable."

Aspects of patient care have a similar tendency to become less orderly and more random if left alone. Constant monitoring and constant feedback are essential to maximal efficiency. Considering the analogy to systems governed by chemical thermodynamics, we should not be surprised by this tendency. Physicians act as critical catalysts in superior medical care. The need for rigorous control is recognized by physicians who must continually check on themselves and others to ensure proper handling of even routine matters. We cite the analogies of the space program and the second law of thermodynamics to emphasize that the tendency for a system to become more disorderly is universal and constant. The physician must therefore be ever alert not only to medical but to nonmedical problems in practice.

THE PHYSICIAN AS MANAGER

How can physicians intervene to correct the tendency for the system to become disorderly and thus less efficient? Joseph Gonnella sees the physician as a manager, constantly monitoring the patient's care to ensure that everything is proceeding as it should and attending to each problem as it occurs. Almost all physicians interviewed acknowledged that numerous difficulties arise in medical practice that are unrelated to medical knowledge, and almost all made conscious efforts to combat them.

HISTORY AND PHYSICAL EXAMINATION

Most physicians guard against an incomplete review of systems during the physical examination by following an outline, preprinted form, or checklist, even though they may know it by memory. Others have a nurse or secretary scrutinize the chart after the examination and return it to the physician, noting any omissions. Physicians who use checklists may also write occasional notes on the progress sheet, such as "Next time do pelvic examination."

Warren Williams had his office staff go over his charts for important oversights in the history-taking or physical examination. As an experiment, he discontinued these procedural audits only to find that in two to three months his workups again had some omissions. The second law of thermodynamics is always operating.

Overbooking patients' appointments increases the risk of rushed examinations, omissions, and inadequate recordings. Similar problems ensue when the patient or physician is late for an appointment.

LABORATORY DATA

Laboratory Studies Unordered, Unperformed, or Unreported

Most physicians use a checklist of possible laboratory studies as a reminder of relevant examinations to order, but the temptation to over-order from such a list must be resisted. Other physicians set aside charts on difficult patients for review at the end of the day, call patients back for further tests, or write notes on progress sheets to order certain tests. Still others ask new patients to return to review their laboratory reports with them, and at that time note any needed tests that were not done.

To discover any unperformed or unreported laboratory studies, physicians can advise patients of the tests ordered and, at the next visit, ask them what was actually done. Was blood drawn or a roentgenogram taken? Having the office staff check tests ordered and completed can also minimize laboratory omissions. Writing laboratory orders in a specific place in the patient chart, such as the left margin, facilitates checking. Some physicians review each day's laboratory reports and ask patients either to call or to schedule another visit to receive the reports.

Lost Laboratory or Radiology Reports

Since loose data are liable to become lost, all laboratory reports should be filed in the patient's chart promptly or kept in a special box for the physician to review and initial before being filed. A master file of all laboratory reports is useful in case of a misfiled or lost report. Some laboratories and departments of radiology have a policy of sending a second report on all significantly abnormal studies, or a staff member will telephone the physician to ensure that a seriously abnormal study has not been lost or remained unnoticed. A backup report on "critical findings," such as suspected cancer, can prevent medical disasters. Ideally, all serious findings should be called in to the physician's office as well as reported in writing.

Failure to Note or Act on Abnormal Laboratory Results

A report that contains a single abnormal result seems most likely to be overlooked. Various techniques can help physicians avoid oversights, such as a red "Alert" stamp on all abnormal laboratory findings or highlighting of abnormal studies and leaving the laboratory sheets on the physician's desk until he reports the results to the patient.

Many physicians require their initials on all laboratory data before the office assistant places reports in patients' charts. Other physicians look over the chart for recent laboratory and roentgenographic reports while they are seeing the patient on a revisit, to make sure that abnormal studies are followed properly. Partners sometimes review one another's hospital charts before a patient's discharge to ensure that all abnormal results have been noted.

Flow Sheets

The advantage of a flow sheet, which can be generated by a computer, is that you can see the data at a glance. "When it occupies four or five pages," said Telfer Reynolds, "the benefit of the flow sheet is lost. A flow sheet for a liver patient contains results of the major studies needed to treat liver diseases, just as that for a fluid-and-electrolyte patient has the fluid and electrolyte data. The flow sheet also has a couple of columns for important clinical information. For a general internal medicine patient, the flow sheet should be adaptable, with blank spaces for physicians to write in whatever they want to follow."

MEDICAL RECORDS

Incomplete or Illegible Records

Physicians avoid forgetting pertinent facts by making notes during the patient visit, but illegibility can cause problems, particularly if their writing deteriorates as they become busier, more rushed, or older. Many physicians dictate their records for later transcription. Physicians generally agree that charting can be improved in most practices. Discipline and determination may provide the only solution, although the monitoring of records, particularly in the hospital, has lessened the deficiencies.

Consulting the Wrong Chart

Consulting the wrong chart does not happen often, but physicians should check the patient's name on the chart at each visit. A safeguard used in some offices is to have patients record their names, dates of birth, and telephone numbers at each visit and then to match that with the information in the chart. Writing the name of the patient on every progress sheet is also helpful, and when more than one patient has the same name, the charts can be labeled in a way to alert the physician, nurse, and file clerk.

Lost or Misfiled Records

Patient records are more likely to be lost or misplaced in group practice than in solo practice. Computerized appointment systems are said to be an aid in this regard. In most clinics, charts are not supposed to leave the building or to be out of file overnight. Outcards can be inserted into the file to indicate where the record is at all times. Misfiling is more likely to occur in hospital practice, but medical record administrators can help immensely.

LACK OF FOLLOW-UP OF PATIENTS

At the end of each day, Murray Salkin's nurse gives him the charts of patients who missed their appointments. He evaluates the records and gets in touch with patients with serious problems. Cathleen Caton uses an FTKA (failed to keep appointment) stamp to denote patients who do not show up or who cancel appointments. Some physicians use a card file to ensure following up patients with certain diseases, and others have a secretary keep a separate list of seriously ill patients and their diagnoses to minimize loss to follow-up. Still others send cards to remind patients of a follow-up visit and, if the condition is particularly serious, they may telephone or e-mail the patient. In addition to contributing to poor care, lack of follow-up can cause an inaccurate perception of results. (See Chapter 10 about sending follow-up questionnaires or letters to patients.)

PATIENT NONCOMPLIANCE: FAILURE TO FILL A PRESCRIPTION OR FOLLOW DIRECTIONS

Physicians should never assume that patients are following instructions. Instead, they should ask their patients on each visit how they are tolerating their medications, if they have finished their supply, and other questions to determine if treatment is being followed. Seeing chronically ill patients every few weeks allows the physician to note symptoms and tolerance to drugs, to adjust dosage, and to encourage compliance. A special form for medications can be kept in the chart, to be updated at each visit when therapy is discussed with the patient. William Hart has his patients list their medications and dosage, to be reviewed on each visit. He reemphasizes the need for medication, explains the reason for the schedule, and relates the possibilities of drug interactions and adverse effects.

A good physician–patient relationship facilitates compliance. When Page McGirr finds that a patient is not complying with prescribed treatment, he restates the medical need, warns of the consequences of omission, and enlists the patient's cooperation, avoiding intimidation. Talking to other members of the family can also be useful.

Noncompliance can be a serious problem in patients with chronic diseases, such as diabetes, hypertension, and mental illness. As long as patients are feeling well, they may not exercise the self-discipline necessary for long-range health preservation. Follow-up visits may be needed to reinforce the importance of treatment and to provide encouragement.

Misunderstanding instructions is a common cause of patient noncompliance. Making the instructions simple, having patients repeat them, and writing them out reduce such misunderstandings. Some physicians keep a copy of written instructions as a reminder of what was communicated, and others ask the patient to bring all medications to the office. Elderly patients, in particular, need additional attention, written instructions, and more frequent office visits.

Inattention of the Patient

Patients, of course, need to give their full attention during conferences with the physician. You may need to ask distracting children or other relatives to remain in the waiting room when the patient is called in to see you. On the other hand, enlisting the aid of a spouse or relative can often help the patient understand. It is your responsibility to individualize your explanations and instructions to the patient's needs, to be extremely careful in delivering them, and to use language the patient understands. Roger Stickney likens a good physician to a good teacher who can hold the attention of a class.

Patient Denial

Patients who are frightened and distracted by anxiety often fail to recognize or accept a serious diagnosis. The patient may use a psychological defense to reject what he does not want to hear. The physician may give a clear description of the patient's problem and its possible solutions or prognosis, only to find that the patient has not absorbed, or has totally misconstrued, what was said. The physician may therefore have to rephrase the information and even schedule another appointment to ensure that instructions are being followed. Pressing for complete patient understanding immediately is not always wise, since denial can offer the patient psychological protection initially. Where education is essential to the patient's well-being and longevity, however, a thoughtful, compassionate, articulate, and attentive physician can usually deliver the proper message.

FACTORS LIMITING PHYSICIAN EFFECTIVENESS

Inattention of the Physician

Perhaps the most significant barrier in the physician–patient relationship is failure to give full attention to the patient. It may be necessary to reduce the patient load in order to provide adequate time for patients. Patients are receiving the physician's full attention, according to Steven Hamman, when they are allowed to tell their full story while the physician actively listens before asking specific questions. The ability to listen and filter carefully is a great asset in medicine. Fred Turrill warned that "Some physicians look at their patients and make a snap diagnosis without giving the patient time to say everything he has to say. Listening may teach you something new about a disease, and the patient will always feel better for having been heard out." Paul Bohannan, communications specialist, recommends paying attention to what is being said instead of planning your next statement while the patient is speaking. Try to discipline yourself to give full attention to your patients, including their "silent messages" and body language.

Sometimes the messages will not be so silent. "The late Conrad Wesselhoeft of Harvard Medical School told a classic story," said Francis Moore, "and the moral was simply that the physician has to think of a diagnosis before he can make one, and listening carefully to the patient is often the most important part of the examination. He illustrated the point with the account of a man who lived on an island in Boston Harbor and was stricken with a disease which made it difficult for him to open his mouth. The physician ministered to him, giving all the pukes, purges, and perspiring agents fashionable at the time, and confiding to the patient all the various diagnoses that came into his mind, ranging from diphtheria to glandular fever, quinsy sore throat, and epileptic seizures. Finally the patient, dying and hardly able to open his mouth, muttered, 'Doctor, don't you think I might have lock-jaw?' To which the physician replied, 'Doggonnit, my good man, why didn't you think of that before?' "

Many of us are so busy asking the patient questions that the patient can never tell a complete story. Kenton King recalled that "The resident staff at Washington University customarily saved the most puzzling and perplexing case on the ward for presentation to the Chief about once a month. Accordingly, Dr. Carl Moore was brought to the bedside of an elderly lady with neurologic findings, as well as abnormalities in many other systems. About 20 house officers were gathered around the bed. A young, eager, well-meaning resident presented the case in a rather dull and rambling manner. When he finished, everybody looked at Dr. Moore, who turned to the patient and asked: 'Ma'am, what do you think your diagnosis is?' She replied, 'Well, when I visited Dr. Wintrobe about 20 years ago in Salt Lake City, he said that I had pernicious anemia before he started treatment.' Dr. Moore, realizing that it all fit together, said, 'My dear lady, why didn't you tell these doctors?' To which she replied, 'I tried to, but they told me to be quiet and answer their questions.' "

William Bardsley is convinced that interest in, and attention to, patients are sharpened by the physician's own good health, proper diet, adequate exercise, and adequate sleep. Interest is also enhanced by a certain amount of teaching and medical student discussions; otherwise, constantly listening to patients' complaints can become tedious and stressful. Occasionally, something about a patient may arouse resistance in the physician. If the physician cannot resolve the matter, the patient should be referred to a more compatible colleague.

Distractions Diverting Attention from the Patient

Telephone calls should not be allowed to interrupt the physician–patient conference unless they are extremely important. Many physicians try to take calls between patient visits, whereas others leave an opening in their morning and afternoon schedules to accommodate calls. When the physician must interrupt a patient interview to take an urgent call, it is best to leave the consultation room and to return afterward, ready to be fully attentive to the patient. Similarly, patients should be asked to turn off cell phones during office visits.

"I have come to realize that the level of expertise a physician develops may be altered significantly by various factors, including fatigue, poor equipment, frequent interruptions, and emotional disturbances," said Francis Buck. "I now try to examine my most difficult diagnostic problems in the morning hours when I am mentally alert and most efficient."

Rushing Through an Examination

Cotton Feray allows a certain number of appointments for acute problems, a certain number for physicals, and a certain number for follow-up appointments. The receptionist asks patients what problems they are having, and Feray provides her with a list of patients who need longer appointments because of multiple problems. By allowing certain slots for physicals and other examinations, he never has to do a complete physical and Pap smear in a 10-minute slot. He schedules acute problems in the morning and all office surgery in the afternoon.

Some physicians schedule patients to arrive 15 minutes before their appointments, but they, too, have an obligation to be prompt. If you find yourself rushing through examinations, you need to plan your schedule more efficiently. To accommodate unexpected events, some physicians schedule "catch-up" periods.

Physician Denial of Significant Data

Occasionally, physicians may psychologically deny significant data or fail to absorb what a patient is saying because they do not wish to accept the evidence that the patient has a life-threatening or socially unacceptable disorder. A long physician–patient relationship may intensify the resistance. The physician must, however, recognize that venereal disease, cancer, child abuse, AIDS, and other serious disorders exist and, regardless of any personal discomfort, should look for them during the evaluation.

Acting on Insufficient Data

Some believe that pressure to reduce the cost of patient care has encouraged physicians to act on insufficient data. It puzzles Roger Stickney that some patients seem to prefer his treating them on instinct rather than factual data. But there is no substitute for a thorough physical examination and penetrating analysis of the medical history and symptoms. To avoid acting on inadequate data, Page McGirr asks two questions: (1) "Do I have enough data on this patient to make everything clear to another physician should I become ill or go on vacation?" and (2) "If the case ends in death or legal action, will my data support my actions?"

COLLEAGUES

Strained Relationships Within the Health Team

Unfortunately, strained and even destructive relationships can develop among physicians or other health professionals attending a patient, just as they can between any two human beings. Resolving the problem at the earliest possible moment serves the patient's interest best. Avoidance or delay usually worsen the situation. In Osler's words, "[W]hen any dispute or trouble does arise, go frankly, ere sunset, and talk the matter over, in which way you may gain a brother and a friend."[11] The willingness of the physician to listen carefully to all concerned is crucial, and frequent team meetings can maintain rapport.

Reporting of Errors and Omissions

"It is a major responsibility of physicians," Richard Reitemeier believes, "to report to the proper authorities all significant errors of commission and omission by the professional staff." Because physicians do not always do this, either for want of time or fear of criticism, simple, remediable problems may accumulate and become chronic. Reitemeier relates three incidents involving personal or institutional responsiveness in identifying and reporting problems. The first occurred when, during the middle of a hot summer, reports of prothrombin time at a hospital were unexpectedly high. Residents on the service had stopped believing the reports or using those data. Neither the residents nor the attending physicians supervising them, however, had investigated the cause of the abnormal prothrombin values. "When I came on the service," said Reitemeier, "I verified that the prothrombins were clinically inconsistent and then advised Walter Bowey, head of our coagulation laboratory. Bowey sent a technician to draw blood from a patient whose prothrombin time we knew should be normal. He gave part of the blood to the laboratory at the hospital and took the rest to the laboratory at the clinic, where a normal prothrombin value was reported. The sample processed at the hospital, transported in the regular fashion to the laboratory, was reported as abnormal.

"Upon investigation, it was discovered that the technicians assigned to draw blood from patients throughout the hospital often did not return to the laboratory for two to three hours. During that time the tubes with the blood samples were kept in racks on their carts, and the prothrombin became degraded as a result of the summer heat. Bowey simply provided each cart with a styrofoam container filled with dry ice to hold the blood samples, and the problem was immediately corrected. In addition, the incident led to a review by the laboratory of all studies affected by the ambient temperature.

"The next incident occurred when I saw a sturdy, tough Wyoming rancher weeping at his bedside on the morning he was to have colon surgery. He had had some 22 enemas in the preceding two and one-half days and told me that he was simply demoralized and could not endure having another one. Several months earlier the gastrointestinal surgeons had complained that the patients' colons were not completely free of feces at operation. This spurred the nurses performing routine preoperative preparations to subject patients to increasing numbers of enemas. A lack of communication among nursing supervisors resulted in an occasional comment about the inadequacy of the preparation, which led, in turn, to an effort to cleanse the colons completely. Large amounts of total body sodium and potassium may have been needlessly washed from these patients. A meeting with each group involved led to the conclusion that each patient needed only a few enemas for cleansing, and a much more humane and comfortable procedure was put into effect.

"The third example occurred while I was Chairman of Medicine. I kept hearing complaints that, although we might be able to put a man on the moon, we could never successfully collect three-day stool samples from a patient. I asked the administrative assistant in the Department of Medicine to solve the problem. He assigned two young men with Master's degrees in business administration to find out what could be done. They discovered that no one felt personally responsible for the collection or handling of the samples. The administrative assistant implemented a program that included methods to identify the samples clearly and specify directions for transferring the material to the responsible party. For the first time in the history of the institution, we had successful three-day collections of stools."

Solutions

Clement McDonald, recognizing man's limited ability to process information, designed a computer program with protocol-based reminders for physicians.[12] Physicians received computer-generated suggestions once a week for two months. As a result, they detected, and responded effectively to, twice as many clinical events and data as previously.

Monthly meetings for clinic and hospital staffs to discuss problems in practice due to systems difficulties and not lack of scientific knowledge should allow physicians and other healthcare professionals to identify, confront, and solve many of the problems outlined in this section.

* * * * *

The tendency for a complex system to go from a state of order to a state of disorder is a serious and frustrating reality in medical practice. A lost laboratory report can sometimes be more devastating to good patient care than a lack of medical knowledge. Computer reminder-and-monitoring systems can help prevent omissions, oversights, and inattention to abnormal findings and can thus lessen disorder in practice. Without such assistance, physicians must themselves constantly monitor and manage the care given their patients.

As Peter Mere Latham wrote: "[I]n medicine . . . it requires as much labour and time fairly to lay hold of an error, and uproot it, and have done with it, as to learn and settle a truth, and abide by it."[13]

REFERENCES

1. Block A. *Murphy's Law and Other Reasons Why Things Go Wrong.* Los Angeles: Price Stern Sloan; 1982: 11–12.

2. Williamson JW, Alexander M, Miller GE. Continuing education and patient care research: physician response to screening test results. *JAMA.* 1967; 201:938–942.

3. Starfield B, Scheff D. Effectiveness of pediatric care: the relationship between processes and outcome. *Pediatrics.* 1972; 49:547–552.

4. Morehead MA, Donaldson R. Quality of clinical management of disease in comprehensive neighborhood health centers. *Med Care.* 1974; 12:301–315.

5. Brook RH, Stevenson RL Jr. Effectiveness of patient care in an emergency room. *N Engl J Med.* 1970; 283:904–907.

6. Gonnella JS, Goran MJ, Williamson JW, Cotsonas NJ Jr. Evaluation of patient care: an approach. *JAMA*. 1970; 214:2040–2043.

7. Blunder of the year: NASA tangles with the metric system. *Science*. 1999; 286:2238.

8. Kranz G. *Failure Is not an Option. Mission Control from Mercury to Apollo 13 and Beyond.* New York: Simon & Schuster; 2000:204.

9. Kohn LT, Corrigan JM, Donaldson M, eds. *To Err Is Human: Building a Health System.* Washington: Institute of Medicine; 1999.

10. McDonald CJ, Weiner M, Hui SL. Deaths due to medical errors are exaggerated in Institute of Medicine report. *JAMA*. 2000; 284:93–95.

11. Osler W. The master-word in medicine. *Bull Johns Hopkins Hosp*. 1904;15:7.

12. McDonald CJ. Protocol-based computer reminders, the quality of care and the non-perfectability of man. *N Engl J Med.* 1976; 295:1351–1355.

13. Latham PM. General remarks on the practice of medicine. In: Martin R, ed. *The Collected Works of Dr. P. M. Latham.* London: New Sydenham Society; 1878:382.

COMMENTARY

• • •

Dr. Don Harper Mills received his M.D. degree from the University of Cincinnati and his J.D. degree from the University of Southern California. During 40-plus years of experience evaluating medical malpractice claims and sorting out practice problems that precipitate these claims, he has published professionally in the medicolegal field. He was the principal investigator for the California Medical Insurance Feasibility Study, a seminal project that laid the groundwork for Harvard's New York Study on medical adverse effects. Dr. Mills was Co-director of the California Hospital Association's Event Notification System, a program calculated to capture adverse events as they occur. At the Medical School, he participates in ethics rounds with upper class students. He is a Past President of the American College of Legal Medicine and of the American Academy of Forensic Sciences.

The Physician's Art of Self-defense

Don Harper Mills, M.D., J.D.
Clinical Professor of Pathology
Clinical Professor of Psychiatry and Behavioral Science
Keck School of Medicine, University of Southern California
Los Angeles, California
Medical Director, Octagon Risk Services
Long Beach, California

Despite the flood of reform legislation 25 years ago, malpractice issues remain unresolved. The primary focus has been on cost control, which, in some states like California, has been remarkably successful. Lawsuits are still being filed, however, and they are still very personal. Even in nonmeritorious cases, the physician is unduly stressed by the accusations and by the need for self-defense. This will not change so long as we have the present (fault) system of liability. The remaining remedy, therefore, is to become skilled in the art of self-defense (AOSD). Don't confuse this with defensive medicine, which is considered to be an irrational response to liability threats; it involves rational approaches, which I shall outline here.

YOUR PATIENT'S KEEPER

You may have read a lot about the physician–patient relationship, but it may not have been emphasized that even when you treat another physician, your special knowledge, training, and experience give you an advantage. You need to assume at all times that the patient knows less than you do about his condition and about your plans to manage it. Since there is no way you can fully inform the patient medically and scientifically, it is important to take adequate time to talk with your patients and let them react to your observations and recommendations. You are in the driver's seat. The advent of managed care tends to cloud that concept, but only slightly. Notwithstanding the restraints of managed care, you still have the primary obligation to serve your patients, including being your patient's keeper, at least medically and surgically. Don't defer to a patient's decision that contravenes your best judgment for the patient's well-being. Be sure you explain fully; then if the patient rejects your opinion, at least you have gone the extra mile your responsibility requires. This is a major element in AOSD.

DUTY TO WARN

Suppose you prescribe a sedative-acting antihistamine drug without warning of the dangers, and the patient proceeds to drive a bus, falls asleep at the wheel, and crashes into a pole, injuring the 15 passengers. They sue the bus company and the driver, but, during discovery, their lawyers learn that the driver had just started taking a certain antihistamine drug without knowledge of its sedative effect. You will be the newest defendant. You have an obligation to people whom you have never seen but who may be adversely affected by your patient's falling asleep at the wheel. The only way to protect these people is to warn the driver. You cannot prevent your patient from driving, but you are obliged to give warnings. If that warning is violated and injuries occur, you will not be a culpable defendant in any lawsuits.

A similar warning is required for patients who have newly diagnosed seizure disorders and for whom drug control has not yet been firmly established. In most states you are required to report these patients to the drivers licensing bureau. That agency usually revokes or otherwise restricts the patient's driving license until medical management can ensure driving competence. During the interval between your report and the agency's response, the patient should be advised of the danger of driving. If you have failed to warn the patient in that interval, you may have the same liability exposure as in the antihistamine case. Again, you have no authority to force the patient not to drive. All you can do is warn.

In either instance, your documentation of the warning is vital and becomes an integral part of AOSD. Remember that juries view physicians no better than patients, giving all people equal status in credibility assessment. If you contend that you warned the patient about the dangers of driving and the patient contends that you did not, the jury may believe either you or the patient. But if you have documented the warning, your credibility rises substantially above the 50/50 level. Documentation is not part of defensive medicine, but is a rational, vital element of AOSD.

Warning the patient of the danger of refusing your recommendation is also a rational requirement of your more informed position in the physician–patient relationship. Although you may believe that the new consent procedures (described later) allow the patient to accept the medical and surgical consequences, they do not relieve you of ensuring a full understanding of those consequences. Any patient who refuses your medical recommendations should be given written instructions documenting the refusal, as well as advice concerning alternative care. For instance, a diabetic patient with an infected foot ulcer needs hospitalization for intensive wound care and intravenous antibiotic coverage, but has refused for personal or financial reasons. You cannot force the patient to be hospitalized, nor should you abandon him. Rather, you should warn him of the dangers of ignoring your counsel and suggest alternative care, even though it may not be the best. If the problem is financial, you can direct the patient to a government hospital for care. If that is refused, the patient may choose the best outpatient care available, and you should outline it in your instructions. Remember, however, that you are not bound to care for this patient under such restrictions; your legal obligation is to resolve the problem or give the patient notice to seek care elsewhere. If he remains under your care, documentation of the decision-making process is mandatory, that is, you might have the patient sign a statement for your office record outlining your recommendation, the refusal, and the alternative remedies available. This does not constitute a consent in the strictest sense, but it certainly establishes that the patient recognized the serious consequences that were discussed and accepted responsibility for them. Those who practice AOSD well often use their office and hospital charts as communicating devices. As discussed later, this applies to interphysician communications as well as physician–patient communications.

The duty to warn extends to cautioning the patient to be alert to possible adverse effects of treatment (drug reactions, postoperative infections). If a drug you have prescribed can cause a significant rash (as in Stevens–Johnson syndrome), the patient should be advised to call you immediately should a rash appear. If he fails to report the rash promptly and continues taking the drug, one can infer that you failed to warn the patient. If you prescribe a drug that can produce liver toxicity (like isoniazid), you should instruct the patient, verbally and in writing, to watch for jaundice or other manifestations of hepatic toxicity and to notify you immediately, noting these instructions in your office record. You must assume that patients will not remember oral instructions once they leave your office and that if you fail to give written instructions or to document them in your records, the patients will say that you did not give oral instructions. Juries of nonphysicians tend to believe that physicians are obligated to look out for their patients, and AOSD demands that you know that. Of course, if your patient does notify you as instructed, you must react with the best medical advice; failing to discontinue the drug is indefensible.

The duty to warn also applies to instructions for follow-up care. If a return visit is required, you must advise the patient of the date before he leaves the office or clinic. If the patient fails to appear at the appointed hour and the condition is relatively minor, it may be disregarded. If, on the other hand, the follow-up is essential and the patient fails to appear, your office staff must color-code or otherwise tag the chart for immediate follow-up by telephone, facsimile, postal mail, or e-mail. You might consider setting aside charts of difficult patients for review at the end of the day. Occasionally, you might want to call a patient that evening to check on the patient's progress, or you might write a follow-up letter. Such actions are becoming more difficult in the controlled atmosphere of managed care, but they remain positive elements in AOSD. The bottom line of this discussion is that a patient's noncompliance may not free you from a lawsuit.

CONSENT FOR TREATMENT

The movement toward autonomy and the patient's right to choose does not contravene the principle that your more informed position in the physician–patient relationship creates special obligations. Your duty to decide what is best for your patient includes the duty to describe what is wrong, what should be done, what benefits may ensue, and what adverse effects may occur. Once you have made your recommendations, the patient must have enough information to say "no" or to choose some reasonable alternative. If the answer is "no" and your recommendation is important, AOSD requires trying to convince the patient to change his mind. The autonomy movement does not extinguish your duty to try to convince patients to do what you think is best for them.

Lawsuits arising from postoperative or medicinal complications may allege lack of informed consent or negligence in the performance of the procedure or the prescribing of the drug. If the patient's attorney fails to prove that your negligence caused the adverse outcome, a second arrow in the bow is to try to prove you failed to communicate with the patient—that there was no informed consent. The consent problem, therefore, is not a medical practice problem. In most states, the patient does not need to have an expert physician show that you were negligent for failing to disclose the necessary information to permit a valid consent. All that is necessary is to show the court that the missing information was material to the decision to accept your recommendation. If, for example, you recommend a subtotal gastric resection for benign gastric disease, you must disclose the risk of injuring the spleen during the procedure. If you recommend a thyroidectomy, you must disclose the risk of injury to the recurrent laryngeal nerve and the parathyroid glands. If you fail to make these disclosures, the patient may later contend in court that he would not have consented to the procedure had he known the truth about the consequences. You still have the opportunity to show the jury that what you intended to do was vitally necessary for the patient's well-being—that a reasonable patient would have consented to the procedure even had you made the proper disclosures about the adverse consequences. If the case is medically clean (no negligence in the decision to perform the procedure or in the way it was done), the decision is usually for the defense, even if the jury believes complete disclosure was not made for a valid consent.

Such a favorable decision does not obtain with misdisclosures. If you underplay the risks of the procedure by saying, "It's simple" or "It's no more dangerous than crossing the street," you may be held responsible for the adverse outcome because a jury will be told that your minimizing the risks influenced the patient's decision to proceed and be subjected to the real risks. Misdisclosures almost always result in a verdict for the prosecution. The AOSD requires you to understand the difference between nondisclosure and misdisclosure. Defense against nondisclosure still requires showing that your management was otherwise above reproach. If the medical aspects of the case are not clean, you will not win the consent issue, even though it is only a nondisclosure problem.

JUDGMENT DECISIONS

Most malpractice lawsuits that turn sour for the defense are the result of the physician's poor judgment, not technical malperformance. The first critical focus in the lawsuit deals with the decision to perform the procedure or to prescribe the drug. "Were there adequate medical or surgical indications?" is a medical, not a legal, question. By acting without adequate indication, you expose the patient to the unnecessary risk of an adverse outcome or drug reaction. You cannot justify this exposure by telling the patient that such an outcome may happen, that is, consent is no defense for an unnecessary procedure. A patient who comes in with pharyngitis, asks you for penicillin, and receives it may have a viable lawsuit if he suffers a significant adverse reaction to that drug. There may be reasons for overusing oral antibiotics, including diagnostic uncertainty and even the perceived threat of litigation, but the latter factor is irrational at best. The patient with streptococcal pharyngitis who is given penicillin may have the same adverse outcome, but at least the issue of the need for the drug has been settled by the medical facts.

The second judgment issue focuses on contraindications: Should the patient not be given the drug at this time? Should the operation not be performed today or on this patient? Even for streptococcal pharyngitis, penicillin should not be prescribed for a patient who is allergic to it. Such a case leads into the issue of asking about drug sensitivity and documenting the answers. How are charts flagged in your office? Is someone assigned to monitor the sensitivity history once you have prescribed a particular drug? These are critical elements in AOSD.

If you injudiciously tamper with your records, be sure to notify your attorney at the outset. With critical retrospection, it may be possible to explain away your alterations. But if not, at least you will not compound your problem in deposition or on the witness stand by claiming that the records are real and proper. Remember that there are expert document examiners in every major community who decide the authenticity of record entries. Don't try to fool them; the more you try, the worse it looks.

Is this something you can do, or should you call in a consultant? You decide daily whether you are competent to do what you intend to do. Assuming you are trained to do well what you intend to do, do you do it often enough to maintain your judgment and dexterity? The past decade has seen a growing list of procedures that require specific volumes to avoid increased risks of adverse outcomes. A recent study analyzed repair of abdominal aortic aneurysms performed between 1990 and 1995. The mortality rate was 2.5 percent at hospitals where more than 100 operations were performed, but 4.2 percent at hospitals with fewer aneurysm operations. Surgeons doing 10 or more procedures had a mortality rate for aneurysmal repair of 2.8 percent to 3.8 percent, but those doing only 2 to 9 procedures had a rate of 4.9 percent.[1] You need to know what procedures are volume-sensitive and when volume-sensitivity also applies to the hospital. Additionally, surgical research has created a new field of minimally invasive procedures. If these were not part of your original training, you need to establish adequate credentials to perform them. "See one, do one" is not the best approach.

Even "performance" problems involve judgment. When do you convert a laparoscopic-assisted gallbladder operation to an open one? What measures do you take to prevent injuring a ureter or the bladder during a pelvic operation? What measures do you take to ensure the integrity of the ureter or the bladder before closing the incision? Lawsuits arising from such injuries during operation are lost more often because of delayed diagnosis and repair than because of the operative injury. Disclosing the risk of ureteral injury to the patient for consent purposes does not absolve you of liability. Nothing is further from the truth. You still have the responsibility of deciding that the procedure was necessary, that you were competent to perform it, that you took precautions to prevent the injury, and that you did what was needed to discover that the injury occurred and to ameliorate the outcome, if possible. Recognition of these additional issues is a critical part of AOSD.

You are allowed to be wrong about a patient's diagnosis, but only if the missed diagnosis or nondiagnosis is reasonable and founded on adequate data (historical information, physical examination, and special diagnostic procedures indicated). Failure to consider the white blood and differential counts in deciding between appendicitis and viral enteritis has resulted in liability when the diagnosis was wrong. Similar outcomes have occurred in cases regarding meningitis and pneumonia. Lawyers like these cases because, in retrospect, the jury will realize that you made a mistake in the diagnosis (you diagnosed viral encephalitis and so failed to prescribe antibiotics for an actual bacterial meningitis), and the burden shifts to you to justify having been wrong. The AOSD requires you to consider the adequacy of the data in each instance. Some people consider this defensive medicine at its worst, requiring excessive tests and procedures. That is a misconception. You should know what the data require for most of the diseases you treat. You need not go beyond those data; indeed, if you do, you may be exposing yourself to liability for unnecessary procedures. The AOSD requires that you know the difference between doing all that is necessary and not doing what is unnecessary.

COMPLICATING CONSULTATIONS

You and your consultant must know who is going to do what. If he makes recommendations but does not write orders, you are required to follow up. If you expected him to write the orders, but failed to notice that he did not, the patient will suffer, and so will your defense. Such a physician–physician communication breakdown is a totally indefensible, but remarkably common, problem. Many hospitals have established guidelines to cover consultant responsibility, and you need to learn precisely what the hospital protocol requires. Don't leave to chance your commitment to the patient.

Curbstone consultations are another matter. Be careful about relying on the off-the-cuff opinions of colleagues who have not had the opportunity to evaluate your patient's complete data, and avoid putting those consultants' names in the patient's chart without consent. If a colleague asks your advice in the dressing room, you may certainly offer generalized statements, but be sure to state you need to see the patient before speaking with certainty. That will either lead to a formal consultation or terminate the discussion.

Sending specimens out for laboratory analysis and having imaging studies performed are consultations of a sort. You need to ensure that abnormal results are noticed. This requires a system to get these results before your eyes, to prompt you to call a patient back or to advise the patient on the next visit. I regularly see instances in which abnormal data enter charts (office or hospital) without the attending physician's awareness. The patient suffers in such a system breakdown. Finally, I strongly urge the creation of flow sheets, by hand or computer, to provide sequential laboratory or x-ray data at a glance. Trends are much more readily recognized in this way.

GUIDELINES

Today, there are guidelines and guidelines. You need to differentiate the good from the bad for the conditions you usually treat. Most will not be introduced into direct evidence against you, but will be brought in by opposing experts who will claim you did not follow standard procedure in arriving at a diagnosis or treating a particular condition. On cross-examination, that expert will buttress his contention about the standard of practice by citing certain guidelines. This enters the guidelines into evidence through the back door. It is your responsibility to be as informed as possible about guidelines applicable to your practice. Review them and decide whether your practice will abide by them; if not, formulate a statement rationalizing your differences and put them in a special file. Then, if you are accused of violating the standard, you will be able to show that you thought about it at the time this patient was being treated and decided on alternative treatment for the reasons stated in your rationalization.

This brings us to a discussion of the drug package insert, prepared by the manufacturer and published in the *Physician's Desk Reference*. For drugs you administer, you should be fully aware of the contents of the package insert, since in most states the insert applicable to your patent's drug can be introduced into evidence against you. The contents do not establish the standard of practice regarding a particular drug, but may be considered by a jury in deciding what the standard of practice is. If you deviate from recommended usage, you need to document the reasons (as with guidelines). Clearly, AOSD requires you to be prepared with the type of medical documentation you may need if a patient should suffer adverse outcomes.

You have the right, medically and legally, to use a drug "off label," but, again, you need to know that your usage is "off label," and you must be able to support the "off label" use with appropriate citations. Like the rationalizations discussed previously, these citations need not be in the patient's chart, but may be kept in a separate file.

MANAGING ADVERSE OUTCOMES

How you handle poor results often determines whether you will face a lawsuit and how it will be resolved. If you clam up, requiring the patient to go to a lawyer to find out what really happened, you can expect the worst. You have been told over the years not to confess, because your statements to the patient or to the family can be used against you in a subsequent lawsuit, but you can talk to a patient and explain what happened without becoming confessional. Indeed, many cases are resolved in subsequent mediation, without the full litigation process, merely by a discussion of what happened. Even that procedure, however, is enough to cause you considerable stress. The AOSD requires you to communicate adequately with the patient about what happened, and even why it happened, if necessary. And it may reduce your stress to say occasionally that you are sorry. You do not need to tinge your remarks with guilt by saying "It's my fault" or "I shouldn't have done that."

The AOSD may require you to reevaluate your status with patients now and then. While making money is a business, treating patients is not. Your advantageous position *vis-à-vis* patients obligates you to protect and guide them through the highly technical and judgmental aspects of modern healthcare. My discussion of these issues may have seemed provocative at times, but with good cause.

SYSTEM AND PERSONAL ERRORS

Patients are sometimes injured in hospitals, not by physicians, but by system management problems. Delays by hospital personnel in following orders or in getting patients to the operating room can have devastating adverse outcomes. You need to be alert that such shortcomings might affect one of your own patients. Your only recourse may be to report the problem to the department head or chief of staff. Failure to do so may lead to your own liability if your patient is mishandled. Sometimes AOSD requires you to rattle someone else's cage.

REFERENCE

1. Dardik A, Lin JW, Eng M, Gordon TA, Williams GM, Perler BA. Results of elective abdominal aortic aneurysm repair in the 1990s: a population based analysis of 2335 cases. *J Vasc Surg*. 1999;30:985–995.

14

Organized Medicine and Lifelong Learning

• • •

> The AAMC believes that specialty societies and specialty boards are best able to assist physicians in their efforts to maintain their clinical competence.
>
> JORDAN J. COHEN, M.D.[1]

Physicians in the United States have unprecedented educational resources from county, state, and national medical organizations, and particularly specialty societies. County societies sponsor computer bulletin boards, chat rooms, legislative updates, and, often, short reviews of important medical studies. State associations provide in-depth information on current state and national medical legislation and ethics, and may offer help and advice to impaired physicians and those with other such problems. Dennis Wentz addressed the issue of organized medicine: "Despite diminishing membership, city, county, and state medical societies still serve a valuable purpose. Unlike the major specialty societies, which convene a single annual meeting, city and county medical societies meet at least monthly and promote collegiality to all members. In an address to the Canadian Medical Association, Osler highlighted these assets: 'By no means the smallest advantage of our meetings is the promotion of harmony and good fellowship. Medical men, particularly in smaller places, live too much apart and do not see enough of each other. In large cities we rub each other's angles down and carom off each other without feeling the shock very much, but it is an unfortunate circumstance that in many towns the friction, being on a small surface, hurts; and mutual misunderstandings arise to the destruction of all harmony. As a result of this may come a professional isolation with a corroding influence of a most disastrous nature, converting, in a few years, a genial, good fellow into a bitter old Timon, railing against the practice of medicine and his colleagues in particular.'"[2]

The American Medical Association (AMA) has taken the lead in establishing quality standards for continuing medical education (CME). In 1955, the AMA began evaluating institutions offering "postgraduate medical education," as it was then known, and the major postgraduate/CME activities that met the standards were listed in *The Journal of the American Medical Association* (*JAMA*). Now, a major change is underway, with CME encompassing lifetime learning for all physicians in a rapidly changing environment. In September 1999, the AMA's Division of CME became the Division of Continuing Physician Professional Development, a change that may dismiss the notion that continuing medical education is limited to lecture courses and conferences. Physician development comprises many concepts beyond teaching and learning, including emphasis on professionalism, patient outcomes, population-based medicine, office management, and physician leadership.

The National Medical Association (NMA) began in 1895 as a major provider of continuing medical education for African-American physicians. Its culture-sensitive educational activities at annual scientific assemblies and at regional, state, and local society meetings stress diseases common to African-Americans. The annual assembly includes 25 specialty programs with a nationally renowned faculty from such institutions as Howard University, Meharry College, and Morehouse College. William Matory, Director of Continuing Medical Education for NMA, believes that "The cultural atmosphere provides African-American classmates, friends, and former teachers with opportunities for leadership in a particularly salutary environment."

NATIONAL MEDICAL ORGANIZATIONS

Most specialty societies were founded to foster quality medical care by setting standards and providing education. The American College of Physicians (ACP), for example, was founded in 1915 to uphold the highest standards in medical education, practice, and research for internal medicine. The American Academy of Orthopaedic Surgeons (AAOS) formally endorsed a lifelong commitment to continuing education as essential for its fellows, issuing an "Advisory Statement" in 1991 (updated in 1996) on the "Commitment to Excellence: Maintaining Skills and Knowledge Through Lifelong Learning." The American Academy of Family Physicians (AAFP), founded in 1947 to promote and maintain higher standards for family physicians providing continuing comprehensive healthcare, was the first to set standards for, and to require, CME for its membership. Its three-pronged approach includes producing a variety of CME formats designed to meet members' needs and preferences, maintaining detailed records of individual members' CME activities, and, in 1948, establishing its own system of identifying and accrediting programs relevant to family physicians. This system will soon incorporate evidence-based medicine into CME accreditation for family physicians.

Medical societies have fulfilled their pledge to support their members by providing more quality educational products and opportunities. Changes are evolving so rapidly that the educational products described here may be improved and retitled within a few months or years, but the principles and commitment to lifelong learning will remain. Physicians should take advantage of the extraordinary opportunities now available.

All specialty societies have annual sessions featuring a wide variety of learning formats, including lectures, panel discussions, debates, scientific and technical exhibits, poster exhibits, and multimedia education (videotapes and computer instructional programs). Meet-the-professor sessions permit fairly close contact with experts. Often available are hands-on training in computer skills and practice sessions on clinical skills, such as physical examinations, skin biopsies, arthrocentesis, and the opportunity to "work up" a live standardized patient. All annual sessions provide extensive commercial exhibits of state-of-the-art diagnosis, therapy, and practice management for many conditions. The American College of Cardiology's Annual Session includes "Spotlight Sessions," with intensive instruction in such subjects as echocardiography, interventional cardiology, and clinical cardiology, and ends with a wrap-up discussion of "Meeting Highlights." Annual meetings of many specialty societies include late-breaking reports of clinical trials.

Since the wide variety of offerings at the annual session can be overwhelming to new attendees, they should select in advance which sessions to attend and make an hour-by-hour schedule to prevent wasting significant time wandering around a large convention center. The Web sites of many specialty societies now allow scanning and creating a personalized meeting schedule. Reading the abstracts, usually provided in advance, and framing specific questions to ask are helpful. If your questions are not answered during the formal presentation, there is usually time to question the speaker during a designated period or directly after the session. For maximum profit, take notes and review them at the end of the day to ensure legibility and comprehension. Discussing content with a colleague at the meeting or after returning home will further solidify the newly acquired information.

From 1991 to 1999, The American College of Physicians operated a "College within the College," which used small groups to enhance learning. Eight to 10 physicians would meet each morning of the annual meeting and determine which sessions each member would attend. At lunch and in the early evening, members of each group would discuss the presentations they attended, giving each the advantage of multiple sessions. Moreover, the collegiality thus established converted a large, sometimes impersonal, meeting to a friendly and enjoyable activity. Physicians can, of course, form their own informal groups to share information and interact with colleagues.

Specialty societies have expanded their educational activities beyond their flagship annual session. In addition to regional meetings organized jointly by the society staff and local physicians, most societies publish a peer-reviewed journal. Many offer audiotapes (pioneered by Audio-Digest) and videotapes, as well as self-assessment programs of study material and test questions in print or on compact disks (CD-ROMs). The American Academy of Orthopaedic Surgeons offers a dozen self-assessment programs—one in general orthopedics and several in specialized topics, such as the shoulder and sports medicine. The American College of Physicians–American Society of Internal Medicine (ACP–ASIM) has supplemented its printed Medical Knowledge Self-Assessment Program (MKSAP) with an Audio Companion featuring a general internist discussing highlights of the program with a leading subspecialist. Self-assessment programs, which provide an opportunity to keep abreast and to review basic principles, provide excellent preparation for recertification board examinations.

Many societies provide interactive programs on CD-ROMs: the physician is presented a case study and allowed to answer questions by selecting diagnostic and therapeutic choices. Also available are audiovisual libraries containing slides, audiotapes, and videotapes.

The American Academy of Ophthalmology (AAO) produces *Focal Points*, a subscription print series of practical applications of research, and *Ophthalmology Monographs*, a text series on clinical skills in specialized topics. The AAO also cooperates with other specialty societies to produce teaching materials for medical students and practicing primary-care physicians. The American College of Obstetrics and Gynecology offers numerous educational opportunities to enhance the development of healthcare professionals in all aspects of women's healthcare.

Some societies have learning centers at their headquarters. The Heart House of the American College of Cardiology in Bethesda, Maryland, has exceptional audiovisual capabilities, as well as specially designed chairs with built-in response systems that allow physicians to answer multiple-choice questions. The AAOS conducts surgical skills programs at its headquarters, where physicians can practice techniques using cadaver specimens or bone models with the hand tools and power tools provided. The Orthopaedic Learning Center was jointly developed and funded by the AAOS and the Arthroscopy Association of North America, which coordinate scheduling their respective courses, primarily on weekends. The AAOS is beginning virtual-reality demonstrations and investigating the development of a knee arthroscopy simulation that would provide experience indistinguishable from the actual procedure.

Medical societies are embracing the Internet to disseminate information to physicians as well as the general public. Numerous formats are offered, including case presentations with discussion as well as didactic lectures, often from the annual meeting. Frequently, societies offer monographs, short quizzes, and online CME. The AAOS offers various images: plain radiographs, CTs, MRIs, and arthrograms. The Academy of Family Physicians emphasizes the "Case of the Month." The American Academy of Pediatrics (AAP) Web site presents specialty news, guideline endorsements, treatment recommendations, and AAP policy statements on many diagnostic, therapeutic, and societal issues related to pediatric care. The American Academy of Ophthalmology's Web site features an Online Education Center that offers short courses, self-assessment cases, selected annual meeting lectures, and reviews of recent research in major ophthalmology topics. The American College of Physicians–American Society of Internal Medicine offers Clinical Problem Solving Cases for CME credit, *Annals of Internal Medicine* online (http://www.annals.org), and a Web site for patients (http://www.doctorsforadults.com). It is a safe bet that societies will continue to expand online educational opportunities.

The American College of Cardiology is exploring methods to assist individual physicians in self-directed, practice-oriented education, including the development or adoption of tools to help define and address educational needs. Databases are being developed to help physicians pose specific clinical questions at the point of care and retrieve brief answers from practice guidelines and other sources. Other information, such as case studies, self-assessment questions, journal articles, and slides from lecture presentations, will also be available. The goal is to provide brief answers to immediate questions as well as in-depth study materials that the physician may review at another time.

These are just a few examples of effective educational products and aids available from medical societies. The programs are directed by practicing and academic physicians with the help of the societies' experienced, full-time staff members. In recent years, societies have become more involved in political and ethical issues affecting their specialty, but the dedication to aiding physicians in lifelong learning is intensifying, not waning. Future directions posited by the American Board of Medical Specialties and the consequent planning activities of several member boards indicate that recertification will emphasize the lifelong learning of individual physicians.

REFERENCE

1. Cohen JJ. Association of American Medical Colleges Memorandum #00-32, issued 2000 Jul 31.

2. Osler W. The growth of a profession. Presidential address, Canadian Medical Association, Chatham, Ontario, 1885 Sep 2. *Can Med & Surg J.* 1885;14:129–155.

REFLECTIONS

• • •

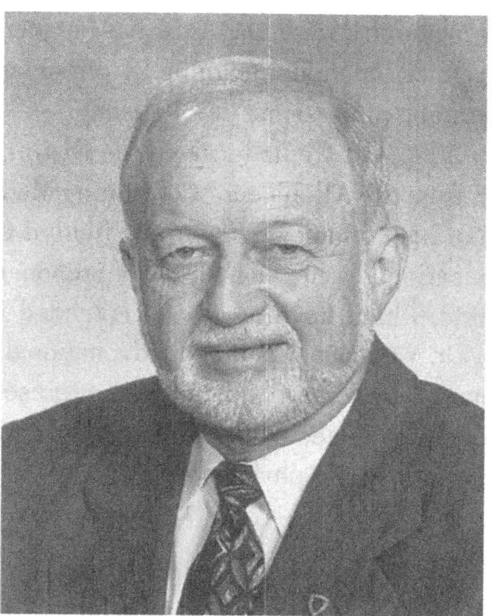

The first benefit of medical society membership is to provide collegial camaraderie, to get us connected with peers and associates outside our usual sphere of interaction.

DENNIS K. WENTZ, M.D.

Dr. Dennis Wentz has had a lifelong interest in the values and standards of medicine. Stimulated by his professors at the University of Chicago, he trained in internal medicine and gastroenterology but moved from clinical and academic pursuits to a career in medical management. He strongly believes that physicians must hold senior administrative positions in academic medical institutions and that they must be educated to fill such roles. After further studies in health systems management, Dr. Wentz became the medical director of two university hospitals and a senior administrator in another academic center. In 1988, he accepted an invitation from the American Medical Association (AMA) to lead its program on Continuing Medical Education (CME), later renamed Continuing Physician Professional Development (CPPD). Using the mechanism of the AMA Physician's Recognition Award, the AMA has broadened the concept of CME to recognize individual learning by physicians in the larger context of continuing professional development.

In January 2002, Dr. Wentz received the Distinguished Service Award in CME from the Alliance for Continuing Medical Education in recognition of his lifelong service to the field of CME as a CME professional, a national policy maker, and a proponent of collaborative CME efforts, which have now been extended internationally. More recently, Dr. Wentz has spearheaded a national effort to create awareness among physicians and industry representatives of the ethical guidelines developed by the profession to address the issues of gift-giving by industry to physicians.

Medical Organizations and Professionalism

Dennis K. Wentz, M.D.
Director, Division of Continuing Physician Professional Development
American Medical Association
Chicago, Illinois

> [N]o physician has a right to consider himself as belonging to himself; but all ought to regard themselves as belonging to the profession, inasmuch as each is part of the profession; and care for the part naturally looks to care for the whole.
>
> WILLIAM OSLER[1]

As a medical student, and even as a house officer, I rarely considered belonging to organized medicine. None of my professors mentioned it. But I was dutiful and perhaps a bit excited when Theodore E. Woodward, Professor of Medicine and my mentor at the University of Maryland, encouraged me to accompany him to a meeting of the Baltimore City Medical Society. At that time, the meetings consisted of a scientific program followed by a reception, responsibility for the scientific program alternating between the University of Maryland and Johns Hopkins medical schools. Because the meetings were at the headquarters of the Medical and Chirurgical Faculty of Maryland, I saw for the first time the extensive and historically important library of the Faculty and the frequency with which members used it. The portraits of famous Maryland physicians hanging in the hallways were both fascinating and humbling. But it was my initial exposure to the practicing physicians, as well as the tough questions and high quality of the scientific discourse, that impressed me most.

Thus, when I joined the faculty at the University of Maryland, it wasn't difficult to decide to join the medical societies, even though the dues seemed high to a young assistant professor. Although my objectives may have been unclear, my membership proved salutary. Particularly at the monthly meetings, I benefited from getting to know my colleagues and learning what all the real issues were, not just those in academia. Although the scientific programs were good, I inevitably learned more in the hallways than in the sessions. Society activities brought new knowledge about the practice of medicine: I came to understand, and even influence, our organization's policies. Osler was correct when he said: "No class of men need friction so much as physicians; no class gets less. . . . [T]he medical society is the best corrective, and a man misses a good part of his education who does not get knocked about a bit by his colleagues in discussions and criticisms."[1]

The first benefit of medical society membership is to provide collegial camaraderie, to get us connected with peers and associates outside our usual sphere of interaction. Whether in a general medical society, where we can learn from all the medical specialties, or in our own specialty societies, the sharing of information, ideas, problems, and opportunities is a significant part of continuing education.

The second benefit of a medical society membership is to keep us aware of new developments and new information at the cutting edge of medicine. Without a constant dose of such information, no one can deliver the quality of healthcare required by colleagues and patients. To those who discount continuing education's impact, ask yourself: Are you practicing the medicine taught in formal education and training five years ago? Has any clinician failed to make significant changes in daily practice as a result of new knowledge and skills?

A third benefit of our medical societies is a commitment to professionalism, including the promotion of standards of education and quality assurance to society at large. In this regard, acknowledgment is due the prestigious journals sponsored by medical societies. Physicians, on average, report reading five to seven hours a week, much of it in medical journals, a key source of continuing education. Increasingly, societies are turning to the Internet to disseminate information. In print or online, these publications inform physicians of new medical developments.

Another important contribution of the medical societies can be best identified as advocacy. In the radically changing environment of medicine over the past 20 years, societies have interceded on behalf of practicing physicians locally and nationally.

Medical societies provide instruction in leadership, negotiation, and management skills. The American Medical Association (AMA) critically reviews the scientific aspects of medicine, and, through its Institute of Medical Ethics, has sponsored major educational programs in end-of-life care. The AMA Council on Ethical and Judicial Affairs determines the code of ethics for the profession.

The aggregate output of our medical societies on behalf of all of us who practice medicine is considerable. The rest of the world looks to this country for the ideal in educational and practice standards.

REFERENCE

1. Osler W. The functions of a state faculty. In Bryan CS. *Osler. Inspiration from a Great Physician.* New York: Oxford Univ Press; 1997:50.

15

Women Physicians

• • •

Man may work from sun to sun,
But woman's work is never done.

ANONYMOUS

TIME PRESSURES FROM MULTIPLE ROLES

The Association of American Medical Colleges reported that in 1977–1978 women graduates of U.S. medical schools represented 21.4 percent of the class; by 1999–2000, that figure had risen to 42.5 percent. If this upward trend continues, women will constitute the majority of the medical profession within the next few decades.

Unless the roles of men and women change dramatically, women physicians will continue to have more difficulty than men in finding time for continuing education. Because women often have multiple roles as physician, wife, mother, and homemaker, they must set priorities, especially in assigning time for education, sometimes at the expense of recreational activities. Fortunately, a balancing trend is occurring in the United States, with men taking a more active role in household duties and child-rearing. And more working couples with children are relying on outside help from relatives or nannies.

The techniques and resources to facilitate lifelong learning in medicine are the same for men and women. In this chapter, women physicians describe how they manage their multiple duties.

Jacqueline Miller believed that early in her career she faced a larger problem than women have today, since mores have changed somewhat. But when she questioned younger associates and friends who work in other occupations, she concluded that women with homes and families generally have more responsibilities than their husbands. "Even when the husbands help," she explained, "the daily responsibilities for the home and the family continue to rest largely with the wives. A woman physician's attention is divided between practice and home, whereas a man's primary concern is his practice and only secondarily duties in the home. This situation may lead women to feel conflicted, and the stress becomes more acute when they have children who are having problems."

Time is the major problem women physicians face, according to Marjorie Price Wilson. "They do more than full-time housewives in the same socioeconomic circles. When they enter medicine, women often do not abandon any of the traditional roles of mother and household manager. As I look back on my life, I realize that although my husband shared the time with the children, I actually spent more time than he did with them while never compromising my professional duties. His life would have been the same if I had been a full-time housewife. I maintained a fairly traditional lifestyle at home; even with a great deal of good help, I still managed the 'helpers' and the household. Most women who assume multiple roles, regardless of their profession, perform them all with great intensity. Some professional men, on the other hand, may feel a greater intensity about their profession than their family responsibilities."

Laurel Weibel traces the difference between men and women physicians in this regard to the fact that few women can go home from their medical offices and relax—read journals, listen to the radio, or watch television. "There are always meals to prepare, children to counsel, and after-dinner chores to do. Even when there is an evening meeting to attend, the family must first be fed. And in the morning, babies have to be bathed and fed, or lunches have to be made."

This "time-vise" has troubled Eileen Duggan. "Being locked into a schedule makes me feel as if I am compressing my professional and private spheres too much. Medicine can be extremely seductive, especially to someone who likes to think of herself as indispensable. Because of the wear-and-tear on my physical and mental health, I have had to set priorities in my work. Mornings with my children are special times, and so I do not attend early rounds, even though my associate does. I make my commitments at work very specific and manageable. I also schedule three to five meetings each year for education. Most are two- or three-day meetings and are inspiring and invigorating. Getting away for a fresh perspective is necessary, I believe. Women physicians should not begrudge paying part of their earnings to another person to do housework. My friends who insist on doing their own housework seem dissatisfied with themselves unless it is done perfectly."

Women physicians are vulnerable to interruptions by husbands, children, and household responsibilities, and this vulnerability makes it difficult to establish a "do not disturb" period. Whereas men physicians face interruptions from medical emergencies, women face interruptions from multiple sources.

There is still great reliance on women for housecleaning, cooking, laundering, and shopping, observed Lailee Bakhtiar. "Few husbands want their day interrupted by household chores. A live-in housekeeper can help with some of these tasks, but this is only a partial solution. Housekeepers quit, children get sick, and the final responsibility for organizing usually falls on the wife. Organization, strength, and a spouse willing to share duties can all help."

Karin Jamison also sees multiple roles as a major problem. "Add to the list any personal interest the woman has outside of medicine and her family, and the demands on her time and energy pose a real conflict. Only the housekeeper role can be delegated, not that of the 'homemaker.' A responsible male physician will also have conflicts if he takes his roles as father, husband, son, sibling, friend, and neighbor seriously, but the role of physician is superimposed on the roles of husband and father, since a traditional aspect of both the latter has been to be a good provider. So he does not experience the same 'shortage' of time or the same degree of inner conflict. For a woman physician, fatigue is a constant companion."

Motherhood complicates the matter. Lailee Bakhtiar sees flexibility and physical well-being as two desirable qualities of a woman physician. "A pregnant woman can work until delivery, and her husband can be supportive, loving, and helpful, but the man married to a woman physician pays a toll as her professional life and the size of their family grow. The difficulty in striking a balance probably accounts for the high divorce rate among women physicians. An extended family, with a solid bond among parents and in-laws, can help with problems arising from the mother's absence when she is at meetings or work."

During pregnancy, Linda Shortliffe had some physical incapacitation, but it did not affect her daytime work. "I worked up to the time of the delivery and was not bothered much by pregnancy, but I was not as efficient in reading and writing in the evenings. I took four weeks off after delivery and found it difficult to return to work after that. Being physically present in the hospital during the day was not a problem, but the chronic fatigue from rising every two to three hours for nursing was. It was difficult to find opportunities to freeze breast milk during the first several months after I returned to work. During that time, many routine home chores, such as laundry, cooking, grocery shopping, and housecleaning, were taking valuable time from our baby. As a result, we employed a live-in 'nanny' and delegated some of the household chores to her so that we could have more time with our child and still fulfill our professional responsibilities."

Interruption of Practice by Childbirth and Child-rearing

For six years, while Karin Jamison's children were in high school, she closed her private practice and worked only two days a week at an Air

Force Base outpatient clinic. "Because I was free of the heavy responsibility of a solo family practice, I was able to attend many medical meetings. The patient contact at the Air Force Base helped me maintain my clinical skills, although I had no acutely ill patients to care for at that time. When I returned to private practice, I wanted to do emergency medicine and so took some intensive courses in that field. I also studied a great deal on subjects for which I knew I would have responsibilities."

When Jacqueline Miller had a child just a few weeks after she completed her residency, she stayed away from work for a year. "I enjoyed my child and did not keep up with medicine, so I found it very difficult when I went back. I don't think I did any of it quite right. I would now recommend that a woman do everything possible to maintain her intellectual activities and her contact with medicine. You can get out of touch in a year. One thing that helped me catch up was that I had not yet taken my clinical pathology boards. I settled down and prepared myself for them, spending the better part of a year in intensive study. I did my studying after the baby went to bed. During that time I had household help and considered it a wise investment."

Kit Chambers sums up her successful career as an anesthesiologist: "I did not marry until seven years after graduation from medical school; I was out of residency and getting ready to take anesthesia boards. Having a husband in academic medicine prompted me to enter private practice because academic salaries were less than adequate at that time. I had expected my working hours to be more flexible than they were, but my work in the group practice was a joy. Several coworkers were of my age and had similar training. The San Fernando Valley population was increasing by 1,000 a day, so the demand for medical services was high. We worked long hours at 10 hospitals, and attended University of Southern California or University of California at Los Angeles weekly Grand Rounds. The group was well-organized, and everyone except the older physicians was Board-certified.

"Before our first child was born, I hired a nanny who stayed with us for three years. A wonderful lady became our substitute grand-

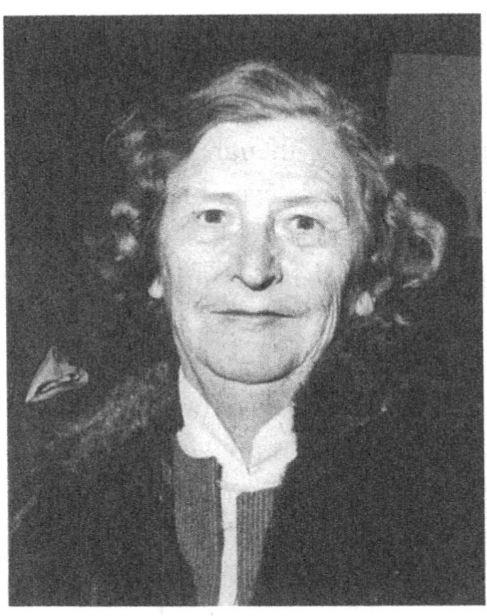

An understanding husband is of inestimable help to the woman physician.

Dame Sheila Sherlock, M.D. (1918–2002)
Former Emeritus Professor.
The Royal Free Hospital, London, England

mother, filling in for the nannies when necessary. Our last nanny left us when both children were teenagers, and I stopped working so I could assume the childcare and carpooling. I have never regretted the time that I was a stay-at-home mother.

"When the children were away at college, I returned to work in the County Health Services. It was not easy. Anesthesia had continued to change rapidly, with an amazing array of new agents, techniques, and equipment. I was fortunate to have several mentors who helped me.

"I cannot think of another profession that gives such a sense of service to humanity and continuous personal satisfaction for doing your best in your daily work. The patients reward you with gratitude and trust. Pediatric patients are a bonus. It also helps to have good health and boundless energy. Support from your husband is essential, and I was fortunate to have that. We took the children on vacations to medical meetings, which they described as magical times. Neither child considered having two working parents a problem, but were pleased to have another adult available for care and counseling."

Because Barbara Buchanan's third child had a congenital anomaly requiring surgery and a prolonged recovery period, she took off six months from medicine. "I never thought it was difficult to 'keep up' during the months I took off, or to 'catch-up' once I started practicing again. If anything, I had more time to read journals and books during that time."

Some women physicians do not take time off for childbirth. Susan Tully went back to work within a couple of weeks after her children were born. "I paid people to care for the children and was never out any longer than my scheduled vacation."

ENLISTING SUPPORT

"The first thing a young woman physician with a family needs to acknowledge," in Jacqueline Miller's view, "is that she cannot do everything herself and do it as well as she would like. Physicians in general, and women physicians in particular, are perfectionists, and it is difficult to acknowledge that you are not going to be superb in all your efforts; there is simply not enough time. You must accept your need for help. My own solution has been to recognize that I will not have as much spendable income as I might expect because I must employ help. Economizing on household and babysitting help is a mistake. The woman physician may also want to spend a few more hours a week at the office or hospital than a man, since she can do some of her studying there. I can get a lot done from 5:00 to 6:00 p.m., or from 5:30 to 7:00 p.m., whereas when I go home, I get little or no work done. Sharing the responsibilities at home with others as much as possible is very helpful."

Success in juggling multiple roles depends on the ability to delegate, according to Joan Hodgman: "Some things require the woman's full attention, whereas some can be performed by others. I firmly believe in child labor at home, so my daughters always had household chores. More important, however, most household tasks can be performed by employees. I was fortunate in having a graduate of the University of California at Berkeley as a housekeeper for 21 years. As the children grew, she drove them to after-school lessons and other activities. Admittedly, I was fortunate, but I paid her twice as much as my colleagues paid their helpers, and she was worth pearls and rubies. My husband complained about her salary until one Saturday when I left him home with our year-old daughter. After six hours of trying to paint some furniture while caring for one small child, he never complained again. Good household help meant that I could go to the hospital reassured that all was well at home."

Of paramount importance to Alice Bessman, when one's children are young, is strong family support (grandparents) or reliable full-time help—someone to be home during the illnesses of children, at the end of the school day, and for errands. "After my training, I did not work full-time until the youngest child was in junior high school. Until then, I worked half-time or less."

Career women need to have realistic expectations for the home, according to Bernice Brown. "To me, being a career woman means settling for standards at home that are not the highest but are acceptable. I try not to look in corners or under beds." Genevieve Burk agreed: "To attempt to satisfy one's mother-in-law regarding household duties is folly. Mine once expressed dismay that I did not save my grease to make soap! Set priorities and stick to them."

Gail Clark identified three major parts of her solution: "(1) a true partnership with your husband at home concerning *all* duties (house and children), (2) working in an academic setting where lectures and day-to-day conversations with interns, residents, and colleagues keep you in touch with prevailing ideas in your specialty, and (3) setting your priorities and realizing that you cannot be an A-1 wife, mother, *and* physician everyday, but that your best should be satisfactory for you, your family, and your patients' well-being. You are not an island, and there is backup all around you if you will accept it."

"Those who combine marriage and medicine have a very difficult time meeting the needs of both," said Ruth Bain. "Some do it, but it isn't easy. It requires an understanding husband who is willing to share what is usually seen as women's duties." Dame Sheila Sherlock agreed: "An understanding husband is of inestimable help to the woman physician."

Joan Hodgman concurs, "It is often said that behind every successful man is a helpful woman. Conversely, behind every successful married career woman is a confident husband who takes pride in her success and helps with the housework."

For Maureen Sims, "Choosing a housekeeper is very important and deserves top priority. I would advise my colleagues to interview several candidates and be prepared to pay top dollar for the type of services they expect. Above all, you must be able to communicate effectively with the housekeeper. Many unpleasant situations with long-term ramifications can develop if inappropriate choices are made, especially in the early developmental phases of child-rearing. In such cases, if difficulties cannot be resolved, it may be necessary to dismiss the housekeeper and start over. If your own employer is not understanding, it can lead to frustration. Fortunately, my boss and my colleagues had been in similar situations and understood.

COLLEGIAL RELATIONSHIPS

"I enjoy the exchange of ideas and discussion of interesting cases with colleagues in the surgery lounge," said Laurel Weibel, "and have never felt excluded because of my sex. I am frequently assigned to committees to investigate female problem-physicians because 'You're not so prone to be vindictive or biased' or 'You can be the devil's advocate.' "

Jacqueline Miller has obtained support from belonging to a collegial group. "If you are in a group, you never feel alone, and you learn

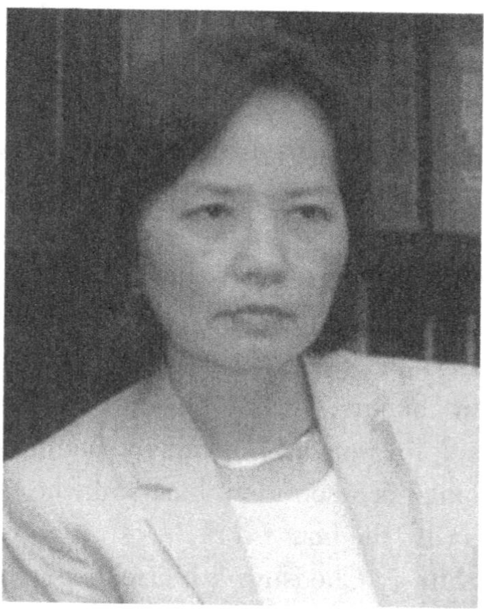

Trying to do my best forces me to be curious, to reevaluate constantly, and to learn.

LINDA D. SHORTLIFFE, M.D.

Professor and Chairman, Department of Urology
Stanford School of Medicine, Stanford, California

how to have a productive relationship with your peers. I have practiced with only an occasional woman physician, so I have had little experience with the 'old girl' network. I have not felt any direct prejudice from men, although on occasion I have observed some reservations about women in medicine. If you sit back and relax, however, it goes away."

Linda Shortliffe, practicing in the male-dominated specialty of urology, has not had any specific collegial difficulties. "My best professional relationships have been with residents with whom I have worked. Probably the most important professional advantage has resulted from interactions with a male faculty mentor, who, fortunately, appears to have overcome the traditional ideas about women in surgery."

In Ruth Bain's experience, you become a full participating member of the 'old boy' network by doing your best at every committee or other assignment. "Some young women seem convinced that they will not be accepted or allowed to participate in organized medicine; that simply is not true. We tend to find what we look for; in expecting problems, many young women create them."

"Although career, marriage, and children impose great stresses on a woman's time and energy," Joan Hodgman strongly recommends joining, and being active in, medical organizations. "As my family duties declined, I was able to assume more responsible roles in medical organizations. This has proved most rewarding, not only educationally, but also in allowing me some influence on the profession I love and in expanding my circle of colleagues in the community, state, and nation."

THE SINGLE WOMAN–PHYSICIAN

Kit Chambers observed that "Single women can devote more time to their work and have more leisure time to develop hobbies." Marjorie Price Wilson agrees: "The single physician can plan more effectively. When you have a family, you must set priorities; that is the dilemma. On the other hand, the single woman may miss the joys of having children and a family." Although unmarried men and women should be able to organize their continuing education more efficiently, motivation is a highly individual matter, and they may not always do so.

SATISFACTION FROM MULTIPLE ROLES

The time demands described by the women physicians interviewed lead to the question: "Is it worth it?" The following represent typical responses from our interviewees.

"Looking back over 50 years of my medical career," Joan Hodgman reminisced, "I have found it extremely rewarding. My friends ask why I am still working, and I can honestly answer that I am working for fun. Earlier in my career, the care of individual infants was my focus. At this stage, I am conducting research about pathophysiology and treatment of groups of infant patients. I also enjoy working with students and young physicians-in-training. Some of their enthusiasm rubs off. One of the unsung benefits of a medical career is the opportunity to continue working in a stimulating environment after the earlier demands of marriage and family have been met."

"Professional activities such as clinical teaching and participation in professional organizations expose you to new experiences, people, ideas, and aspects of life outside medicine," said Bernice Brown. "If you believe that we have only one 'go-round' in life, it makes sense to pack in as much as possible and make it as meaningful as possible in the time we have. Being a professional woman leads to a hectic, busy, often overextended life, and a woman physician must strive to save moments for herself so she does not become a machine. A medical career is fulfilling and stimulating, but being a homemaker and having children are also fulfilling, although when the children grow up and lead their own lives, it creates a void for the woman who has dedicated herself solely to her children. A profession, on the other hand, can provide a feeling of self-worth, of making a contribution to society, and of keeping the brain cells working.

"A real source of pleasure in being a physician, wife, and mother is that your children and husband are proud of your accomplishments and let you know it now and then, in sometimes amusing or offhand ways. They do not treat you like a 'has been' or someone not to be reckoned with, as many children seem to treat parents. Once, after I repaired a deep laceration on my 13-year-old daughter's ankle in a backwoods place where we were vacationing but where there were not good medical facilities, she turned to me and said, 'Say Mom, you're not a half-bad doc.' "

The human element is the most rewarding factor in the medical career of Kit Chambers. "I enjoy helping and caring for people. Allaying their anxiety is a large part of my contact with patients, as well as explaining what they can expect from me."

For Beverly Gregorius, the practice of medicine is the best thing that ever happened to her—with the exception of marrying her husband and having her daughter. "One cannot have a better mood-elevator, energizer, or ego-builder than seeing patients. They are always glad to see me and are fond of me as their physician. I can't imagine anything more interesting, exciting, and fulfilling than the practice of medicine."

When Karin Jamison's four children were grown and almost out of college, she was practicing from 24 to 48 hours a week in an emergency room. "This was far and away the happiest time in my professional life because the sometimes agonizing conflict between the legitimate demands of my family and my medical career was over. The benefit of the busy life women physicians lead is that they can realize their intellectual, physical, emotional, and creative potential in a way few others are privileged to do. I would here acknowledge that our dear husbands play a vital part in facilitating this. And, if one has an intrinsic interest in medicine and people, all the effort is richly rewarded."

Linda Shortliffe has enjoyed several benefits from the lifelong associations made through her medical career: "It is gratifying to attend meetings and recognize old friends and acquaintances with whom I can discuss research ideas or academic problems. In addition, there is a fulfilling relationship with residents and young people. Perhaps the most important satisfaction is a constant association with new ideas, and later seeing those ideas turned into action. It is exciting to see hypotheses become research protocols for experimental studies and later have them accepted as facts or routine treatments. Participating in the evolution of ideas is most gratifying."

Shortliffe reports a number of changes in her life since the publication of the first edition of this book. In 1995, she assumed the chairmanship of the Department of Urology at Stanford and was divorced in 1997. She believes that all events influence her thinking and her approach to learning: "Over the past few years, I decided that my impetus for learning is not that I work in medicine, but rather a simple desire to perform to the best of my ability, unlimited by 'good enough' as a goal. Trying to do my best forces me to be curious, to reevaluate constantly, and to learn. I have been told that 'nothing is ever good enough for you,' and that may be correct. Just because I have found 'an answer' does not mean that I will stop looking for, or learning about, other or better answers. I believe that people and conditions can always improve, usually through new information. From this perspective, I am optimistic about, not dissatisfied with, conditions and people. My original goals have always been limited by childhood ideas. As I have changed, readjusted my goals and plans, and taken some risks to accomplish my responsibilities, I have constantly required new information. Watching my residents, faculty, and others, I have learned that inflexibility is probably the greatest impediment to continued learning. The most dogmatic are the least likely to continue to learn or contribute to learning. The correct answer at one time may later be wrong."

As Jacqueline Miller looked back over the past several decades, which included years of postgraduate training and practice, she found that she had been extremely happy in her choice of medicine as a profession. "Each day has been stimulating and interesting, full of intellectual challenges and interesting cases. My professional associates and companions have been intelligent, motivated by concern for their fellow man, and compulsive in their desire to excel. This kind of association is well worth the sacrifices. The most difficult problem is the inability to do as much as you would like for and with your family, which leads to a pervasive sense of guilt. The variety of experiences from combining a marriage and family with a career is nonetheless a satisfying life."

In Alice Bessman's view, academic advancement should not be the physician's only goal. "An oft-heard dissatisfaction is that women do not advance as rapidly as their male colleagues. In many cases, however, outside distractions may limit productivity. The contributions to the social structure in general and to the family in particular should more than outweigh this lack of academic advancement. My satisfaction from having contributed to increased medical knowledge and to the replenishment of the younger generation of physicians is satisfaction enough."

* * * * *

Since many women physicians have more diverse responsibilities than men physicians, they may feel time pressures more acutely. Organization of time and development of efficient study methods are therefore even more critical for women in medicine. All the women physicians we interviewed agreed that it is mandatory to rely heavily on outside or extended family help for household tasks and child care. A woman physician who marries would do well to discuss with her prospective husband the time difficulties that are certain to occur so as to come to a mutual agreement in advance. If the woman physician plans carefully, sets realistic goals for each of her roles, and accepts competent household help to permit the best use of her time, a medical career can offer her great opportunities for service and fulfillment. This rich professional life can go hand-in-hand with an equally rewarding personal life, one enhancing the other.

REFLECTIONS

• • •

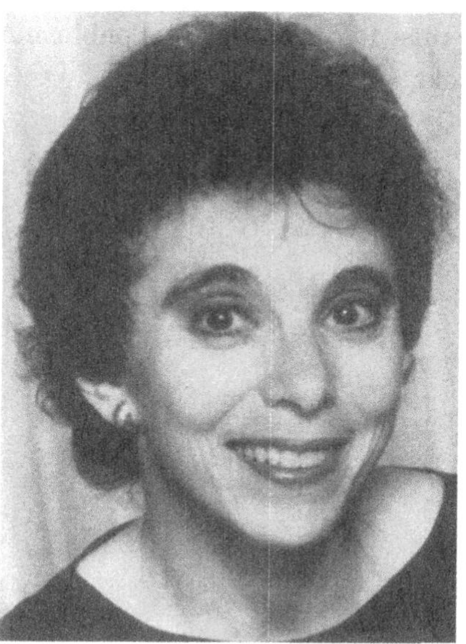

I always wanted to pull my own weight, never to receive concessions because I am a woman.

NORA GOLDSCHLAGER, M.D.

Dr. Nora Goldschlager, Associate Chief, Division of Cardiology and Director of the Coronary Care Unit, ECG Laboratory and Pacemaker Clinic at San Francisco General Hospital, received her M.D. degree from New York University School of Medicine, her residency training in internal medicine at Montefiere Hospital Medical Center and Henry Ford Hospital, Detroit, Michigan, and her cardiology training from Wayne State University in Detroit and the Presbyterian Hospital/Pacific Medical Center in San Francisco. She has received honors as a gifted teacher and cardiovascular specialist.

Dr. Goldschlager has served on the editorial board of the *American Journal of Cardiology, American Journal of Geriatric Cardiol-*

ogy, and the *Journal of Interventional Cardiac Electrophysiology*. A Fellow of the American College of Cardiology and American College of Physicians and a member of the Council on Clinical Cardiology of the American Heart Association, she is the author or coauthor of more than 147 peer-reviewed publications, 15 book reviews, and 10 books.

Triple Careers: Physician, Wife, Mother

Nora Goldschlager, M.D.
Professor of Clinical Medicine
University of California at San Francisco
San Francisco, California

Since the age of seven, I have wanted to be a cardiologist, and my ambition never wavered except for two weeks in college when I thought perhaps I would get a Ph.D. in philosophy and then teach. I married a medical student who liked independent women, and we postponed having children until my fellowship was almost completed, since I did not want to go out on night call when I had babies at home. I was pregnant during my second (and, in those years, last) year of fellowship and was not received favorably by the other fellows who would have to take up the slack when I delivered. The women were ruder than the men regarding my absence. I took three weeks off to have my first baby and was grateful to get back to work; a nurse for the baby and then a live-in housekeeper helped considerably. I took only two weeks off to have my second baby, again grateful to get back to work.

In the early 1970s, long maternity leave was not an issue; most of us did not take it, or, if we did, we were prepared to leave medicine for a prolonged period. I always believed that the more time off new mothers took, the more justified would be the questions about the propriety of our role in medicine. In that sense, things are now much improved, reentry into medicine being common and not especially penalized. The ability to leave the field for a period seemed specialty-dependent in part; if, for example, your specialty was critical care, it was more difficult to leave. I always wanted to pull my own weight, never to receive concessions because I am a woman. And I never wanted to deal with the resentment resulting from a prolonged absence to have and rear children.

Having reliable housekeepers was mandatory for continuing to work. In my case, it helped my two daughters become independent much earlier than their peers. My unrealistic fears of fire, trauma, and dog bites were actually guilt for leaving my children at home. When I asked them, at ages 12 and 14, if they regretted my absence when they came home from school, they replied: "No! If you hadn't gone to work, we would all have needed therapy!" I was grateful that they bore me no malice. Interestingly, some nonworking mothers, whom I would have relied on for carpooling when I was working, were so resentful that they did not want to participate in carpooling, even though I made myself available for entire weekends.

My career in academic cardiology has been extremely rewarding. While many in practice are retiring early or taking immense pressure from managed care, I continue to love what I do (clinical cardiology, with 60 percent education of house staff and physicians). Unlike many of my colleagues, I do not envision retiring until I have to.

I have not encountered the glass ceiling and have been promoted on schedule at all levels of academic rank. Not once have I experienced unfair treatment or discrimination. Maybe I did not recognize it when it existed, but why search for it? Making issues of slights—real or imagined—is unproductive and distracts from important activities. I have always advised the house staff, "Do what you love and be good at it, and you will be rewarded."

How do I keep up? I prepare talks and keep them current, and that means reading medical publications. Can I keep up in all fields? Definitely not. But so long as you have consultants and a friendly, nonthreatening atmosphere in which to ask questions, you can keep reasonably abreast. Having an area or two of expertise, by the way, will lead to being sought out for your opinion.

When you begin your career, you have to do everything, check everything, micromanage a great deal, and be frazzled if you take pride in your performance. But if you enjoy your work, it will still be worthwhile. Somewhere in your late thirties, you begin to have a better perspective, and your life settles down. But nobody ever promised you a rose garden when you went into medicine.

REFLECTIONS

• • •

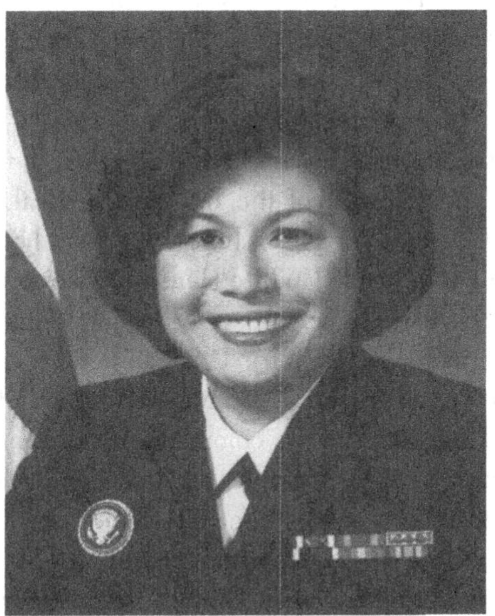

Dr. Mariano was in the Medical Unit [of the White House], and I had the highest regard for her. She was a tireless worker, always available, and often gave me the best of counsel.

PRESIDENT GEORGE HERBERT WALKER BUSH

Dr. Connie Mariano was born in Sangley Point, Philippines, to a Navy steward and his dentist wife. She received a B.A. cum laude in biology from Revelle College at the University of California at San Diego in 1977 and an M.D. degree from the Uniformed Services University School of Medicine in Bethesda, Maryland, in 1981. After an internship in internal medicine at San Diego Naval Hospital in 1982, she was assigned as the General Medical Officer onboard the *USS Prairie*, a destroyer tender, where she served as the sole physician for a ship's company of 750 men and women. She developed a mass casualty training program that earned her ship the title of "Benchmark Ship in Mass Casualty Control" for two consecutive years during her tour. After completing her internal medicine residency in 1986 at the Naval Hospital in San Diego, Dr. Mariano was assigned to the Naval Medical Clinic in Port Hueneme, California, where she was the only internist serving a community of more than 75,000 healthcare beneficiaries.

In 1991, Dr. Mariano became Division Head of General Internal Medicine and Director of the Internal Medical Clinic at the Naval Hospital in San Diego. In June 1992, she became the first military woman to be named White House Physician when she was selected as the Navy White House Physician under President George H. W. Bush. In February 1994, under President Clinton, she was promoted to Director of the White House Medical Unit and Senior White House Physician, commanding a 21-member tri-service healthcare team responsible for worldwide comprehensive medical care to the President, Vice President, and their families. She has served three sitting American presidents.

In February 2000, President Clinton awarded Dr. Mariano the presidential appointment of Physician to the President. She was promoted to Rear Admiral (lower half) on July 1, 2000, the first Filipino-American to become Admiral in the United States Navy. She is currently the highest ranking Asian-American woman in the armed forces of the United States and is also the first graduate of Uniformed Services University School of Medicine to achieve flag rank. Admiral Mariano's decorations include the Defense Distinguished Service Medal and the Joint Service Commendation Medal, among others.

Journey to the White House: A Passion for Medicine and People

E. Connie Mariano, M.D.
Rear Admiral, Medical Corps, United States Navy (Retired)
Former Physician to the President and
Commander, White House Medical Unit

I have been blessed throughout my life with numerous opportunities to learn. Education has always been the cornerstone of my survival and achievement. I was born in the Philippines to a Navy steward and his wife, a dentist. When I was two years old, my family moved to Pearl Harbor, Hawaii, where I learned to speak English and quickly acquired the lifelong practice of adapting to a new environment. For our family, home was wherever the Navy sent us; we moved every two or three years throughout the United States and overseas to Taiwan. My father finally retired in San Diego, California, where I completed high school and college. Instead of the traditional medical school, my Navy upbringing led me naturally to select the Uniformed Services University School of Medicine. In 1977, I was one of 15 women in a class of 65 students, the second class to enroll in the nation's military medical school. On the first day of medical school, we underwent battlefield training. Instead of short white coats and small black medical bags, we donned camouflage fatigues with Army boots and wielded M-16s. The first week of medical school looked more like a scene from the sitcom "MASH" than from "Marcus Welby, M.D."

Medical school provided me with superb clinical training and the unique perspective to become a career Navy medical officer. In 1982, after an internship in internal medicine, I was assigned as the general medical officer aboard the Navy destroyer tender, *USS Prairie.* For the first time in Navy history, women were being assigned to ships. When I reported aboard *Prairie,* only a handful of women officers were assigned to a ship's company of 650 men. A few months later, the first enlisted women crew members came aboard.

As a woman officer and the only physician on the ship during this historic time, I learned many lessons about leadership, military organizational structure, and acute-care medicine. The crew came to "sick bay" for medical care and sometimes just to "check out the new doc." Making it possible to do my job well was the shipboard medical department, consisting of 15 hospital corpsmen led by a seasoned senior chief who served as my division officer and mentor. My first few months on the ship taught me that before the crew would accept me, I would have to prove first and foremost that I was a good physician.

There is nothing like an extended sea cruise to test your clinical skills. There is a period during a seven-month Western Pacific deployment when the nearest medical facility is seven days sailing time away. During such a voyage, the ship's physician maintains a close eye on the crew, prays frequently, and relies solely on the skills of good history-taking and physical diagnosis.The *Prairie*'s Captain once assured me that he would turn the ship around and return to port if I needed to get a sick sailor ashore. Reversing the ship's course, however, would not be a trivial matter, but a major undertaking. As ship's doctor, not only was I responsible for the lives of all crew members onboard, but if a patient were too ill for treatment in my sick bay, I was responsible for advising the Captain to evacuate the patient to another facility. This responsibility bore directly on the ship's course and the overall mission.

Fortunately, I enjoyed many quiet nights at sea. I relished the moments when I would sit in my small stateroom, reading medical journals and chapters from the *Scientific American Medicine* series that I brought with me on the cruise. I would use the evenings to prepare lectures for my corpsmen. Whenever the corpsmen would evaluate a patient in sick bay, we would quickly look up the disease in the *Merck Manual* or in my *Harrison's Internal Medicine.* Our shipboard lecture series focused on the patients we saw every day.

After my two-year tour as ship's doctor, I returned to the Naval Hospital in San Diego to complete my residency in internal medicine. Compared to my tiny sick bay, the large teaching hospital seemed luxuriously appointed with technology and expertise available to treat patients. The rigorous training consisted of countless hours at the bedside and in the library. Learning was obtained directly from patients, grand rounds, morning report, journal club, bibliographic searches, and required reading material for subspecialty rotations.

Following residency, I was assigned to the medical clinic that supported the Navy's Construction Battalion ("Seabee") Center. During my four-year tour there, I provided outpatient and emergency medical care to a large, diverse community. I enjoyed a busy internal medicine practice and continued to teach corpsmen. My own education continued as I attended grand rounds at the local hospital, participated in annual review courses in internal medicine, and maintained my journal reading.

After completing my tour at the medical clinic in 1990, the Navy assigned me to be the division head for internal medicine at the teaching hospital in San Diego where I had earlier trained. I returned to attend on the wards and to continue teaching residents, interns, and medical students.

My career path was to veer dramatically in 1991, when, as one of six Navy candidates, I was nominated for the position of White House Physician. Following an interview at the White House, I was selected for this honor. I reported to the White House in June 1992, and served in the White House Medical Unit during the last seven months of the

Bush administration. When President Clinton was inaugurated in 1993, he did not bring a personal physician with him to the White House. In 1994, he named me as his personal physician and promoted me to Director of the White House Medical Unit.

My original assignment to the White House was to be two years. President Clinton extended my tour to four years to allow me to serve throughout his first term of office. With his reelection, I was asked to remain until the end of his second term. An original two-year stint ended in January, 2001, with an eight-and-one-half year incredible, historic journey for me.

I could not have planned or predicted this career path. I have been blessed with amazing opportunities. Recalling that I came to this country speaking no English, I am living testimony to the fact that education leads to opportunity. As I reflect upon my career, every step that allowed my education to expand both professionally and personally has moved me closer to the position I held at the White House.

When I was aboard ship, I was asked to be a member of a panel of officers who would select the Sailor of the Quarter. As the only woman among the panelists, I endured my male officer colleagues asking all the male enlisted candidates, "What do you think about women on board ships?" When the one and only female candidate came before the panel, I asked her, "What do you think about *men* on board ships?" The candidate laughed, gave an excellent answer, and was selected Sailor of the Quarter.

How has being a woman affected my career? One might further ask: How has being a Filipino woman affected my career? Throughout my professional life, I have always "stood out." In medical school, I was the only Asian-American woman in my class. In internship, I was one of two Asian-American women. In my internal medicine residency group, I was the only woman. Onboard ship, I was the only physician. As one of two women physicians at the Navy's Construction Battalion Center, I was conspicuous in maternity clothes during my two pregnancies.

Being a woman at this time in American history has allowed me to stand out in positive and beneficial ways. I believe that if you are going to be "standing out," you might as well be "outstanding." Often people will notice upon meeting me that I am not the typical American physician. But when the dialogue begins, I believe people do not think of me in stereotypical terms. Instead, through communication and familiarization, the people I meet will know me for the person I am.

In June 1992, President George Bush was told that the new White House Physician selected by the Navy was a Commander, a specialist in internal medicine, and a woman. I was that Navy Commander who would be the first military woman White House Physician. The only other woman physician who had served in the White House was Dr. Janet Travell, a rehabilitation medicine specialist who was President Kennedy's personal civilian physician.

When President Bush learned that a woman physician was to join his all-male team of physicians, he wanted to know only two things about her: (1) Was she athletic? and (2) Did she have a sense of humor? As it turned out, President Bush's inquiries showed considerable wisdom.

First, White House Physicians have to be in good physical condition to follow the President of the United States all over the country and all over the world. The presidency demands superhuman levels of energy of its occupants. White House physicians must be able to walk briskly as they "shadow" the President, be ready to jump on and off moving vehicles, climb onto helicopters, scramble up stairs to a waiting airplane, and do all this while lugging around a 40-pound medical bag.

And what about a sense of humor? As a White House Physician, if you do not learn to laugh, you may want to cry. A sense of humor—the ability to laugh at yourself and with (not at) others—is vital to that job.

As Physician to the President, I was responsible for the medical care of the leader of the free world. With this responsibility came the obligation to seek the "world's best" care for my patients. This meant that medicine was never practiced in a vacuum. Whenever I or my patients had a question beyond my immediate knowledge or specialty, I actively sought second opinions for guidance.

The Internet and information explosion have helped patients gather medical knowledge independently. As a result, I have often seen patients in clinic who showed me the latest information from the Internet or a newspaper article. It is vital for me to know what information my patients are getting from cyberspace and newsprint. In my position at the White House, not only did I maintain my journal reading, but I also read at least three different newspapers a day.

I was fortunate to have a panel of excellent consultants for current information and advice. The medicine I practiced had to be consistent with the medicine practiced by my colleagues at respected medical institutions. White House medicine must be state-of-the-art medicine. Many of my consultants were the world's experts in their respective fields, and I frequently received the benefit of one-on-one training from them. Continuing medical education (CME) is vital to the practice of state-of-the art medicine. All members of the White House Medical Unit must participate in CME courses every year. I attended or participated in at least three conferences a year. In addition to receiving continuing medical education, White House Physicians also teach. My teaching responsibilities included proctoring medical students at the Uniformed Services University School of Medicine, as well as serving as instructor for courses in advanced cardiac life support and advanced trauma life support.

The White House Medical Unit consistently draws data from information technology resources. Its mission involves a large amount of travel, with heavy reliance upon current health advisories and information on medical facilities. For overseas travel, the Unit uses computer-based information systems, such as *Travax,* as well as the network of contacts with state departments and the Centers for Disease Control.

My passion for the profession of medicine has always been fueled by my love of people. Practicing medicine at the White House gave me a unique opportunity to serve my country. My feelings about my

White House responsibilities are captured in the following poignant letter written in 1961 by Admiral Joel Boone, physician to President Hoover, to Dr. Janet Travell, physician to President Kennedy: "I hope, Doctor, you will enjoy thoroughly your new life of vital service to our country in a position of transcendent responsibility only second in importance to the Presidency because you will be the one to keep him fit and physically and mentally well so that he can carry on his incomparable tasks in this volatile world. . . . You will be faced with serious demanding obligations; however, you will be a most privileged person in your profession. I found the White House to be a house of joy, sorrow, and tragedy. It always has been such."

16

Professionalism

• • •

> Medical professionalism is more than first-rate knowledge, proficiency, and dedication. It requires compassion, integrity, and the highest ethical standards, free of the shackles of profit as a priority.
>
> Phil R. Manning, M.D., and Lois DeBakey, Ph.D.

The lexical definition of professional is: having or showing great skill; expert; following a profession, especially a learned profession; conforming to the standards of professional behavior; an occupation, such as law, medicine, engineering, that requires considerable training and specialized study. In medicine, professionalism connotes not only knowledge and skills, but character as well, specifically compassion and ethics.

Of late, those within and without medicine seem to believe, correctly or not, that physicians evince less professionalism than previously. To Robert Moser, "Professionalism is first cousin to humanitarianism and ethical behavior. It is what we used to call 'character' (before that fine word was appropriated by actors and comics). It applies to all professions: jurisprudence, medicine, legislation, engineering."[1]

A number of factors have influenced contemporary medical professionalism. Words, for example, have a potent, if sometimes intangible, effect on attitudes, behavior, and actions. Michael and Lois DeBakey have addressed this insidious issue: "Today patients are called 'consumers,' physicians are 'providers,' and health care is a 'product'—all terms of commerce, not of a profession, and certainly not of a humanitarian profession. The new vocabulary, and its obvious intentions, are grossly inappropriate. Physicians do not provide inanimate commodities, as salespeople and service people do; they treat human beings. They deal with our most precious possession—our health and well-being—and to apply rules of commerce to such activities is unsound, indeed disastrous."[2] The onerous restrictions and regulations imposed by managed care, they point out, have wreaked havoc on the quality of healthcare.[3,4] "Instead of being allowed to focus primarily on the patient's health problems," they lament, "physicians must now expend much of their time complying with unreasonable paperwork, avoiding specious litigation, and awaiting a decision regarding treatment from a faceless nonphysician 'authority' at a remote point who has never seen the patient, but consults a computer for the 'guidelines.' . . . [M]any HMOs have gag rules prohibiting a physician from telling patients when the HMO rejects a procedure he deems necessary."[2]

"When a physician cannot be honest with a patient," they contend, "the relationship is compromised, and the patient is victimized. Many HMOs reward physicians with a bonus on the basis of how much care they deny patients and punish them if they exceed a certain cost for health care. Thus, the overriding dictum is to save money for corporate officers, not to provide quality health care to patients."[2] This, the DeBakeys assert, is the goal of business, and should never be that of the medical profession. Finally, they plead "for a single code for all politicians, bureaucrats, managed-care executives, health-care professionals, and others, who themselves may one day be patients: *Primum non nocere.* First do no harm."[2]

Although concerned about the current status of medical professionalism, Robert Moser envisions a brighter future: "The hard fact is that over the years most of us did become complacent. Many lost some sensitivity. (How often have you heard 'quality of life' discussed on teaching rounds?) We also suffered a lapse of intellectual discipline. In our naive zeal to 'leave no stone unturned' on behalf of our patients, we neglected the realities of fiscal responsibility. In our benignly paternalistic fashion, we did things our way for a long time. And that is how the unwelcome nose of the managed care camel succeeded in creeping under our tent. Undoubtedly, managed care has imposed a renewed sense of fiscal discipline on medicine. But as it exists, it has excessive warts. Major modifications are already evident; we will retain the good ones, but we are obliged to abandon those that have caused grief." In an editorial in the *Southern Medical Journal,* Moser wrote: "[W]e must fight for our individual patients testing the limits of whatever constraining envelopes that bind us. I do not advocate dishonesty, but I do believe in taking action when the constraints imposed seem unfair or unreasonable. If we are driven by the 'system' to provide less than optimal care, we must seek other options, external to the system, as we protest most vigorously for change. To do less is truly to 'capitulate.'"[1]

Thomas Lincoln reminds us that "Healthcare is not first and foremost a consumer industry, as viewed from the physician's or patient's perspective. Although the financial costs are often supported by insurance, all serious medical care is a personal patient investment in time, sometimes with pain and anxiety, and commonly with discipline, the physician serving as an active participant and advisor. One does not 'consume' an artificial hip or a cardiac vessel bypass."

Moser hopes that "Ultimately, a system will evolve that will eliminate the unsavory profit motive, and those infamous mantras 'obligation to shareholder' and 'incentive and disincentive' will be purged from the medical lexicon. Once this is accomplished, the intangibles of compassion, caring, and patient advocacy—elements intrinsic to our self-fulfillment—will re-emerge. These virtues must, of course, always be coupled with the best possible medical science. We will survive this dark night of the soul of medicine to enjoy a truly enlightened partnership with those for whom we care."

Professionalism not only serves our patients best, but also preserves our passion for medicine. The invited thoughts on this subject from Jordan Cohen and Kenneth Shine follow this chapter in their "Reflections."

REFERENCES

1. Moser RH. A few thoughts about professionalism [editorial]. *South Med J.* 2000;93:1132–1133.

2. DeBakey ME, DeBakey L. Should physicians unionize? *The Wall Street Journal.* 1999 Jul 7;CIV(4):A22.

3. DeBakey ME. Winds of change in medicine. *South Med J.* 1993;86:1316–1317.

4. DeBakey ME. A surgical perspective. *Ann Surg.* 1991; 213:525–526.

REFLECTIONS

• • •

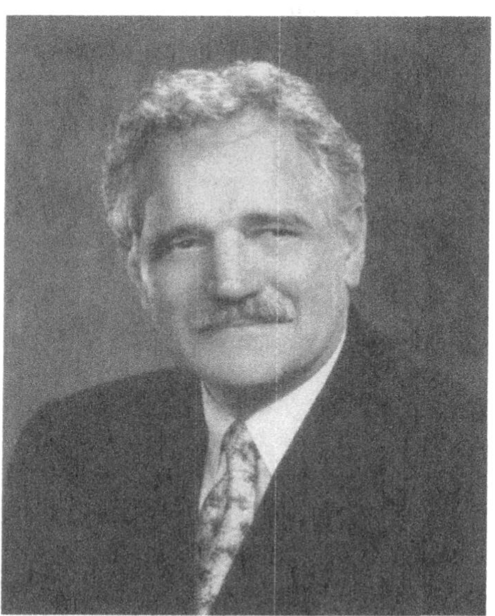

Professionalism, the commitment to subordinate our self-interest to the interest of our patients, is the foundation of trust upon which our social contract rests.

JORDAN J. COHEN, M.D.

Dr. Jordan Cohen, who leads the Association of American Medical College's support and service to the nation's medical schools and teaching hospitals, received his M.D. degree from Harvard Medical School. During an almost 40-year career in academic medicine, he has held faculty positions at Harvard Medical School, Brown University, Tufts University School of Medicine, the University of Chicago Pritzker School of Medicine, and the State University of New York at Stony Brook. He has served as Chairman of the American Board of Internal Medicine and the Accreditation Council for

Graduate Medical Education, and has been a Regent and Vice Chairman of the Board of Regents of the American College of Physicians. He is the author of more than 100 publications and is an Editor of *Nephrology Forum*.

Requisites for Physicians: Competence, Service, Trust

Jordan J. Cohen, M.D.
President, Association of American Medical Colleges
Washington, D.C.

What, precisely, defines a profession? That not only medical students, but practicing physicians as well, are uncertain of the meaning of professionalism in medicine[1] is troubling, particularly when turbulent market forces threaten to distract us frequently, if not permanently, from our mission. How can we safeguard the values of our calling if we are not entirely sure what they are?

A profession is defined by its specialized body of knowledge, its organized activities for continuous advancement, its responsibility to regulate itself, its pledge to public service above personal gain, and its implied contract with society. In medicine, the pledge to societal good is particularly sacred because our mission affects life itself. We hold the lives of others in our hands; they trust us with their health, and the moment we take the Hippocratic Oath, we vow to prove forevermore worthy of that trust. No small commitment, and one that I fear is in danger of being lost in the financial dissonance pervading today's healthcare system. The concept of professionalism, powerful though it may be, is not so deeply rooted in American medical history as to be immune from contemporary forces. Far from it. In *Social Transformation of American Medicine,*[2] Princeton economist Paul Starr recounted what a fledgling concept this is. Professionalism, hinging as it does on an exceedingly lofty principle, is thus altogether too fragile for us to take for granted.

Too often of late, people in need of healthcare are called "healthcare consumers" rather than "patients." Admittedly, "patient" implies illness, and some people who seek wellness care and other services from medical professionals are not ill. Moreover, for some, the word "patient" evokes the notion of "patiently" waiting for a physician to get around, finally, to seeing him for all of five minutes. But "healthcare consumers"? If the people we treat are consumers, what does that make physicians? Salespeople? Retailers? Is the care, the guidance, the expertise we provide just another commodity to be traded? Unfortunately, in today's market-driven economy, with rising costs squeezing the entire healthcare system, the answer may be "yes." And we physicians may well have contributed to the commercialization of medicine by allowing the erosion of the core values of professionalism, which elevate medicine from a nine-to-five job to a calling in the service of healing.

Inculcating professional attitudes and values in medical students and residents through curricula and practical experience is at the heart of the Association of American Medical Colleges' Medical School Objectives Project (MSOP),[3] which identifies four major attributes of a good physician:

- altruistic, compassionate, and truthful;
- well informed in the scientific basis of medicine and the normal and abnormal functioning of the body;
- skillful in communicating with and caring for patients;
- dutiful in working with others to promote the health of individual patients and the broader community.

MSOP also identifies objectives for medical school education, objectives designed to instill and reinforce traits that can be honed both to withstand the rigors of a professional life and to compel adherence to the norms of professionalism. Among these traits are old-fashioned words like honesty, integrity, altruism, compassion, and respect.

I am encouraged that more and more medical schools around the country are adding specific topics to their curricula that focus on teaching and measuring professionalism, no longer assuming that medical students will absorb professional values by osmosis. But it will profit us little to bathe aspiring physicians in the precepts of professionalism if, when they receive the coveted M.D. and complete their residencies, we turn them out into a healthcare system that has become cavalier in its commitment to professionalism. That is the point where the community of practicing physicians must retake the reins. In order to value our profession, we must not only profess but also practice its values. And how do we do that?

Many factors that have contributed to a decline in medical professionalism can serve as an impetus to reinvigorate professional values. The current backlash against managed care provides an opportunity for physicians to reassert their traditional role as advocates for patients and as servants of society. An alignment of interests among patients and physicians can be a powerful motivator for rectitude, rather than for expediency or profit. In a number of communities, thoughtful people with concerns about how their healthcare is delivered have become involved with their local hospitals, clinics, and medical schools to promote nonhierarchic patient- and family-centered care, with patients and family as partners rather than passive recipients of a physician's wisdom. Such a partnership can reinvigorate professionalism by constantly reminding physicians about the needs, the lives, and the priorities of the people they serve.

I urge practicing physicians to reexamine constantly their commitment to public and community service, a fundamental ethic of professionalism. How much time do you devote to uncompensated care? Countless opportunities exist for physicians to reconnect with the central values of their profession by volunteering at shelters for the homeless and for battered women, treatment programs for addicts, and walk-in clinics for adolescents and pregnant women, among many others.

In addition, physicians should pursue continuing medical education that examines and refines their commitment to professionalism. Courses in medical ethics and other aspects of professionalism can be just as vital to your lifelong learning as the study of the latest developments in gene-mapping, oncology, or psychopharmacology.

I wholeheartedly agree with the recommendation of Richard and Sylvia Cruess that physicians assume responsibility for their local and national associations. In "Renewing Professionalism: An Opportunity for Medicine," they state that if physicians and medical schools and organizations fulfill the obligations implicit in their contracts with society, the morality inherent in medical professionalism will predominate, and optimal healthcare will result.[4]

Professionalism, the commitment to subordinate our self-interest to the interest of our patients, is the foundation of trust upon which our social contract rests. And maintaining mutual trust in the physician–patient relationship is, to my mind, the only way to assure the public that medicine is fulfilling its sacred obligation. No laws, no regulations, no patients' bill of rights, no fine print in the insurance policy, no watchdog federal agency can substitute for trustworthy physicians who care.

Fending off the powerful forces of commercialism and placing our confidence in the tenets of professionalism will require considerable courage. Taking a strong stand may be risky, but the larger risk is to lose sight of what we are defending. We are not fighting to protect the medical profession because it is "our turf" or because we want to preserve our autonomy or, even worse, protect our incomes. The issue for us, as physicians who care, is the welfare of patients. In this age of Health Maintenance Organizations (HMOs), Preferred Provider Organizations (PPOs), Physician/Hospital Organizatins (PHOs), gatekeepers, and utilization reviews, *we must* be the ones our patients can trust.

REFERENCES

1. Shaw G. A calling, not a nine-to-five job: teaching tomorrow's physicians what it means to be a professional. *AAMC Reporter.* 1998;7:10–11.

2. Starr P. *Social Transformation of American Medicine.* New York: Basic Books, 1982.

3. Anderson MB, Cohen JJ, Hallock JE, Kassebaum DG, Turnbull J, Whitcomb M. Learning objectives for medical student education—guidelines for medical schools: Report I of the Medical Schools Objectives Project. *Acad Med.* 1999; 74:13–18.

4. Cruess R, Cruess S, Johnston S. Renewing professionalism: an opportunity for medicine. *Acad Med.* 1999;74:878–884.

REFLECTIONS

• • •

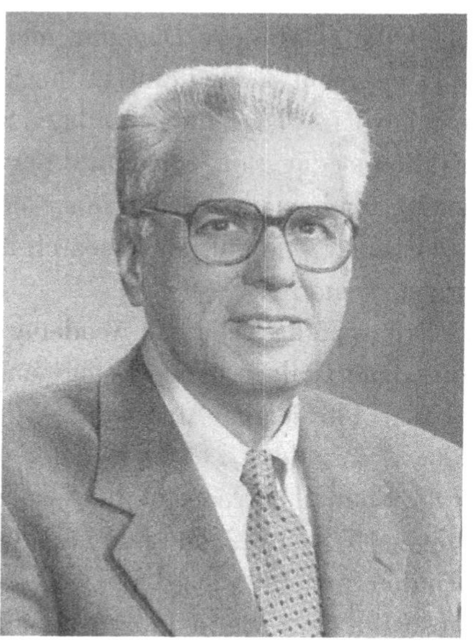

> Medicine offers the physician a profession in which art, science, compassion, and communication provide some of the richest human experiences anyone can have.
>
> KENNETH I. SHINE, M.D.

Kenneth Shine, M.D., Founding Director of the RAND Corporation's Center for Domestic and International Health Security, has served as President of the Institute of Medicine, National Academy of Sciences, and Professor of Medicine Emeritus at the University of California, Los Angeles (UCLA) School of Medicine. He is UCLA School of Medicine's immediate past Dean and Provost for Medical Sciences.

A cardiologist and physiologist, Dr. Shine received his A.B. from Harvard College in 1957 and his M.D. from Harvard Medical

School in 1961. Most of his advanced training was at Massachusetts General Hospital, where he became Chief Resident in Medicine in 1968. Thereafter, he was Assistant Professor of Medicine at Harvard Medical School. In 1971, he became Director of the Coronary Care Unit, Chief of the Cardiology Division, and, subsequently, Chairman of the Department of Medicine at the UCLA School of Medicine. As Dean at UCLA, Dr. Shine stimulated major initiatives in ambulatory healthcare education, community service for medical students and faculty, mathematics and science education in the public schools, and construction of new research facilities funded entirely by the private sector.

Dr. Shine is a Fellow of the American Academy of Arts and Sciences and the American College of Cardiology and Master of the American College of Physicians–American Society of Internal Medicine. In 1988, he was elected to the Institute of Medicine. He was Chairman of the Council of Deans of the Association of American Medical Colleges 1991–1992, and was President of the American Heart Association from 1985 to 1986.

Dr. Shine's research interests include metabolic events in the heart muscle, the relation of behavior to heart disease, and emergency medicine. He participated in efforts to prove the value of cardiopulmonary resuscitation after a heart attack and in the establishment of the 911 emergency telephone number in the multijurisdictional Los Angeles area. Dr. Shine is the author of numerous articles and scientific papers on heart physiology and clinical research.

"That Was Frank's Doctor"

Kenneth I. Shine, M.D.
Founding Director
Center for Domestic and International Health Security
RAND Corporation
Santa Monca, California

Frank* was a distinguished academic administrator, responsible for a leading professional program at a major university. I had participated in his care for over a dozen years, during which time he underwent two cardiac coronary artery bypass operations and multiple other procedures. He now had profoundly depressed cardiac muscle function and a marginal cardiac output. He and his wife discussed with me the various options available at this stage of his chronic illness. We talked about experimental medical therapy, cardiac transplantation, taking a cruise to interesting places, and a variety of other options. After some thought, he turned to me. "My wife and I both believe that my work is the most important part of our lives, and what I would like from you is to do everything you can to help me function in my profession until the time I die. I don't want to be in the hospital or have additional operations. I want to be allowed to continue to work."

*a pseudonym

In spite of his dire prognosis, he worked for another four years. I pushed the limits of medical therapy to the point that he would get dizzy from standing in the sun for more than two or three minutes. But the treatment kept him functioning and out of the hospital. He worked a full day before he collapsed one Friday evening at dinner. Although a surgeon in the restaurant resuscitated him, it later became clear in the coronary care unit that if he recovered, he would be badly damaged neurologically. After several days of careful observation, his family and I agreed that he should be removed from life support so that nature could take its course. The memorial service was a remarkable event, replete with mayors and scholars, a senator, and many other dignitaries. Everyone going through the receiving line was identified by the other mourners. When I reached his wife, she hugged and kissed me. I consoled her, and as I walked away, someone asked her who I was. She said nothing about my being a Professor, Dean, Provost, or Chief of Cardiology. She simply replied, "That was Frank's doctor."

Professionalism means competence. Patients and their families expect their physicians to be well informed and to be able to provide the most effective healthcare available. Patients expect their physicians to know the limitations of their professional competence and to seek consultation or referral when that will provide the best possible treatment. Professionalism means not being threatened when a patient or a family asks for a second opinion. Professionalism means lifelong learning and continual education. Frank lived and worked for four more years because he received excellent care.

Professionalism is about trust, about creating circumstances in which patients and families can be open and honest with their physicians and in which physicians reciprocate in kind. Trust is about believing that the physician will describe all the options fairly and honestly and will make recommendations based solely on the patient's best interests, not on those of the physician, insurer, managed-care organization, or any other entity. Trust requires openness. A professional cannot accept any limitation on discussions of the patient's condition, prognosis, therapeutic choices, or other options. Frank and his wife trusted me with their most private hopes, fears, and aspirations and made good choices for themselves.

Professionalism means integrity. Integrity implies not only truth-telling, but avoidance of conflicts of interest, such as referring patients for laboratory studies or procedures in which the physician has a commercial interest, receives payment for referral, or participates in procedures without being identified to the patient.

Trust and integrity require observing the confidentiality of patient–physician communications. Frank was entitled to continue his career in the knowledge that whatever I knew about his condition would not be communicated to others, except at his instruction and with his permission.

In medicine, professionalism also means being concerned about the public health. This concern creates some of the most difficult dilemmas for physicians. The law requires reporting of certain communicable diseases in the interest of the health of the community. When the physician identifies tuberculosis, syphilis, gonorrhea, or hepatitis, reporting is required, and the physician's obligation is clear. Much more challenging is the dilemma in which the patient is infected with human immunodeficiency virus (HIV) and has not advised a spouse or other sexual partners. In this situation, without legal requirements for reporting, it is even more important to build trust so that patients understand their responsibilities to others.

In the past, physicians were compensated primarily on a fee-for-service basis. Before the introduction of Medicare and Medicaid, physicians often adjusted their fees according to a patient's ability to pay, and, particularly in rural communities, they were sometimes compensated in nonmonetary ways. There was a strong tradition of caring for the poor through volunteer services. Later, Medicare provided healthcare for Americans beyond the age of 65 years, and Medicaid covered many of the poor, particularly young mothers and children. Volunteerism then declined. Fee-for-service identified the patient's interest with that of the physician, but there was the risk of unnecessary tests and procedures (performed by physicians knowingly or innocently) that increased the physician's personal income and raised the specter of a conflict of interest. Controlling healthcare costs was not considered an obligation of the physician. Even if additional treatment had minimal incremental value, it was often recommended.

As more and more technology became available, healthcare costs began to grow at unsustainable rates, so that by the early 1990s, close to one-seventh of the gross domestic product was being expended on health. Despite these high expenditures, there was little evidence that the overall quality of health in America was substantially better than that found in other countries that spent only 50 to 60 percent of the American expenditure. Unwilling to adopt a strong federal governmental solution, purchasers of healthcare turned increasingly toward managed care, in which market forces were supposed to help constrain costs. In this environment, patients are cared for either in capitated systems in which physicians or institutions receive a flat fee per patient per year to provide care or through systems of providers receiving discounted fees. In such systems, physicians are rewarded for doing less and are constrained from referring patients for specialty consultations.

Professionalism requires that physicians always seek appropriate care for their patients, even in the face of financial limitations imposed or of incentives to provide less care. Patients must also be fully informed. Trust and integrity require that patients understand the conditions under which their physicians are compensated. Professionalism means advocating systems of care that provide the best possible results for patients in a responsible, cost-effective manner.

At the same time, professionalism is knowing when enough treatment is enough. Having accomplished his goal of working until the end of his life, Frank's family did not want to see him live in a persistent vegetative state, nor did I. After careful consultation, support systems were removed, and Frank passed away.

Medicine has a code of ethics that covers not only how professionals interact with patients, but how they accept responsibility for their own behavior and that of their colleagues, including evaluating the care given by others, identifying incompetent practicing physicians or those with substance-abuse problems or improper behavior. A physician's failure to deal with a colleague's unprofessional behavior undermines the trust and integrity essential to a profession. Patients rely on physicians to apply the peer-review process to medical staffs through their medical society or state licensing board. A profession that fails to police itself loses public confidence and invites outside control.

In the current rapidly changing environment, the relationships between physicians and their patients, as well as physicians and their colleagues, are undergoing substantial stress. The fundamental principles of a profession, however, including competence, trust, integrity, responsibility, and accountability, are essential. No personal distinction that I have received has ever quite measured up to Frank's wife's explanation: "That was Frank's doctor." Medicine offers the physician a profession in which art, science, compassion, and communication provide some of the richest human experiences anyone can have.

Afterword

• • •

On the basis of our extensive interactions with highly skilled physicians, we have certain recommendations for you as clinicians. One is that you understand the **need for two kinds of lifelong study:** (1) general and (2) specific, patient-oriented study. By reading, listening to audiotapes, attending conferences and symposia, viewing daily medical news from reliable Internet services, and conversing informally with experts and colleagues, you will become alert to new developments and can obtain a nucleus of understanding upon which to build. Toward that end, editorials in leading medical journals are particularly useful. Most newspapers and weekly magazines report medical news fairly accurately, if briefly. So with just a little effort, you can be aware of recent medical developments and with the current state of the art. Although essential, this is not enough. You will also profit from nurturing your intellectual curiosity and from assuming personal responsibility for answers to specific questions arising in your practice. Such answers require framing the question precisely and, often, accessing pertinent medical information as well as consulting colleagues.

Electronic databases have significantly simplified searching for medical publications, which, in turn, helps optimize the care of your patients. The possibilities that the computer offers for information retrieval, especially though the Internet, seem almost limitless. Technology will undoubtedly continue to facilitate and expedite access to accurate, pertinent information. With current print and electronic information sources, there is no justification for being uninformed.

We do better what we do daily. You will therefore practice better medicine if you engage in daily study and daily evaluation of your performance. You need to acquire the discipline and diligence to **read and study every day** and, because of time limitations and the flood of mediocre publications, to **screen articles critically for pertinence and validity.** Current medical textbooks provide a quick source of relevant information, although they are, by nature, somewhat dated. A personal file of articles you have found useful in your practice, indexed either manually or on a computer, is extremely efficient in satisfying information needs. Because electronic databases are increasingly easy to access, there is little excuse for failing to obtain the most reliable current information. If you do not wish to access the information databases yourself, medical librarians can fulfill almost any such request provided you delineate your needs carefully. Choosing one or two medical subjects for intense study, moreover, will heighten your intellectual satisfaction, engage your curiosity, prepare you to serve as a consultant, and thus enhance your self-confidence.

Participating in the **collegial medical network** permits you to benefit from shared experience. Not only is this interaction an excellent way to learn, but the camaraderie and sociability contribute to fulfillment. Teaching is an added stimulus for learning, and even if you are not affiliated with a medical school or teaching hospital, you can profit from informal teaching sessions with your colleagues, other members of your healthcare team, and your patients. You can eliminate ineffective and inefficient practice habits by inviting peers to observe you periodically, even during your routine clinical activities, such as taking a history or performing a physical examination or clinical procedure.

Our fervent hope is that all clinicians will adopt simple methods of practice analysis to effect corrective changes in their practices. Billing data can be used to maintain statistics on clinical problems seen, drugs prescribed, and laboratory studies ordered. By indexing your medical records by problem or diagnosis, you can examine your cumulative experience. Keeping notes by hand or computer on lessons learned from instructive cases is equally beneficial. Lessons learned from the study of practice are reinforced and expanded when discussed with well-informed colleagues. Hospitals, medical societies, and medical schools can help physicians evaluate their experience by advocating standards, encouraging discussions of the validity of published material, and offering guidance in effective methods of practice analysis.

We also encourage you to be attentive to the **changing social and ethical issues** in medicine. Here again, it is wise to remember the two approaches: (1) general, for a framework upon which to build, and (2) specific, including consultation, for solutions to problems particular patients present.

Although you need to be well informed, many problems in practice are unrelated to medical knowledge, but are caused by omission, administrative or personnel inefficiency, lost data, or failure to react to data obtained. These problems must constantly be combatted. With patient care becoming more complex and with stronger emphasis on the team approach, greater entrepreneurial involvement, and more regulation to contain medical costs, systems problems will probably multiply. To improve the quality of medical care, you must become a more skilled manager of patient care rather than abrogate these responsibilities. In the words of Hippocrates: "The physician must be ready, not only to do his duty himself, but also to secure the co-operation of the patient, of the attendants and externals.[1]

Mastering many of the learning techniques and objectives that we advocate in this book will help you achieve the competence promoted by the Accreditation Council for Graduate Medical Education (ACGME) Outcome Project (Sept. 28, 1999). Such competence will enrich residency training and may become a part of the certification and maintenance of certification processes. The specific knowledge, skills, and attitude to be required of residents are here modified in these six components:

- **patient care** that is compassionate, appropriate, and effective for the treatment of health problems and the promotion of health;
- **medical knowledge** about established and evolving biomedical, clinical, and cognate (epidemiological and social–behavioral) sciences and the application of this knowledge to patient care;
- **practice-based learning and improvement** that involves investigation and evaluation of their own patient care, appraisal of assimilation of scientific evidence, and improvements in patient care;
- **interpersonal and communication skills** that result in effective information exchange and teaming with patients, their families, and other health professionals;
- **professionalism**, as manifested through a commitment to carrying out professional responsibilities, adherence to ethical principles, and sensitivity to a diverse patient population;
- **system-based practice**, as manifested by actions that demonstrate an awareness of and responsiveness to the larger context and system of healthcare and the ability to effectively call on system resources to provide care that is of optimal value.

If you approach the clinical puzzles in medical practice as intellectual challenges; if you acquire the habit of reading and discussing with colleagues the steady flow of new medical information issuing from scientists and scholars; if you evaluate your clinical results regularly, framing precise questions and obtaining answers to the questions arising in practice; and if you view each patient not as a clinical case; but as a fellow human being whose unstated fears, anxieties, and dependence associated with illness also require attention, you will be rewarded with professional satisfaction and personal enjoyment, and you will assuredly *preserve the passion* for medicine that led you into this noble humanitarian profession.

PHIL R. MANNING, M.D.
LOIS DEBAKEY, PH.D.

REFERENCES

1. Hippocrates. *Aphorisms.* With an English translation by W.H.S. Jones. New York: G.P. Putnam's Sons, 1931, Vol IV, p. 99.
2. ACGME· Outcome Project [homepage on the Internet]. Accreditation Council for Graduate Medical Education; c2001. Available at: http://www.acgme.org/outcome/comp/compFull.asp.

Interviewees and Correspondents

• • •

Nancy Abdou
Stephen Abrahamson
Michael Ackerman
James Aiyarrow
Bobby R. Alford
Clarence P. Alfrey
Horace J. Anderson
Gary J. Anthone
Susan S. Anthony
Henry Aranow, Jr.
Juan A. Asensio
John Martin Askey
J. B. Aust
Ruth Bain
Carol A. Baker
Duke H. Baker
Lailee Bakhtiar
Oscar Balchum
James J. Ball
Edwin V. Banta, Jr.
Barry Barber
Richard Barbers
Emil Bardana, Jr.
William Bardsley
Marloe Bareis
R. Bareis
Anne L. Barlow
Octo G. Barnett
Jeremiah A. Barondess
Howard S. Barrows
Jacques Barzun
Robert Beck
Garry G. Becker
John S. Beedie
Paul B. Beeson
Roy Behnke
John G. Bellows
Howard Belzberg
Jack Benhayon
William M. Bennett
J. Alfred Berend
Kenneth Berge
Stanley Berman
Betty Bernard
Clarence J. Berne
Thomas V. Berne
Maurice Bernstein
Michael Bernstein

Charles A. Berry
Alice N. Bessman
Peter Best
John E. Bethune
Daniel C. Bird
Marjorie Bird
Gordon L. Black
Courtland Blake
David Blankenhorn
Andrew Bliss
Harry A. Bliss
Melvin A. Block
Marsden S. Blois
Daniel K. Bloomfield
Baruch S. Blumberg
Morton Bogdonoff
Paul Bohannan
Eli L. Borkon
Louis G. Bove
Francis L. Bowler
Marjorie A. Bowman
Tom Bradley
Major W. Bradshaw
Robert M. Braude
Mark Braunstein
Eugene Braunwald
Donald F. Brayton
Thomas H. Brem
Cedric Bremner
D. J. Brennan
Gayne Brenneman
Sandra Bressler
Jeannie Brewer
Garry Brody
Dorothy Brooks
Arnold L. Brown

Bernice Z. Brown
Janis Brown
Sallye P. Brown
F. Charles Brunicardi
Barbara Buchanan
Francis S. Buck
Charles S. Burger
J. H. Burgess
Genevieve Burk
Joan Burns
Thomas W. Burns
George Herbert Walker Bush, President
Peter Butler
Richard Byyny
C. A. Caceres
Arthur A. Calix
Thomas Callister
J. T. Campbell, Jr.
Richard M. Caplan
Tor Carlsen
David B. Carmichael
Susan T. Carver
William J. Casarella
William B. Castle
Cathleen Caton
M. E. Chaffin
Katherine R. Challoner
Kit Chambers
Wallace L. Chambers
Schumarry H. Chao
Robert Cheshier
Arthur C. Christakos
Norman Christiansen
Gail Clark
J. Philip Clarke

D. Kay Clawson
Clifton R. Cleaveland
Steven G. Clemenson
Linda Hawes Clever
William A. Clintworth
Nancy Coates
Walter S. Coe
Jordan J. Cohen
Bradford Cohn
Lawrence H. Cohn
Morris Collen
Russell F. Compton
Marilyn Cook
William M. Cooper
William G. Corey
Mitchel D. Covel
Susan Covel
David G. Covell
Joyce W. Craddick
Cheryl M. Craft
Jean A. Creek
Peter F. Crookes
Harold D. Cross
Martin H. Crumrine
Robert Cullin
Martin Cummings
Hiram Cury
David J. Dahl
David C. Dale
W. Andrew Dale
Walter J. Daly
William H. Daughaday
Nicholas Davies
David A. Davis
Lawrence Davis
William D. Davis, Jr.

Pamela Day
Catherine D. DeAngelis
John De Angelis
Michael E. DeBakey
Vincent A. DeLuca, Jr.
Tom R. DeMeester
Demetrios Demetriades
Scott Deppe
Vincent DeQuattro
N. A. Desbiens
Kenneth Diddie
Preston V. Dilts, Jr.
Richard L. Dobson
James E. Doherty
John Donald
James Dooley
Doris Doran
T. E. Doszkocs
J. Douglas
Dan Dover
Andrew Dow
Edgar Draper
F. Dubeck
N. L. DuBlurg, Jr.
Eileen Duggan
Harriett P. Dustan
James M. Duvall
Donald Dworken
Eileen Eandi
Allan J. Ebbin
Robert E. Ecklund
William H. Edwards
Richard H. Egdahl
Roger Egeberg
Hans E. Einstein
Robert S. Eisenberg
Marvyn L. Elgart
Neil Elgee
George J. Ellis
Mark L. Entman
Henry L. Ernstthal
Daniel Essin
T. N. Evans
Alison Ewing
Saul Farber
Gerald Farinola
Richard G. Farmer
Aaron Feder
Daniel B. Federman
James F. Feeney
Ralph D. Feigin
Arthur W. Feinberg
Donald I. Feinstein
Theodore Feit
William C. Felch
Alan W. Feld
Steven Feldon
Benjamin Felson
Cotton Feray
Thomas B. Ferguson
Daniel Ferrigno
Richard Field
William R. Fifer
Harry W. Fischer
Joseph Fischer
Winthrop Fish
Charles Fitch
Edmond B. Flink
Timothy Foley
Michael Fordis
Arthur Fox
Raul Fraide
Boy Frame
Richard Friedman
William F. Friedman
James F. Fries
K. O. Fritz
John Fry
Atsuko Fujimoto
Ronald K. Fujimoto
Sherrilynne Fuller
Jack J. Fulton
William B. Galbraith
Augustin A. Garcia
Norman H. Garrett, Jr.
Paul J. Geiger
John P. Geyman
Ray W. Gifford, Jr.
Nelson J. Gilman
Robert J. Glaser
Arnold W. Goldschlager
Nora Goldschlager
Charles Goldstein
Robert M. Goldwyn
Joseph Gonnella
Lillian Gonzalez-Pardo
Brian W. Goodell
J. F. Goodman
Alan L. Gordon
Babs Gordon
Antonio M. Gotto, Jr.
Arthur E. Grant
Lawrence A. Green
Robert Green
Stephen B. Greenberg
Norton J. Greenberger
Robert Greenes
Lazar J. Greenfield

Beverly June Gregorius
Ward O. Griffen, Jr.
Janet Grignon
James A. Grimes
Paul Griner
David S. Gullion
Rolf M. Gunnar
Warren G. Guntheroth
Michael Hagen
Jeffrey A. Hahn
Daniel Hamaty
David A. Hamburg
Jean Hamburger
James T. Hamlin, III
Steven Hamman
C. Rollins Hanlon
Richard J. Hannigan
Louise Hart
William Hart
A. McGehee Harvey
Paul Harvey
W. Proctor Harvey
James N. Haug
Robert M. Hayes
H. Ralph Haymond
R. Brian Haynes
L. Julian Haywood
Katherine Hecht
Robert Hecht
Eugene M. Helveston
Bruce L. Henderson
Robert W. Henderson
Eva H. Henriksen
John Bernard Henry
Lester T. Hibbard
Lawrence Highman
Allen Hinman
Joan E. Hodgman
Daniel Hoffman
Wu Hokwang
John H. Holbrook
Hans Asbjorn Holm
Grace Holmes
Rita B. Hopper
Louis Horlick
Sylvan H. Horwood
Cyril Houle
James D. Houy
Sidney Howard
James T. Howell
Willard J. Howland
J. P. Hubbard
Thomas Harrison Hunter
J. Willis Hurst
F. Ikezaki
James M. Ingram
Thomas S. Inui
Julien H. Isaacs
Nicolas Jabbour
Marcia Jackson
Donald M. Jacobs
Karin E. Jamison
Charles L. Janes
Stephen Jay
Harold Jeghers
Frederick R. Jelovsek
Thomas M. Jenkins
M. Harry Jennison
Wu Jieping
Carol Johnson Johns
Allen H. Johnson
Cage Johnson
J. W. Johnson
Marvin E. Johnson
Harry S. Jonas
Olga Jonasson
Lawrence W. Jones
Albert R. Jonsen
P. B. Jorgensen
Desmond G. Julian
Ralph C. Jung
Charles L. Junkerman
Maurice J. Jurkiewicz
Norman Kahn
Mehwet Kam
Rokay Kamyar
Thomas Edward Kane
W. Kane
Stanley Kaplan
Manny J. Karbeling
Harvey R. Kaslow
Jerome P. Kassier
D. Kassum
Laurence H. Kedes
Gary Kelsberg
Robert Kerlan
Louis J. Kettel
Kaye Kilburn
M. Kenton King
Richard Kingston
David M. Kipnis
Rebecca T. Kirkland
Joseph B. Kirsner
Rodanthi Kitridou
Margaret S. Klapper
Gerald Klatskin
Suzanne B. Knoebel
Malcolm Knowles

Chris Kraft
Richard O. Kraft
Gabriel A. Kune
Gustavo G. R. Kuster
Robin B. Lake
Frank L. Lambert
Richard H. Lampert
F. Wilfrid Lancaster
Donald G. Landale
Tom Landry
Robert A. Larsen
Jeffrey Latts
Peter Lawin
G. Hugh Lawrence
Aubrey Leatham
Joshua Lederberg
Jeffrey S. Lee
Peter V. Lee
Philip R. Lee
John M. Leedom
Wenzel A. Leff
Howard A. Leibman
Thomas J. Lehar
John N. Lein
Michael A. Lemp
Patrick D. Lester
C. Robin LeSueur
Leo L. Leveridge
Ceylon S. Lewis, Jr.
Jerry P. Lewis
Richard P. Lewis
Walter M. Lewis
Fred V. Light
William Liley
Thomas Lincoln
Donald A. B. Lindberg

A. J. Lindgren
Karen Lindsay
G. Littenberg
Nancy M. Lorenzi
William Loskota
Leah M. Lowenstein
Richard Lubman
Robert J. Luchi
Frederick Ludwig
George D. Lundberg
Joseph Lydon
Garrett R. Lynch
George Macer
Donald N. Mackay
Ian R. Mackay
Robert Mager
W. E. Malle
Susan B. Mallory
Robert T. Manning
Charles M. March
N. M. March
Eugenia Marcus
Alexander R. Margulis
E. Connie Mariano
Helen E. Martin
Maurice J. Martin
Ralph B. Martin
Manuel Martinez-Maldonado
Byron J. Masterson
Nina W. Matheson
James L. Mathis
Gastone Matioli
William Matory
Betty H. Mawardi
Paul E. Mazmanian
Andrew McCanse

Margaret McCarron
Robert N. McClelland
Ruth McCormick
Clement J. McDonald
C. E. McDonnell
Walter R. McFarland
Page M. McGirr
Charles H. McKinna
John McMichael
I. R. McWhinney
Sherman M. Mellinkoff
Kenneth Melmon
Robert C. Mendenhall
Pat Mensah
Henry S. Metz
Thomas C. Meyer
David Micaelvitch
William Millard
George E. Miller
Jacqueline D. Miller
Perry L. Miller
William Richey Miller
Don Harper Mills
Donald S. Minckler
Shri K. Mishra
Malcolm S. Mitchell
Dan Mohler
R. W. Montgomery
Pat Mooney
Francis D. Moore
Dean H. Morrow
David H. Morse
Robert H. Moser
James M. Moss
Edward Movius
Richard H. Moy

Cheryl A. Moyer
Donald R. Moyes
John F. Mueller
John H. Mulholland
W. V. Murowsky
Daniel M. Musher
Alvin I. Mushlin
Jack D. Myers
Richard Nabours
Frederick Naftolin
Richard H. Nalick
Stephen Nazarian
William D. Nelligan
Eugene C. Nelson
Janet Nelson
Victor Neufeld
Anita Newman
Edward Newton
Charles H. Nicholson
John T. Nicoloff
Nancy Nielson-Brown
Lilia F. Nikolaeva
Robert A. Nordyke
Jackson Norwood
Celia M. Oakley
Claron L. Oakley
Byron Oberst
Richard L. O'Brien
Alton Ochsner
Frederick C. O'Dell, Jr.
Kunio Okuda
Wesley M. Oler
D. E. Olson
Claude H. Organ, Jr.
Edwin L. Overholt
Irvine H. Page

R. H. Palmer
Robert L. Palmer
P. J. H. Pansegrouw
Theodore Pappas
John Parboosingh
Dilip Parekh
Charles E. Parker
James L. Parkin
Richard P. Parkinson
William W. Parmley
Joseph Paterno
E. Mansell Pattison
Stephen G. Pauker
Beverly C. Payne
Meredith J. Payne
Gee Pei
Jeffrey H. Peters
Ruth K. Peters
Robert G. Petersdorf
Hans E. Peterson
Roger Peterson
Donald Petit
Thomas A. Petro
Ronald J. Pion
Nicholas Pisacano
Lynn Pittier
Gerald I. Plitman
Hiram C. Polk, Jr.
Bernard Portnoy
John Premi
Gretchen P. Purcell
Barbara Quint
George J. Race
Derek Raghavan
Robert C. Rainie
Robert E. Rakel

Rangasamy Ramanathan
Eli A. Ramirez-Rodriguez
Elizabeth Ramirez-Rodriguez
K. J. Rao
Samuel I. Rapaport
C. Thorpe Ray
Joe Redding
Frank Reed
Peter L. Reichertz
J. S. Reinschmidt
Richard J. Reitemeier
Linda J. Rever
Ralph D. Reynolds
Telfer B. Reynolds
William A. Reynolds
Richard D. Richards
Robert Richards
Benjamin M. Rigor
Jesse D. Rising, III
Brooke Roberts
James M. Robertson
Carroll M. Robie
L. Rodney Rodgers
Jonathan E. Rodnick
John Romano
Robert Rosati
Donald H. Rose
Margaret Rose
Noel R. Rose
Robert M. Rose
Edward C. Rosenow, Jr.
Joseph F. Ross
Herbert J. Rothenberg
Edward Rubenstein
Robert Rude
Ian E. Rusted

Robb H. Rutledge
David C. Sabiston, Jr.
David L. Sackett
Paulette Y. Saddler
Alfredo A. Sadun
Murray Salkin
Paul J. Sanazaro
Marilyn Sanders
Jay P. Sanford
Yoichi Satomura
Ragheb Sawires
John L. Sawyers
Andrew I. Schafer
Irwin J. Schatz
Robert Scheig
DuWayne Schmidt
Harold M. Schoolman
Alvin Schultz
M. Roy Schwarz
Hervey D. Segall
Milton M. Seifert, Jr.
R. Rick Selby
Donald Wayne Seldin
Hugh Shade
Edward Shapiro
Om Sharma
Jiaqi Shen
Sheila Sherlock
Kenneth I. Shine
William C. Shoemaker
Edward Shortliffe
Linda D. Shortliffe
Jerry M. Shuck
Ira A. Shulman
A. A. Siddiqui
Jill K. Silverman
Mark E. Silverman
George M. Simpson
Maureen Sims
Marjorie S. Sirridge
S. E. Sivertson
Harold Skalka
David Slawson
Henry Slotnick
J. Orson Smith
Lloyd H. Smith, Jr.
Robert B. Smith, III
Ronald E. Smith
Eric W. Sohr
Bjarte G. Solheim
Jane Somerville
Walter Somerville
Eli Sorkow
Robert D. Sparks
Robert L. Spears
Harold M. Spinka
John A. Spittell, Jr.
Steven Stain
Eugene A. Stead, Jr.
William Stead
Knight Steel
David Steinman
G. Gayle Stephens
Lorin Stephens
W. Eugene Stern
Roger Stickney
Margaret T. Stockstill
Gene H. Stollerman
Daniel C. Stone
Patrick B. Storey
C. F. Stout
John S. Strauss
Oscar Streeter
Jeffrey K. Stross
Patricia J. Stuff
Stephen Sullivan
James M. Swain
Donald M. Switz
Lee R. Talbert
Dorothy Tatter
Clive Taylor
Annabel J. Teberg
Jack E. Tetirick
John Thayer
Joe Theil
Leigh Thompson
George W. Thorn
John Toews
David Torin
Gary Toule
Richard Treiman
Donald Trunkey
Suzanne Trupin
Susan B. Tully
Philip A. Tumulty
Marvin Turck
Fred Turrill
Edmund E. Van Brunt
Stanley van den Noort
Joseph P. Van Der Meulen
J. Van Dyke
John F. Viljoen
Richard W. Vilter
Jean-Louis Vincent
Jan Vleck
Robert Volpe
Kenneth Walker
Gary L. Walkup

Marsha Wallace
Betty Wallerstein
Ralph Wallerstein
Lila Wallis
Alexander J. Walt
Richard F. Walters
Waltman Walters
John Walther
Paul H. Ward
William C. Waters, III
David E. Waugh
Fred A. Weaver
Lawrence L. Weed
Paul F. Wehrle
Laurel Weibel
Max H. Weil
Horst D. Weinborg
John M. Weiner
James M. A. Weiss
Mark W. Weiting
Claude E. Welch
Dennis K. Wentz
Murray Wexler
G. M. Whitacre
G. E. Wiebe
George D. Wilbanks
Hibbard E. Williams
Martha E. Williams
Warren Williams
John Williamson
Robert J. Williamson
Marjorie Price Wilson
Deborah A. Wing
George Winokur
Alice Witkowski
John E. Wolf, Jr.
Francis C. Wood
Thomas C. Wood
Sherwyn M. Woods
Frank Woolsey
Harold Wooster
Eton W. Wright
Kerry E. Wylke
Milford G. Wyman
James B. Wyngaarden
Rosalyn S. Yalow
Sadahiro Yamamoto
Myron Yanoff
J. Young
James B. Young
Lawrence E. Young
Stuart C. Yudofsky
Rex C. Yung
Martin Zane
Christopher K. Zarins
Bruce E. Zawacki
Samir M. Zeind
Israel Zwerling

Name Index

• • •

Subject Index

• • •

Phil R. Manning, M.D.

• • •

Phil Richard Manning has had a long and illustrious career at his Alma Mater, the University of Southern California School of Medicine, beginning in 1954. He was a Professor of Medicine from 1964 to 2002, when he retired. In 1981, he was named Paul Ingalls Hoagland-Hastings Professor of Continuing Medical Education, and until June 2002, he was Associate Dean in charge of Postgraduate Medical Education and Associate Vice President for Postgraduate Affairs.

His interest in medical education was apparent from the beginning of his career, evidenced by a deep involvement in undergraduate and postgraduate instruction, including active bedside teaching, course organization and evaluation, and publications dating back to the mid-fifties.

Dr. Manning has been organizing and directing national and international postgraduate medical programs since 1955. Considered the master of continuing medical education, he has done more to influence this field than any other single person. Some of his more recent efforts have been directed to the role of computers in continuing education, development of the community hospital as a teaching center, and methods allowing the practicing internist, in his or her private office, to keep abreast of ongoing developments.

His Mastership from the American College of Physicians was accompanied by the following statements: "If one were to count achievement in medicine in terms of influencing the thinking and manner of practice of countless thousands of health professionals, Dr. Manning has no peer. He has never lost his own passion for the art and science of medicine and has rekindled it in many others by his example, knowledge, teaching, writing, and research."

Lois DeBakey, Ph.D.

• • •

Lois DeBakey, Professor of Scientific Communication at Baylor College of Medicine in Houston, Texas, received her B.A. degree in mathematics with honors from Newcomb College, and her M.A. and Ph.D. degrees in literature and linguistics from Tulane University. A pioneer in the teaching of biomedical communication, she designed and conducted the first curriculum-approved courses in this subject in a medical school. The success of her oversubscribed courses, including those sponsored by prestigious medical societies, has been attributed to her approach through critical reasoning first and lucid language second, and to her use of cartoons to illustrate illogicalities, infelicities, pomposities, and inadvertent humor in medical publications.

Described by distinguished physicians as "the medical world's great communicator," "the unchallenged champion of the proper use of medical English," and "the preeminent defender of integrity in

American medical letters," Dr. DeBakey is recognized as the leading scholar and authority in this discipline. She has published prolifically in medical and lay periodicals on biomedical communication, medical ethics and socioeconomics, language, literacy, and education. Her definitive edition, *The Scientific Journal*, has been adopted by editorial staffs of major medical journals.

Dr. DeBakey has served on the Board of Regents of the National Library of Medicine, on the Usage Panel of *The American Heritage Dictionary*, as a team leader consultant to the *Encyclopaedia Britannica* health and medical database, and on numerous national and international committees, university accrediting agencies, and government consulting bodies, as well as on the editorial and advisory boards of the *Journal of the American Medical Association* and other prestigious medical journals.

Among honors recognizing her achievements are Phi Beta Kappa, scholastic excellence society; the Golden Key National Honor Society; Distinguished Service Award of the American Medical Writers Association; the first John P. McGovern Award of the Medical Library Association; Newcomb College Distinguished Alumna; and Fellowship in the American College of Medical Informatics.

Dr. DeBakey has been called "the conscience of medical journalism" and has been credited with doing more to bring literacy, clarity, and validity to medical writing than any other person in the country.

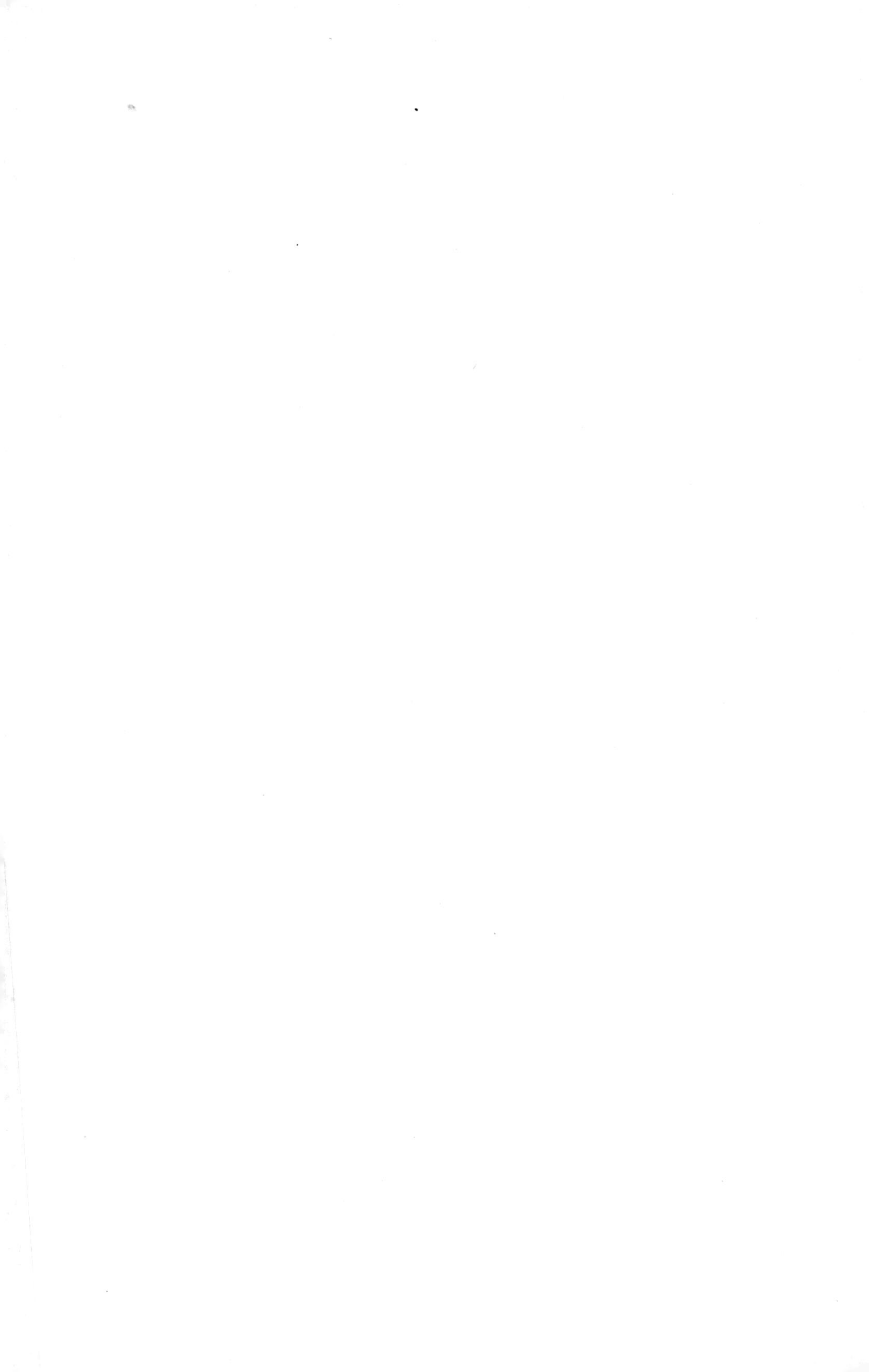